Management of
Adult Neurogenic Dysphagia

Dysphagia Series

Series Editor

John C. Rosenbek, Ph.D.

Management of Adult Neurogenic Dysphagia

Maggie Lee Huckabee, MA, CCC/SLP

University Clinic of Neurology
Ludwig Boltzmann Institute for
Functional Brain Imaging
Vienna, Austria
and
University of Memphis, Tennessee

Cathy A. Pelletier, MS, CCC/SLP

Cathy Pelletier and Associates, Inc.
Freeville, New York

THOMSON

DELMAR LEARNING

Australia Canada Mexico Singapore Spain United Kingdom United States

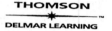

THOMSON
DELMAR LEARNING

Management of
Adult Neurogenic Dysphagia

Vice President,
Health Care Business Unit:
William Brottmiller
Editorial Director:
Cathy L. Esperti

Acquisitions Editor:
Kalen Conerly
Marketing Director:
Jennifer McAvey

Marketing Coordinator:
Chris Manion
Production Editor:
James Zayicek

Library of Congress Cataloging-in-Publication Data
Huckabee, Maggie Lee.
Management of adult neurogenic dysphagia/by Maggie Lee Huckabee and Cathy A. Pelletier
   p.; cm. ---- (Dyspagia series)
   Includes bibliographical references index.
   ISBN-13: 978-1-5659-3731-4
   ISBN-10: 1-5659-3731-7
   1. Deglutition disorders.
   I. Pelletier, Cathy A.
   II. Title   III. Series
   (DNLM1.Deglutition Disorders Deglutition disorders-Thera WI 250H882m   1998)
RC815.2.H83 1998
   616.3'1---dc21
DNLM/DLC
for Library of Congress   98-27474
                                          CIP

Notice to the Reader

Publisher does not warrant or guarantee any of the products described herein or perform any independent analysis in connection with any of the product information contained herein. Publisher does not assume, and expressly disclaims, any obligation to obtain and include information other than that provided to it by the manufacturer.

The reader is expressly warned to consider and adopt all safety precautions that might be indicated by the activities described herein and to avoid all potential hazards. By following the instructions contained herein, the reader willingly assumes all risks in connection with such instructions.

The publisher makes no representations or warranties of any kind, including but not limited to, the warranties of fitness for particular purpose or merchantability, nor are any such representations implied with respect to the material set forth herein, and the publisher takes no responsibility with respect to such material. The publisher shall not be liable for any special, consequential, or exemplary damages resulting, in whole or part, from the readers' use of, or reliance upon, this material.

Contents

Foreword

Interdisciplinary research and clinical practice in dysphagia are expanding rapidly worldwide. Singular Publishing Group, Inc.'s recently created Dysphagia Series was initiated to be the publishing support for that expansion. Dysphagia is an interdisciplinary practice because swallowing and swallowing disorders are complex and the person with dysphagia is more than simply a person who cannot swallow adequately or safely. The best research and clinical practice is being done by groups of physicians, clinicians, dietitians, surgeons, and others with special insight into human swallowing and related behaviors. Research and clinical practice is expanding worldwide because the human toll of swallowing impairment can be so high and its successful management so satisfying. Eating enough and safely is one of life's joys.

The *Dysphagia Series*, when complete, will comprise publications from the most basic to the most advanced. *Management of Adult Neurogenic Dysphagia* by Maggie Lee Huckabee and Cathy Pelletier is for those practitioners with present or future responsibility for treating adults with impaired swallowing. Huckabee and Pelletier are experienced, insightful speech-language pathologists. They have learned what it takes to help dysphagic persons and their caregivers; they know how to work on teams; they know how to combine principles and practices into responsible, effective management; and they know who to ask or where to look for help when a management problem is unique or seemingly intractable.

Management of Adult Neurogenic Dysphagia contains the best of their experience. Their approach to management is not atheoretical for they are not technicians interested primarily in simply completing a task. This book makes clear how tailoring treatment to the physiologic abnormality responsible for the dysphagia is to be accomplished. Nor are they narrowly or obsessively focused on only one approach to management. They define and describe both rehabilitation and compensation, and they specify the criteria as well as the procedures for accomplishing both.

Treatment books are hard to write because practice outruns the data. Huckabee and Pelletier carefully identify what is known and what can only be guessed at. As a result, students and clinicians will learn what to do, why to do it, and with how much confidence by reading this book. They will also learn what a difference doing the right thing can make in the lives of adults with dysphagia. This is a book for the thoughtful among us who want to help. It is unique in dysphagia. No other book is devoted as specifically to management as is this one. It may well become the most dog-eared volume in your library.

John C. Rosenbek, PhD
Editor, Dysphagia Series

Preface

Dysphagia is a relatively new area of expertise within the field of speech-language pathology, with clinical interest and need for these services mushrooming over the past 2 decades. Practicing clinicians, young and old, often struggle to gain the skills they need to provide competent dysphagia services. Most clinicians initially focus on developing the necessary skills and knowledge to make an accurate diagnosis of dysphagia, and rightly so. We need to understand completely the physiology of a swallowing disorder before we can even begin to think about treating it. But once we have diagnosed the disorder, what intervention is best for the patient? How do we decide? What can we do to implement the intervention with success, across various clinical practice settings?

As experienced clinicians practicing in different settings, we found that we were asking these questions and sometimes getting different answers. The definitive answers to these questions are not given in this text, since this information is our next great challenge. The goal of this text is to provide practicing clinicians with a comprehensive resource of what we know and hope to know about how to manage adults with neurogenic dysphagia. We offer a challenge to our friends and colleagues to use this book as only the beginning of rigorous study and critique of our treatment practices. We have so much more to learn.

The first two chapters outline the many issues of trying to manage adult neurogenic dysphagia and offer a unique framework to apply to intervention decisions. Clinicians are encouraged to become a dysphagia coach, similar to an athletic coach, in their assessment and intervention skills. Chapters 3 and 6 comprise a comprehensive review of various intervention techniques, the research behind the technique, and what physiologic disorder(s) may be alleviated with the technique. These interventions are discussed according to the specific physiologic abnormality they are designed to address. This uncommon organization requires clinicians first to identify and understand the physiology behind the swallowing disorder before attempting to apply a technique to treat it. We believe this is an essential prerequisite to any dysphagia intervention. Chapters 4 and 5 offer a complete discussion of the theory of biofeedback and its application as a dysphagia intervention technique with various modalities. Chapters 7 to 9 provide clinicians with a foundation to understand better the complexities involved in diagnosing and maintaining adequate nutritional status in patients with dysphagia and the role they may play within the multidisciplinary approach to management. The special issues involved when patients are dependent on others to be fed are discussed in Chapter 10. The surgical management options available to patients are explained in detail in Chapter 11. Chapter 12 provides specific instructions regarding how clinicians need to document their dysphagia services to meet legal, reimbursement, and ethical requirements. Finally, our last chapter provides a most important, yet often forgotten, viewpoint when management decisions for dysphagia are discussed. Chapter 13 offers the patient's perspective on what it feels like to have dysphagia and to undergo treatment for dysphagia. It is written by one of our patients, and perhaps it is fitting that we let them have the final word.

Chapters 1, 3, 4 and 6 were authored by M.L. Huckabee. Chapters 2, 7 to 10, and 12 were authored by C. A. Pelletier. Chapter 5 was co-authored, Chapter 11 was authored by Mark A. Vavares, MD, Massachusetts Eye and Ear Infirmary, and Chapter 13 was authored by Deborah Dwyer Batjer.

Acknowledgments

I would like to acknowledge the many friends and colleagues who provided me with valuable critiques, references, friendship, and support during the completion of this text: Tom Chavanic, COTA; Sybil Deuso, RDH; Karen J. Dikeman, MA, CCC; Jane E. Donn, MS, CCC; Cheryl Durand; Cheryl Dykeman-Lovelass, RN; Cynthia Elberty, DDS; Eileen Gravani, PhD; Robert Gravani, PhD; Marta S. Kazandjian, MA, CCC; Susan E. Langmore, PhD; Christine G. Matijas, RN, FNP; R. H. Mills, PhD; Neita Stafford, ART; Sarah Stark, MA, CCC; Carol A. Taylor, RN; Cynthia Van Patten-Young, BA; and Diane Wheeler, MA, CCC. A special thank you to Donna Acox, MA, RD, and Margy Gutchess, RD, for their willingness to answer numerous questions and review many revisions of text. To Sharlyn Keegan, MA, CCC: Thanks for listening, covering my caseload, and providing the "wind beneath my wings." This book would not have happened without your support, help, and friendship, personally and professionally.

I am also grateful to the following wonderful professionals who provided me with company pictures or information: Eileen M. Griffin, RD/CDN; Peter Osterdale, Ross Products Division, Abbott Laboratories; Marsha Reeves, National HealthCare, Don Tymchuck, Med-Diet Laboratories; and Nicholas Tsaclas, Pentax Precision Instrument Company.

Deepest admiration and appreciation to our editor, John C. Rosenbek, PhD, for teaching me much more than how to write a book chapter. The lessons I learned from you are lifelong treasures. Many thanks also to Marie Linvill and Candice Janco, for answering never-ending editorial questions and being so forgiving!

Finally, I am indebted to my family who have sustained me throughout many hours of writing. To my husband, David, and children, Jennifer and Jason: Thanks for being my "giving tree." Without your unconditional love, patience, and encouragement, I could not have completed this work. To Jason: I don't have any more words to write. You can come into the computer room now!

Cathy A. Pelletier

Great appreciation is extended to my co-author Cathy Pelletier. To all who read these pages, be assured that author sequencing is an alphabetical issue, not one of merit. Cathy took on this project late in the game and carried the burden when life's intrusions had me perpetually dropping the ball. Without her perseverance at writing and patience with me, there would be no book. Have a margarita on me, Cathy!

Gratitude seems an inadequate word when I think of Jay Rosenbek. His perspectives on book writing, swallowing, poetry, and life are now woven into my own. For this I am tremendously blessed and have most assuredly become a better clinician, academician, and, most important, human.

And last but certainly not least, great thanks to my best buddies, Greg Flamme and Ginny Alexander, who helped me keep perspective and a wee little bit of sanity through a very, very difficult year.

Maggie Lee Huckabee

Dedication

To my grandmother, Elizabeth M. Buffington,
with deep love and admiration.

CP

To William H. Tullis, MD, and
Deborah Dwyer Batjer,
both of whom taught me remarkable lessons about the potential for recovery.

MLH

CHAPTER

▮

Issues in Dysphagia Management

Any book represents the heart, soul, experiences, philosophy and biases of the authors. This chapter presents these biases and the general framework that is followed throughout the text. Specifically, the chapter presents the philosophical approach taken by the authors in developing the text, a framework for intervention that draws parallels between the skills needed by a speech pathologist and those developed by an athletic coach, and some suggestions for critiquing new research in an ever-changing area of practice.

The realm of direct dysphagia management has its origins as early as the 1930s based in the provision of services to patients with cerebral palsy. However, it has only been since the early 1980s that this area of practice has taken on the distinctive multidisciplinary organization of concentrated research and clinical practice. Within this fairly recent time period, the profession has made great strides in defining parameters and variations in swallowing physiology and developing diagnostic procedures. However, given the relative immaturity in the development of the discipline, management practices are affected by several "evolutionary issues" that reflect the ever-developing nature of this area.

THE CHALLENGES OF A NEW PRACTICE AREA

Initially, our research focus has been on defining normal swallowing physiology and recognizing deviations that would fall within the definition of the diagnostic term *dysphagia*. This is unquestionably a critical first step in the development of any field of study and has justifiably consumed the majority of our research efforts. Through these efforts, the profession possesses a continually updating database, which defines "normal" for a broad range of ages and conditions.

Being in a rehabilitative profession, researchers and clinicians in speech pathology have very successfully identified behavioral and nonbehavioral mechanisms to address the deficits as they were identified. However, in some ways it appears that these management strategies were developed as somewhat stopgap measures to address the diagnosis, rather than as a conscientious and thoughtful generation of practice patterns based on physiologic deficits.

It is now time to focus our attention systematically in research and clinical practice to the development of management techniques. In an area that is, by necessity and desire, a multidisciplinary effort, the continued evolution into more systematic and refined management is critical to the speech pathologist's continued role on the team. Our contributions to the dysphagia management team are diverse and certainly include clinical and instrumental diagnosis. However, the unique contribution of the speech pathologist is our expertise in treatment planning and execution. With changes in health care structure and increasing limitations in reimbursement, there is a critical need to maintain our place on the dysphagia team, and subsequently our place in line at the pay window. This can be assured by continuing our efforts at what we are uniquely suited to provide—management services. Through these efforts, we can continue to provide efficacious, but empirically supported, intervention for our patients and maintain our credibility and indispensability in the medical community.

The second evolutionary hurdle that we face relates to terminology. How do you pronounce "d-y-s-p-h-a-g-i-a"? Although this question is posed with a somewhat tongue-in-cheek intent, it nonetheless reflects on a fundamental weakness in clinical and diagnostic practices. That weakness is the ambiguity and miscommunication of terminology both within the profession of speech pathology and across multidisciplinary boundaries.

This could be a fatal flaw. Recognizing this, at the 1995 annual meeting of the Dysphagia Research Society, an entire panel discussion was devoted just to the task of clarifying terminology.

Imprecise terminology can adversely affect both diagnostic and therapeutic efforts. As an example, a clinician in an acute-care facility may perform a videofluoroscopic swallowing study on a chronic care patient on the referral of another clinician. The ensuing report generated from the examination may document "moderate vallecular pooling." The term *vallecular pooling* is used by many. However, one clinician may always infer that term to indicate postswallowing accumulation of the bolus in the pharynx, while another clinician may perceive that terminology to include preswallow collection of the bolus as well. In addition, the severity descriptor of "moderate" could be perceived quite differently by two different clinicians, given their experience in interpreting exams and their subsequent point of reference. Thus, a single physiologic deficit and the associated documentation may be interpreted by two clinicians to reflect two distinctly different physiologic processes.

Therapeutic efforts may also be clouded by imprecise terminology. As an example, DePippo et al. (1994), published a controlled study regarding dysphagia therapy efficacy. In this study, 115 patients with dysphagia secondary to stroke were randomly assigned to three conditions of dysphagia intervention, each with increasing levels of therapist intervention. The results of the study indicated no greater benefit for patients assigned to the group with the greatest degree of therapist intervention than those patients who received only one educational session post diagnosis. However, the therapy provided to those who received intensive intervention was limited to compensatory swallowing techniques and did not include rehabilitative interventions. With a title of "Dysphagia Therapy Following Stroke," and findings that do not strongly support speech pathology intervention, specificity in terminology is critical to circumvent overgeneralization of these findings, both within our profession and beyond to our referral sources.

There is a compelling need, as a profession, to define more succinctly such terms as intervention, rehabilitation, treatment, compensation, and management, and to agree on the use of these terms across disciplines. Our definitions appear in Table 1–1. It is important to point out that the definitions used in this text are not the only definitions, or necessarily even the right definitions. Final determinations across the field will only be derived after discussion and formalization through some organization that subserves the multidisciplinary swallowing community. However, the definitions reiterated throughout the text support the philosophical and practical framework for dysphagia intervention that is offered to the reader.

Table 1–1. Definitions

Terminology	Definition
Compensation	Strategies that provide an immediate but typically transient effect on the efficiency or safety of swallowing. As a rule, if the strategy is not consistently executed, swallowing will return to the prior dysfunctional status. May include, but are not necessarily limited to, posturing, adaptations in rate, route, or nature of oral intake.
Rehabilitation	Interventions that when provided over the course of time are thought to result in permanent changes in the substrates underlying deglutition, that is, changing the physiology of swallowing mechanisms. May include, but not limited to, oral/facial exercises, vocal adduction exercises, breathing exercises, pharyngeal strengthening exercises.
Management	Overall multidisciplinary approach to addressing swallowing impairment. May include services from speech pathology, surgery, otolaryngology, occupational therapy, nursing, nutrition, social services. Addresses not only the physiologic abnormality, but the psychosocial, nutritional, and medical needs of the patient.
Intervention	Specific technique, or techniques, that are targeted toward a specific goal of remediation.
Behavioral Intervention	Interventions or strategies that the patient is actively involved in executing over a prolonged period of time. May include techniques in both the compensatory and rehabilitative frameworks, such as pharyngeal strengthening exercises or posturing changes.
Nonbehavioral Intervention	Interventions or strategies that are typically medically based and alter swallowing physiology outside of the realm of daily patient participation. May include techniques in both the compensatory and rehabilitative frameworks such as vocal fold medialization as a permanent surgical intervention to change the physiology of the mechanism or palatal prosthesis as a nonbehavioral but transient compensation.

PERSPECTIVES ACROSS THE HEALTH CARE CONTINUUM

Traditionally, management books in speech-language pathology have been written with scant attention to differences in the sites where such management is taking place. Recent refinement of what might be called a continuum of health care services—from acute and subacute to outpatient, long-term, and home health care—has forced the retirement of this traditional approach. Implications of this continuum of care must be recognized. These implications include the amount of time clinicians have to work with patients and therefore the activities they can realistically hope to accomplish; the severity and acuteness of patient illness; and patient, family, and staff expectations. Rehabilitation as defined in this book can sometimes begin but seldom be completed in the acute environment, and completion is sometimes impossible even in subacute care, depending on its duration. Chronic care, depending on environment, whether outpatient clinic, home, or chronic care facility, may be hampered by staffing and equipment limitations. Of course such limitations are not inevitable and they do not prevent management of dysphagia.

For clinicians in all settings, it is critical to respect the limitations of patient cognition, endurance, and independence and facility staffing and mission, and to provide realistic recommendations and undertake realistic management goals that can be successfully implemented. Rehabilitation should be provided if there is a realistic expectation that it can improve swallowing physiology. If rehabilitation is impossible or unlikely to succeed then the best compensations need to be introduced.

Regardless of the setting in which the patient resides, any interventional plan that optimizes the patient's abilities, improves quality of life, and maintains medical integrity should be considered an important success. In some cases, this plan consists of realistically recognizing the limitations of the patient, while optimizing swallowing ability and quality of life through behavioral and environmental compensation. In other cases, the optimal plan consists of aggressive rehabilitation and return to full oral intake without compensation. Both approaches are patient dependent, require significant expertise and skill on the part of the clinician, and offer a valuable service.

DIAGNOSIS PRECEDES INTERVENTION

The goal of this text is to provide clinicians from a variety of settings a resource for management of the patient with dysphagia. It is beyond the scope of this text, however, to provide a full review of underlying swallowing physiology, diagnostic procedures, patient clinical evaluation, and an indepth coverage of medical management. It is assumed that the practicing clinician will refer to other very comprehensive texts on these issues (Perlman & Schulze-Delrieu, 1997; Logemann, 1997). A major recurring theme that will surface throughout this text is that effective treatment of any oral pharyngeal swallowing impairment relies on accurate diagnosis and individualization of the treatment plan to the specific physiology, not the symptomatology. This applies to dysphagia intervention practices that are compensatory, rehabilitative, or both, and is crucial to the success of the treatment program. Inappropriate treatment is not efficacious, is not cost effective, and may be contraindicated.

Clarification of physiologic abnormality is not always a simple task and requires skillful evaluation and a clear understanding of swallowing physiology. As an example, premature spillage from poor oral control and delayed pharyngeal swallow may look very similar on radiographic exam, with the presenting symptoms of vallecular or pyriform sinus pooling prior to onset of airway protection and the potential for preswallow aspiration. To further complicate diagnosis, these two physiologic impairments frequently coexist in the neurologic population because of the close proximity of cranial nerve nuclei in the brain stem mediating both functions. However, the underlying physiologic abnormalities for these two deficits are very different. Premature spillage reflects primarily a motor disturbance affecting orolingual control of the bolus, whereas delayed pharyngeal swallow reflects primarily a sensory deficit.

One could ask that if the symptomatology is similar, why not manage them similarly? The answer is that interventions that work well for one physiologic abnormality may not facilitate improvement in the other. For example, chin tuck posturing works quite well for the sensory-based deficit of delayed pharyngeal swallow; however, a patient with the motor-based impairment of premature spillage from poor oral control may exhibit greater oral control difficulties if this technique is implemented. He or she may demonstrate difficulty maintaining the bolus in the oral cavity or working against gravity to propel the bolus over the base of the tongue in this posture. With respect to rehabilitative interventions, oral motor exercises may be prescribed to address premature spillage from poor oral control; however, there is no evidence or philosophical support for this type of intervention as a viable intervention for the sensory-based delayed pharyngeal swallow. Thus, noncritical diagnosis based on symptomotology may result in considerable rehabilitative effort that is not effective or cost efficient.

This is only one example of the need for precise assessment of swallowing physiology. Diagnostic evaluation may include one or more of the following, each of which provides unique information to the swallowing diagnosis: videofluoroscopy, fiberoptic endoscopic assessment of swallowing, manometry, scintigraphy. Surface electromyography, at this point in development, is not considered a diagnostic tool, but may provide the clinician with valuable insights into swallowing behavior. Diagnostic evaluation should address the specifics of swallowing physiology and the effectiveness of compensations for that particular patient. Therapeutic maneuvers should be evaluated thoroughly prior to application. A cookbook approach to dysphagia rehabilitation is inappropriate. In a small percentage of patients, prescription of a chin tuck posture may actually facilitate, rather than inhibit, aspiration. The information gleaned from the diagnostic evaluation is utilized to address the goals of minimizing aspiration risk and nutritional compromise and maximizing quality of life.

A MODEL FOR SERVICE DELIVERY

The role of the clinician in the care of the patient with dysphagia is an important one. In the context of a medically based team, it is often the therapist who can provide adequate time to answer questions, allay fears, and support the patient and family as they learn to advocate for themselves. These skills are undertaken in addition to the role of diagnostician, therapist, and family educator.

Throughout this text, an analogy is drawn between a therapist guiding the intervention of the patient with dysphagia and a football coach guiding the development of an individual athlete within a team. The intent of this comparison is to provide a framework for intervention in which the therapist evaluates, recommends, and teaches, but is not solely, or even primarily, responsible for the outcome. The clinician develops a treatment plan only by evaluating the patient in two ways. First, the patient is evaluated in terms of his or her individual attributes, such as cognition, motivation, and physiology. Second, the patient is evaluated in terms of environmental or contextual attributes, which include the people surrounding the patient and the setting in which he or she will live and eat.

This is similar to a coach who evaluates individual players according to their personal strengths weaknesses and the position they play on the team, and how each player can fit within the team (i.e., environment). How can the team help a player overcome weaknesses and maximize strengths so they can win the game? An important point in this framework is that clinicians must look at patients not solely according to physiologic and cognitive deficits but also to the people they are, the roles they play in their environment, and how the people surrounding them can both help and hurt them. In dysphagia management, as in team sports, the patient is the crux of the outcome, with the support of family and other caretakers critical to success and the speech pathologists serving as a guide through the treatment process.

THE LIMITATIONS OF STATE OF THE ART

The concepts and content of this text are derived, to the extent that they are supported, from a search of the literature regarding swallowing and swallowing disorders. However, as will be very apparent, if the text were only to include information that is substantiated through empirical research, this would be a very short book indeed! It is unfortunate, but perhaps forgivable, that clinical practice often precedes supportive research. Thus, a portion of the text reflects the clinical experiences, and thus, the clinical biases of the authors. For this we make no apology. However, every effort is made to delineate those practices for which we have empirical support from those that are offered in the spirit of clinical practice.

In keeping with the preceding description of service delivery, throughout the rest of this text, the term *Coaching Tip(s)* is used to delineate the advice and suggestions of the authors. Both authors are experienced clinicians, with many years of practice in different settings. Recognizing the value of clinical experience and yet also being humbled by its limitations, the authors share their insights, wisdom, and personal experiences of treating patients with dysphagia. This information is therefore be separated from the scientific data compiled in dysphagia treatment.

There are also some observations that have been derived from clinical practice for which we have nothing but curiosity to offer. Given the purely speculative nature of these observations, they are set aside as "Food for Thought." They are offered to the reader as nothing more than clinical curiosity with the hope that they will not foster confusion, but will tweak the reader's curiosity about those things of which we know very little. Greater yet, their presentation may perhaps lead to discussion that will ultimately bring them out of the speculative realm and into what is known.

CRITICAL THINKING: SEPARATING FACT FROM CLINICAL LORE

Although our empirical data in swallowing treatment is limited, it is fortunate that our progress is rapid and continual in this area. Thus, what may be "state of the art" at the time of publication could be outdated shortly thereafter. However, the opportunities offered by this burgeoning field pose significant responsibilities. The clinician practicing in this area holds a serious responsibility to remain abreast of new developments, critique them wisely, and incorporate them judiciously into clinical practice. Between television reports, newsmagazines, and now computer communications, considerable information and misinformation can circulate quickly. Be wary of what you read and hear. As new techniques and technologies surface in our approach to dysphagia management, particularly those that are potentially invasive, what criteria should be followed before incorporating these into clinical practice?

Suggestions for Critical Evaluation of a Procedure

To evaluate a procedure, consider the following criteria:

1. Where did you hear about it? Most responsible researchers will willingly offer their work for peer review and critique as a necessary step in working toward acceptance. Through the publication process, journal editors with much greater experience in interpreting methodological design and statistical analysis than most of us meticulously review research for flaws that may not be immediately obvious and consequently may be misleading. Thus, research that eventually makes it to press has a much higher chance of presenting unbiased and well-substantiated information. In the late 1980s, two physicists presented through the popular press what was hailed as a revolutionary step toward cold fusion of ions for energy production. Great excitement was generated, but over time other researchers were not able to replicate their findings and determined great flaws and misrepresentations in their theories. They eventually packed their bags and faded away.
2. Critically evaluate even what you read in journals with a keen eye on methodology, underlying theoretical support, and evaluative measures. The establishment of regional journal groups provides a wonderful opportunity for clinicians to stay abreast of current information with the burden for information gathering shared by others.
3. Search the literature for replications of the research that support the technique.
4. Consider the professional and personal implications of use of the technique as being equally important as the possible implications for patient care.
5. Recall your responsibility to the Code of Ethics under which we all practice (see Appendix A).

The burgeoning field of dysphagia imposes one other responsibility on practitioners. That is the responsibility to educate other health care providers and the public about state-of-the-art diagnostic and therapeutic practices in dysphagia. All professionals read and hear information in the media that makes them cringe, sometimes even when they have been the sole or partial source of the information being summarized. Translating professional information for nonprofessionals is difficult and errors are inevitable. Professionals in dysphagia cannot be dissuaded by the possibility of being misquoted or misunderstood, however. Rather they have the responsibility to speak and write judiciously and forcefully when given the opportunity. An informed consumer of health care can be a powerful ally in the struggle to recover from or compensate for a swallowing problem.

John Basmajian, MD, a physiatrist in Canada and one of the premier researchers in motor potentials and rehabilitation, has posed a cautionary comment regarding rehabilitation practices. He comments, "Probably half of what we do in rehab is useless or harmful. Unfortunately I don't know which half that is" (1997). It behooves us to struggle with the painstakingly slow progress of research to figure this out. Our early years of research and clinical practice related to dysphagia management have necessarily focused heavily on physiologic definition and diagnosis. As we begin to elucidate the nature of the disorder, we now are in a position to attend more heartily to treatment issues. In this endeavor, our best intentions to provide innovative care need to be balanced with judiciousness and a critical eye. Although we need to continue to seek alternative therapies for our patients with dysphagia, we must walk with carefully measured steps. It is much wiser to take small, sometimes slowly progressive steps instead of single big steps forward followed by multiple bigger steps back. In many ways, our position as the provider of dysphagia management services is fragile and is vulnerable to the whims of the medical community. As the sophistication of our understanding increases and our use of instrumentation follows, we must exercise great caution in the development of practice patterns.

Our current clinical practices tend to be laden with diagnostic examinations and short-term follow-up but tend to be sparse in long-term follow-up and comprehensive rehabilitation efforts. We have exerted considerable effort to earn our place on the multidisciplinary dysphagia team. Now we need to place equivalent effort in assuring that we maintain and expand this role. This text will serve the clinician as a reference for treatment planning and clinical management such that the quality of our interventional efforts will rival the quality of our diagnostic ones.

2

Framework for Intervention

This chapter discusses a framework for intervention that is based on developing the skills of an athletic coach. Coaches must be able to synthesize pertinent information of their team players so that an appropriate game plan can be developed. Clinicians must also acquire vital skills to diagnose and then develop appropriate intervention plans for their patients. Suggestions on how to determine appropriate intervention options and evaluate their functional outcome(s) are discussed. In addition, clinicians must learn how to evaluate clinically relevant research critically as they search for appropriate interventions.

BECOME A DYSPHAGIA COACH

Once a comprehensive dysphagia evaluation is done, how are appropriate treatment recommendations made? This is an important question. The decision-making process for selecting treatment is complex, since it involves many variables and the variables can change over time. The ultimate challenge is to help patients "treat" themselves so they can learn to effectively improve or cope with their dysphagia. They need to know when and how to adapt their skills, just as players on an athletic team have to adjust their skills during a game.

Definition of a Dysphagia Coach

A dysphagia coach is a clinician who possesses the astute observation, diagnostic, and treatment skills used by an athletic coach with the team. Ylvisaker and Holland (1985) described how a clinician can develop the skills of an athletic coach in the context of cognitive rehabilitation, and how to encourage self-coaching skills in their patients. They skillfully integrated the assessment and treatment of cognitive impairment by comparing the skills of a football coach to those needed by a clinician. Clinicians working in the field of cognitive rehabilitation have found this analogy quite beneficial in its simplicity and application. This analogy is certainly applicable to dysphagia management as well. Table 2–1 illustrates the simi-

Table 2–1. Coaching skills for assessment.

Athletic Coaching Skills	Dysphagia Coaching Skills
Formal	**Formal**
Statistics (height, weight, speed, throwing, etc.)	Review of medical history
	Review of nutritional status Results of clinical bedside evaluation of instrumental exam
Informal	**Informal**
Scout player in actual game	Observe patient in actual eating environment
Evaluate individual attributes Composure under stress Initiative Team spirit/desire	Evaluate individual attributes Self-awareness of problems Interest/motivation in therapy Ability to follow instruction
Interview players coach to learn about the player behind the stat sheet	Interview the patients family, friends and caregivers to learn about the person premorbidly and now
Determine position on team based on entire team needs and the nature of the opposition	Determine how patient could be most successful given setting and situation, present and future

larities in skills required for an athletic coach to assess a certain player, and a dysphagia "coach" clinician to assess a patient.

Coaching Skills for Assessment

Coaching Skill: Gather Pertinent Formal and Informal Information

Clinicians must carefully assess each patient, using formal and informal assessment tools, to collect valuable information on which intervention decisions are made. As this information is collected, it is important to remember that the formal diagnostic "stat" sheet cannot be the only data used to manage dysphagia. Inappropriate decisions may occur if dysphagia intervention plans are based solely on the results of the formal assessment. It is well known the folly of initially criticizing certain team players as being too small for a winning team, who later become the team's most valuable players. In addition, clinicians must evaluate the entire "dysphagia team," the people who will surround the patient during treatment. The amount of support—or lack of support—the dysphagia team can give to the patient will affect the entire management plan.

Components of Formal Assessment. The components of a formal assessment of dysphagia are well documented in the literature. It includes a careful review of the medical history, nutritional status, and the results of the clinical examination and instrumental diagnostic tools. It is important to understand the physiology of the swallowing disorder, not just its symptoms, to determine what type of management techniques might be appropriate. The information collected in the formal assessment is critical and reassessment may be necessary frequently.

A careful review of the medical history involves collecting information regarding the medical diagnosis and course of recovery to the present time. Pertinent medical history information, especially with regard to neurologic, pulmonary, cardiac, and cognitive status, is important to dysphagia management. In addition, it is critical to know a patient's previous and current nutritional status, including mode of intake.

The ability of the clinician to predict a dysphagia diagnosis from a medical diagnosis has recently been questioned. Although it is tempting to group certain clinical and videofluorographic dysphagia features according to medical diagnosis, Buchholz and Robbins (1997) caution against this practice. There are few data to distinguish reliably among the kinds of dysphagia associated with certain neurogenic diseases, such as stroke, Parkinson's disease, and multiple sclerosis. A grouping of dysphagia features according to specific diagnosis is obscured because of the changing nature of severity of impairment and the great variability of premorbid characteristics of each patient. Therefore, clinicians must carefully evaluate each patient for individual swallowing physiology strengths and weaknesses, and not presuppose what problems may exist as inferred by medical diagnosis.

Although the medical diagnosis cannot reliably predict the physiology and clinical problems of swallowing, it can eliminate certain treatment protocols because of the characteristics of the disease. For example, rehabilitative approaches to treat myasthenia gravis are contraindicated since the hallmark of this disease is rapid deterioration of muscle strength with increased use. The application of certain treatment protocols also may rely on the timing of treatment. For some neurodegenerative diseases, treatment may be effective if it is administered in the early stages of progression or timed after taking certain medication (Dooley, Goulden, Gatien, Gibson, & Brown, 1986; Kasarskis, Berryman, Vanderleest, Schnieder, & McClain, 1996; Kelly & Buchholz, 1996; Mazzini, Corra, Zaccala, DelPiano, & Galante, 1995; Strand, Miller, Yorkston, & Hillel, 1996; Willig, Paulus, Laucau Saint Guily, Beon, & Navarro, 1994).

Components of Informal Assessment.   The components of an informal assessment of dysphagia include a comprehensive observation of the individual with dysphagia within his or her living environment and interviews with the primary caregivers and/or family, if at all possible. Ideally, individuals with dysphagia need to be observed in the setting in which they currently live, to assess how well they can eat and function there. If possible, information regarding where the patient will live in the future should also be collected. Thus, discharge planning from a medical facility should occur initially as a dysphagia management plan is developed, in conjunction with the patient, family, and social work service.

Clinicians must evaluate patients' individual motivation and dedication to recover from their dysphagia and complete a careful assessment of the environment and people surrounding them. Clinicians must "scout" their patients and assess their informal attributes and environment as they eat, before a treatment plan is developed. This is similar to a football coach watching a player play in an actual game, before a specific set of drills or plays are developed for that player on the team.

Definition of a Dysphagia Team.   The definition of a "dysphagia team" is different in this framework from what is commonly used in the literature. A dysphagia team in the literature traditionally refers to its diagnostic players, such as a speech-language pathologist, dietitian, nurse, and physician, and so forth (Groher, 1992).

In this framework, the dysphagia team members are the people who will surround the patient and be in close, frequent contact with him or her. An evaluation of the dysphagia team includes an assessment of the physical setting where the patient will be living and/or working, since this is directly related to who will be in contact with the patient during his or her recovery. This is similar to evaluating an entire football team and playing field, according to individual player strengths and weaknesses, and then assessing the team's overall strengths and weaknesses.

Coaching Skill: Synthesize All the Information

The synthesis of the formal and informal information is crucial as a clinician assesses patients' specific strengths and weaknesses within their own environment. The role of patients on the "team," and the ability of the "team" to maximize their strengths and minimize their weaknesses, must be determined before appropriate management plan can be developed.

This type of analysis can lead to quite different management decisions, even when the results from a formal assessment are similar. For example, the intervention decisions of a patient with advanced Alzheimer's dementia living in a nursing home would be quite different from the patient who recently experienced a stroke admitted to a subacute rehabilitation center with plans to be discharged home, even when the formal assessment results of swallowing physiology are the same. The team members are different (family or staff), the living environment is different (home or nursing home), and the prognosis for recovery for the patient (team player) is dramatically different. Two very different intervention plans would be developed for the patient and team members, despite similar impairments of swallowing physiology.

Coaching Skills for Intervention

Coaching Skill: Determine the Goal(s) of Intervention for the Patient

Clinicians must first determine whether the goal(s) of intervention should focus on *rehabilitation* or *compensatory* intervention of the swallowing disorder. Rehabilitation interventions are designed to improve the actual swallowing physiology weakness or impairment. Compensatory interventions are designed to improve the ability to adapt and cope with the disorder. Compensatory techniques may be temporary and adjunct to rehabilitation techniques, or they may be the sole treatment option for safe oral intake. This dichotomy in dysphagia management is crucial for clinicians to recognize since it will aid the development of appropriate intervention goals and recommendations and help patients understand the choices before them.

Effective intervention cannot be symptom driven. It must be based on knowledge of the patient's swallowing physiology, what can be done to treat it, and a critical analysis of a patient's personal attributes and environmental support. This is similar to the way a coach develops an individual player's drills and practice sessions for an upcoming game. A player's unique strengths and weaknesses are assessed in relation to his or her team position and what the team can do to enhance his or her strengths. Decisions are made regarding whether certain weaknesses can be reduced or eliminated through exercise, surgery, or even pharmacologic methods. These decisions must be made by every clinician for their patients as well. Table 2–2 illustrates the comparison of coaching skills for intervention between an athletic and dysphagia coach.

The level of patient involvement and independent practice necessary for certain intervention approaches will also affect what goals are chosen. Many terms have been used in the literature to describe these intervention approaches. In this text, the terms *behavioral* and *nonbehavioral* intervention are used to delineate these differences, but similar terms include *direct* and *indirect,* or *passive* and *active* treatment approaches.

Behavioral Intervention Approaches.   Behavioral intervention requires a patient to participate in a treatment approach, with the continuum of participation ranging from independent use/practice to the absence of resistance and a willingness to try a certain approach, at the very least. For the most part, behavioral approaches are patient driven and, therefore, a certain level of cognition and motivation must be present.

Nonbehavioral Intervention Approaches.   Nonbehavioral intervention requires patient cooperation but not necessarily patient participation, as the approaches themselves allow the patient to adapt to his or her disordered physiology. Although compensatory techniques will not alter the physiology, they can effectively help a patient manage his or her dysphagia to allow oral eating. Caregivers may have the sole burden of implementing compensatory techniques, but the patient ultimately must be able to accept them. Active resistance to compensatory techniques must lead to frank discussions with the patient and team regarding alternate modes of nutrition, which is essentially another form of adaptation to dysphagia. This route should be entertained only after careful consideration of all other options, and it is the option of last resort.

Table 2–2. Coaching skills for intervention

Athletic Coaching Skills	Dysphagia Coaching Skills
Rehabilitation Intervention	**Rehabilitation Intervention**
Individualized intervention plan of isolated drills/exercises designed to eliminate or improve specific weaknesses for a certain team position	Individualized intervention plan of isolated drills/exercises designed to eliminate or improve specific weaknesses of swallowing physiology
Independent player practice	Independent patient practice
Integration of isolated skills to prepare for actual game	Integration of isolated skills to attain patient eating goal
Systematically practice related groups of players together to prepare for a game	Systematically practice limited oral eating in small amounts with certain textures
Full scrimmage to simulate real game stress	Gradually build intake and texture in real eating situations
Surgical approaches	Surgical approaches
Pharmacologic approaches	Pharmacologic approaches
Compensatory Intervention	**Compensatory Intervention**
Specific game plan to compensate for player weakness	Specific interventions to compensate for patient
Maximize player strengths and minimize weaknesses	Maximize patient strengths and minimize weakness
Use the home team advantage such as support of the fans and familiar playing field	Educate and encourage caregivers to provide support and appropriate maintenance of intervention plan

Choosing the Best Intervention Options. All patients should first be evaluated with the goal of rehabilitation, that is, improving physiology, if at all possible. If there is a chance for recovery, clinicians must determine the best options. Behavioral rehabilitation interventions involve exercises aimed at improving the physiology of the swallowing musculature. Nonbehavioral rehabilitation interventions improve the physiology through surgical or pharmacologic methods. Obviously, the use of surgical or pharmacologic intervention to improve swallowing physiology permanently must be considered carefully. A careful review of compensatory approaches should always be discussed with a patient, prior to suggesting surgical intervention or long-term use of medication.

Compensatory intervention can also include components of behavioral and nonbehavioral approaches. An example of a behavioral compensatory approach is volitional airway protection, whereby a patient must actively learn and use this technique with every swallow. On the other hand, a nonbehavioral compensatory approach is some type of prosthetic device used by a patient, such as a palatal lift or even dentures. Many common compensatory options involve both behavioral and nonbehavioral components, depending on the level of patient autonomy in using the approaches. For instance, self-feeding patients are responsible to use the strategies with every meal and, therefore, they are implementing a behavioral compensatory approach. For patients who are dependent on caregivers for feeding, they are involved in a nonbehavioral compensatory approach.

Coaching Skill: Determine the Goal(s) of Intervention for the Team

Clinicians must determine what type of support is required from caregivers (the team) for the patient, given the various settings and situations where the patient will eat. This is similar to an athletic coach assessing the entire team and deciding how to prepare the entire team for an upcoming game. How can the caregivers minimize patients' weaknesses and maximize their strengths to allow success in oral eating? What are the potential problems anticipated from the "opposition"? How can the team adequately prepare for the upcoming game?

Careful evaluation of caregivers and the environment in which a patient will live and eat is important to the success of any treatment protocol. Appropriate maintenance of compensatory strategies, such as diet modifications and correct body postures, may become the responsibility of the caregiver. Clinicians may want to create a "home field advantage" for their patients by preparing caregivers appropriately.

Coaching Skill: Foster Individual and Team Commitment to the Goal(s)

No coach ever goes out on the field and actually plays on the team, although the temptation must be great at times during a losing game. Similarly, clinicians cannot make a patient or dysphagia team comply with an intervention plan, even if they try to be present at every meal. It has been suggested that knowing how to feed a meal does not guarantee compliance in caregivers (Sanders, Hoffman, & Lund, 1992). Anecdotally, patients also have not demonstrated good compliance in using safe eating techniques, despite lengthy patient education on how to self-feed. The reasons for poor compliance in intervention recommendations are many and varied. It does appear that patients and caregivers must understand why the care plan is important before they will comply with the recommendations (Sanders et al., 1992).

Clinicians need to inspire and motivate patients and caregivers to follow the "game plan." Clinicians need to develop the motivational skills of coaches with their teams. The sports literature is full of books describing these skills, based on the success of individual coaches. In addition, personal motivation books are also widely available. Clinicians may want to explore this literature to learn how to motivate their patients and clinicians to follow the care plan.

Coaching Skill: Adjust the Intervention Plan When Necessary

Clinicians need to remain astute observers of a patient and the team, since particular strengths and weaknesses can always change. Just as a football coach may need to adjust a game plan during the game against formidable opposition, clinicians need to remain flexible and alert to make timely adjustments in the intervention plan as well. The patient cannot be the sole focus of intervention. Constant reevaluation of all team members (patient and surrounding caregivers) is necessary to enhance success of the intervention plan. Periodic reevaluation should occur even for those patients initially assessed as poor treatment candidates or who eventually received tube feedings. Reevaluation of these patients may reveal new management options that were not initially possible.

When to Start and Stop Intervention. The criteria used in determining when to try an intervention option and when to stop is complicated and often is a factor of individual clinician training and experience. A combination of rehabilitation and compensatory intervention options may be indicated at times. In these cases, a patient may need to use compensatory techniques to maintain oral eating while simultaneously participating in a rehabilitation program. As previously stated, a careful synthesis of formal and informal assessment data must occur to determine whether a patient is a candidate for intervention.

Rehabilitation efforts may be stopped when a reasonable amount of time has transpired without significant progress on the identified intervention outcome goal(s). Obviously, the definition of what constitutes "reasonable time," "significant progress," and "intervention outcome goal(s)" will vary, according to clinician experience, training and what goal(s) are being measured and evaluated.

Coaching Skill: Be Accountable for the Intervention Outcome(s)

Clinicians are accountable for the success or failure of intervention outcome(s), just as athletic coaches are accountable to their individual players, the team, the fans, and the owners who pay them. A coach may lose an occasional game, but he or she should still demonstrate effective skill at coaching to have a winning season or, at the very least, observe overall team improvement each game.

Clinicians are ultimately responsible for their intervention outcomes. They are accountable not only to patients, their families, and caregivers but also to their employers and the overall health care system. Defining "success" in dysphagia intervention is complicated, however, since the criteria for evaluating success may differ for each patient, team, and health care payer.

Coaching Skill: Seek "Coaching Tips" from Experienced Coaches

Every clinician, and every coach, can benefit from hearing the "voice of experience." The wisdom imparted from an experienced coach or clinician during a time of crisis or confusion regarding the best options to implement, can sometimes make all the difference in outcome. Athletic coaches learn valuable coaching tips by watching other coaches during a game. Clinicians also can benefit from observing experienced clinicians and discussing intervention strategies with them. This does not mean that clinicians should indiscriminately follow the advice of experienced clinicians. In fact, advice from an experienced clinician may actually increase indecision, since experience often teaches there are many ways to manage dysphagia, and no one intervention will always benefit a patient.

OUTCOME MEASUREMENT IN DYSPHAGIA

The development and collection of outcome data has become a national preoccupation, not only in health care, but other businesses as well. Every business is being asked to produce evidence that the monies spent on that product or service is worth the price. Defining what type of evidence is required to demonstrate that dysphagia clinical services are "worth the price" is complicated. The information deemed most critical to show value will differ, according to individual and professional perspectives and objectives. Furthermore, it is a complex task to conduct carefully designed studies to demonstrate the efficacy of treatment in dysphagia (McHorney & Rosenbek, 1998; Miller & Langmore, 1994). This is the greatest current challenge to the field of dysphagia management.

Traditional Outcome Measures in Dysphagia

Clinicians have traditionally viewed outcome measures of dysphagia as a function of physiologic improvement, achieved by the use of rehabilitation and/or compensatory intervention techniques (McHorney & Rosenbek, 1998). These measures have focused on providing information regarding the effect of certain interventions (postures, volitional airway maneuvers, surgery, and so on) in improving swallowing physiology, such as duration of swallow response, percent of aspiration, and so on.

In addition, clinicians have attempted to measure the "success" of dysphagia services by observing various health status indicators that improve or stabilize, given dysphagia intervention. Typical health status indicators include data related to aspiration pneumonia (Martin et al., 1994), dehydration, malnutrition, and death (Schmidt, Holas, Halvorson, & Reding, 1994). Indirect health status indicators, such as the duration and frequency of hospital stays and whether the patient is discharged home or to another health care facility, may also be potentially valuable measures of dysphagia intervention success (McHorney & Rosenbek, 1998).

The Relationship of Health Status to Dysphagia

Health status indicators are assumed to be signs related to the presence of dysphagia. However, this presumption has not been empirically proven (McHorney & Rosenbek, 1998). Due to the presence of many complicating factors typically seen in patients with dysphagia, it is not possible to know conclusively that the observation of a certain health problem, or length of a hospital stay, for example, is directly related to dysphagia. In fact, the diagnosis and relationship of aspiration pneumonia to dysphagia is not even as clear-cut as many clinicians may believe.

Recognizing that aspiration pneumonia is a difficult diagnosis to make in patients, especially the elderly, various criteria have been used in recent studies (Feinberg, Knebl, Tully, & Segall, 1990; Langmore et al.,1998; Martin et al., 1994). In addition, Langmore and colleagues (1998) reported that while dysphagia does increase the risk for aspiration pneumonia, pneumonia does not generally occur unless other risk factors are present as well. In this study, the other important risk factors to consider in a patient with dysphagia are multiple medical diagnoses, multiple medications, the condition of the teeth, and dependence for feeding and oral care. Given these data, and the lack of conclusive data on the relationship of dysphagia to health status indicators, clinicians need to exercise caution when proclaiming positive outcomes due to their intervention. This is not to say that clinicians should not collect and share their positive outcome data, since these data are sorely needed. However, clinicians do need to be aware of the complexities involved in interpreting outcome data.

Functional Outcome Measures

Another form of outcome measurement involves the development and collection of what is termed *functional outcome measures.* This term encompasses many variables and typically is used to measure the feeding and eating skills of a patient. Functional outcome measurement has become the required standard for intervention goals by many reimbursement and accrediting agencies. Unfortunately, empirically tested, data-based scales that accurately measure these complex variables are not yet available. Many scales now exist, but no study has conclusively established even the relationship of dysphagia to eating and drinking skills (American Speech-Language-Hearing Association, 1996; Cherney, Cantieri, & Pannell, 1986; Hillel et al., 1989; Salassa, 1997; Waxman, Durfee, Moore, Morantz, & Koeller, 1990).

The development of functional outcome scales is difficult since there are many variables associated with the treatment of feeding and eating skills. In the long-term care setting, for instance, Medicare requires measurement of the amount of assistance required for eating, in addition to other nutritional parameters. This information aids in determining reimbursement rates to the nursing home (Health Care Financing Administration, 1997). Changes in levels of assistance have obvious cost benefits and, therefore, measurement of a patient's "functional performance" to eat and swallow independently are considered quite valuable.

Another outcome variable receiving attention is the amount of education a patient receives regarding his or her care plan. The Joint Commission on Accreditation of Healthcare Organizations (JCAHO) requires the measurement of patient education and involvement in the development of the care plan and, when necessary, its modification (JCAHO, 1996). It is believed that "functional status and functional outcomes" are maximized when the patient is educated and involved in his or her own self-care and care decisions. Therefore, education for the patient and family is considered an essential part of intervention outcome. The impact of patient education for dysphagia functional outcome is not known at this time. Other variables affecting functional outcome may also include the length of time to eat or drink, the necessity of adaptive feeding equipment, use of compensatory postures and type of diet modification, as well as others (McHorney & Rosenbek, 1998).

Ideal Outcome Measurement

Clinicians need a functional outcome scale that is sensitive to small individual changes over a variety of factors, yet applicable to all possible disorders and settings. The measurement of functional outcomes must also be simple and efficient in design to allow implementation within all settings. A single scale with multiple subtests or a series of functional outcome scales may be the best solution to these problems (McHorney & Rosenbek, 1998).

Quality of Care and Quality of Life Measures

The final two areas of outcome measurement gaining attention are focused on the patients themselves, regarding how they feel about their dysphagia and treatment. Reimbursement agencies and employers are increasingly interested in measuring the amount of patient satisfaction with their treatment (quality of care received) and the perceived benefit of that intervention to the patient's quality of life.

Measurement of quality of care and life issues inherently relies on subjective data and interpretation. This does not mean the data are any less useful or valid. In fact, the importance of measuring these issues cannot be ignored. While these measurements may appear to lack the precision of other scientific research in dysphagia, this has not been validated in other disciplines that routinely conduct this type of research. For example, food scientists have demonstrated that the subjective evaluation used in the sensory testing of foods and liquids can be as exact and reproducible as objective measurements (Bourne, 1982).

Unfortunately, there is a paucity of literature addressing the quality of care and life issues regarding dysphagia (McHorney & Rosenbek, 1998). However, a new scale called SWAL-QOL is currently being developed in Madison, Wisconsin, which is designed to measure the patient's perspective on the quality of life impact of dysphagia (McHorney & Rosenbek, 1998). The information gathered by a tool such as SWAL-QOL may dramatically alter the focus of intervention since patients may hold different viewpoints from their clinicians, regarding what the goals of intervention should be. In other words, a physiologic improvement in swallowing that is not perceived by the patient as improving quality of life may not be a "success" after all. Measurement of quality of life and care issues is sorely needed in the field of dysphagia management.

INCORPORATING RESEARCH INTO CLINICAL PRACTICE

Clinicians need to learn how to evaluate their intervention practices and new ideas for treatment. Athletic coaches continually keep abreast of new approaches to improve a team's skills and play and rely greatly on the medical and sports literature to help them determine the best ways to prepare players for a winning team. Likewise, clinicians must rely on the scientific research in the literature to evaluate dysphagia intervention practices that may be useful for particular patients.

Clinicians are often intimidated by scientific research and feel unprepared to evaluate its value to their daily practice. A couple of excellent articles have recently been written that can help clinicians overcome these feelings of inadequacy (Huckabee, 1997; Sonies & Huckabee, 1995). Huckabee has described a simple and eloquent model for clinicians to use when evaluating clinical research and new ideas within the profession. The components of this model include a careful analysis of the

1. Source of information
2. Methodology of the study
3. Strength of the conclusions
4. Legal and ethical considerations

Source of the Information

Clinicians must identify the source of the information regarding the clinical treatment. Peer-reviewed journal articles are rigorously evaluated by experts in the field and therefore constitute the best source of information regarding treatment ideas and practice. Clinicians need to be wary of information gleaned from the public media, such as television or newspapers, since misinterpretation of the information can often result through these mediums. This does not mean all information regarding dysphagia management should be distrusted when viewed on public mediums. In fact, the general public is generally quite ignorant about current knowledge and practices regarding dysphagia services, and this fact hurts the profession (and public!) greatly. More public presentations regarding dysphagia intervention, based on careful research that has withstood the critic of colleagues, are encouraged. However, presenters must be careful not to overstate the value of the information being shared.

Methodology of the Study

Clinicians need to evaluate the underlying theoretical support for the intervention being evaluated in the study, and the research design used in the study. Why would this intervention be useful in improving dysphagia based on the current knowledge and thoughts regarding dysphagia? Does the research design have a control group so that the intervention being studied can be compared with a similar group that does not receive the intervention?

Efficacy Research

Efficacy research must include a control group to demonstrate that the treatment is responsible for the changes observed. In single case design research, patients can serve as their own control if careful attention is given to the collection of baseline data and observation of a change only when a treatment is applied (Kazdin, 1982; McReynolds & Kearns, 1983). Excellent reviews of efficacy research conducted thus far in dysphagia are available in the literature, and are recommended reading for all clinicians (Langmore & Miller, 1994; Miller & Langmore, 1994).

Demonstrating Effectiveness of a Treatment

Clinicians need to remember that efficacy research is not the same as demonstrating the effectiveness of a treatment. This has important implications as reimbursement agencies are evaluating the cost effectiveness of dysphagia services. The effectiveness of a treatment is based on demonstrating a positive change in a patient in the clinic (Rosenbek, 1995). Cost effectiveness is a simple calculation of comparing how much money was needed to achieve this positive effect. Caution needs to be applied when discussing the effectiveness of a treatment in the clinic and its cost effectiveness compared with its demonstrated efficacy. Clinicians need to be careful not to describe a treatment as efficacious, unless some type of comparison control was used in the data collection. If a treatment has been proven efficacious in the literature, then the criteria for proving effectiveness (also called efficiency) are not as stringent. The strict experimental controls used in efficacy research are assumed sufficient to assume efficiency as well, given competent clinical practice (Rosenbek, 1995).

The Use of Normal Volunteers and Patients with Dysphagia as Subjects

In dysphagia research, an interesting question has arisen given the subjects used in evaluating treatment approaches. Should treatments be evaluated on subjects with dysphagia only? How should data be evaluated when normal volunteers are used to demonstrate the effect of a treatment approach? If a change occurs in normal volunteers, should patients with dysphagia also be expected to demonstrate similar changes? Should the underlying theory of a treatment be based on normal physiology or abnormal physiology? These are difficult questions, especially since the understanding of normal and abnormal swallowing physiology is still not completely understood. This is a great challenge for the profession, but one that is exciting. Clinicians are encouraged to ponder these excellent questions as they read and critically review the literature.

Strength of the Conclusions

What did the data actually demonstrate? Did the data confirm the underlying theory or not? Did the authors base their conclusions on their data and subjects, or did they try to generalize the data beyond what they studied? Practicing clinicians often have the greatest trouble evaluating the strength of a study's conclusions, since it requires some basic knowledge of research design and critical skill to make sure the conclusions fit the results reported.

The skill of evaluating study conclusions is one that can be developed and strengthened through a variety of methods. Dysphagia study groups are springing up across the country, comprised of local colleagues who share an interest in improving their clinical skills. Group discussions of treatment articles at these study groups may help all participants learn this skill. In addition, attendance at advanced workshops that will critique current research or contacting a local university for workshops in this area may also help. Finally, just reading the literature may also improve critical analysis skills, since the information gained from reading research articles can increase understanding and, eventually, increase clinical questions. It is the ability to question an article's conclusion that identifies growth in critical analysis skills.

Legal and Ethical Considerations

Research conducted with human subjects must be approved by a human subjects safety review committee prior to funding. This safeguard was legislated into effect by government as a protection of all human subjects that agree to participate in a research project. The risks and benefits of participation in the study must be clearly documented and explained in all research subject agreement forms. All subjects are informed they are free to remove themselves from the study at any time.

It is recognized that all treatment, including the choice of no treatment, includes a risk of harm. This is readily apparent in dysphagia intervention where the establishment of a control group of patients may constitute a legal and ethical dilemma. If subjects do not receive what is commonly believed to be essential treatment, harm may occur to those subjects. In the most serious scenario, this practice could be considered professional negligence since it deviates from what is considered standard clinical practice (Scott, 1994).

All treatment options, including the choice of no treatment, involve risk. There is no treatment that is risk free, since all risk decisions involve a comparison of the risks and benefits of each option (National Research Council, 1989). Clinicians must carefully evaluate clinical research and ideas that have not survived human subjects committee review. The relative risks and benefits of the treatment need to be critically assessed before embracing the new treatment idea. Use of the model described to evaluate clinical research will help clinicians make prudent legal and ethical treatment decisions.

CONCLUSION

The skills of an athletic coach are desirable in clinicians who manage dysphagia. Clinicians need to develop coaching skills for assessment and intervention, being mindful that they are accountable for their actions. The ability to collect and weigh the formal and informal assessments of a patient, within their particular environment, is similar to the skills coaches use as they evaluate individual players and then, the overall team. A dysphagia team, in this framework, refers to the people who surround the patient with dysphagia and directly impact the success of the intervention plan.

Intervention options can be divided into two main areas: rehabilitation and compensatory options. Rehabilitation techniques usually require active patient participation and are specifically designed to improve or eliminate the physiologic dysphagia impairment. Compensatory techniques may or may not require active participation by the patient, and are designed to help a patient adapt or cope with the physiologic impairment. The level of awareness, motivation, and physical/cognitive attributes a patient can apply to improve the dysphagia can influence treatment options. Clinicians must continually reassess these factors to make timely adjustments to the intervention plan. Clinicians need to develop skills to motivate and inspire patients and their caregivers to follow the care plan, using the techniques coaches use to motivate a team to win.

The criteria used to define success in dysphagia intervention are currently under investigation. This is the next great challenge for the profession. The development of outcome measures in dysphagia is sorely needed, as patients, families, and payers question the value of dysphagia services. Clinicians are encouraged to seek the advice of an experienced clinician during difficult management decisions, recognizing the limitations of anecdotal experience, and also the value of wisdom from the "voice of experience."

Clinicians are encouraged to use a simple model to learn how to evaluate clinical research critically and incorporate it into practice. Clinicians need to evaluate an intervention idea based on four components: the source of the information where they learned of the idea, the methodology used in the research design, the strength of the conclusions, and the legal and ethical considerations in using that intervention in clinical practice.

3

Rehabilitation of Dysphagia

This chapter provides definitions, supporting research and techniques for swallowing rehabilitation and differentiates these techniques from compensatory techniques. When appropriate, instructions, teaching techniques, and short-term objectives are included. As with compensatory techniques section, the maneuvers are presented based on the physiologic abnormality that they are considered to address, rather than the symptom.

DEFINITIONS AND EXPECTATIONS

Rehabilitate:"(a) to restore to a former capacity; (b) to restore to a condition of health or useful and constructive activity"(Webster, 1995). Some of this book's chapters will outline mechanisms by which the patient and clinician can improve airway protection, caloric intake, and, subsequently, quality of life through effective compensation for a recognized disorder. Thus, the goal of intervention is to facilitate safer, more efficient oral intake in the context of a disordered system. Although these approaches to dysphagia management do not negate Webster's definition, they tend to fall short of the intent. The clinical focus of intervention through compensation is to render a disordered system functional and safe, not to restore physiology. However, the clinical focus of rehabilitation of swallowing is to improve permanently the physiological substrates such that the significance of the disorder is minimized or eliminated and the disordered system operates more efficiently. Certainly, the effects can be varied.

Rehabilitation at its most promising offers a patient with dysphagia the opportunity for oral intake without compensation or nutritional limitation at a level approximating preinjury function. In a patient who is severely disordered, rehabilitation may improve swallowing physiology to a level such that behavioral compensations may be successfully applied, thus allowing for at least limited oral intake. In either case, function is not only maximized, it is optimized by providing a long-term physiological shift.

PHYSIOLOGY LEADS TO SYMPTOMATOLOGY

Effective rehabilitation of dysphagia relies on accurate diagnosis and individualization of the treatment plan to the specific physiology. As pointed out earlier in this text, there is an important distinction between dysphagic physiology and dysphagic symptoms. Often during a diagnostic swallowing examination, the swallowing symptoms are more static and thus more easily observed. The physiology that leads to the symptoms is unfortunately a dynamic process and thus requires a more critical eye. It is fairly easy for even a novice clinician to observe vallecular pooling at some point in the swallowing process. However, the underlying etiology of this residual can be varied and thus treatment would be varied. If the pooling were present before onset of the swallow, two underlying physiological deficits would be suspect. First, the patient may demonstrate poor oral control of the bolus with premature spillage into the pharyngeal space. On the other hand, this symptom may represent a delayed pharyngeal swallow secondary to poor neurosensory feedback and thus an untimely pharyngeal response. As the first physiologic abnormality is motor-based and the second is sensory-based, rehabilitative approaches will differ markedly. Yet another interpretation of this symptom is reduced base of tongue to posterior pharyngeal wall approximation, paired with reduced pharyngeal stripping. This would likely be the case when the pooling is present postswallow, for which we would more accurately use the term *residual*. Inappropriate treatment due to inaccurate identification of physiology, regardless of the good intentions supporting it, is not efficacious, not cost effective, and may indeed be contraindicated. Thus, rehabilitation of swallowing should be preceded by critical diagnostic evaluation. Given the necessity of planning treatment based on physiology rather sympto-matology, this chapter is organized accordingly, focusing on rehabilitation of physiological deficits, not management of symptoms.

The following text provides what little empirical research is available in reference to physiologic justification and efficacy. However, as discussed previously, a book based only on proven fact in this area would be a short one indeed. It is unfortunate that clinical practice almost always precedes scientific support. Thus, as is the case frequently in clinical practice, a por-tion of the information offered to the clinician is based on anecdotal infor-mation gleaned from clinical practice, with a smattering of clinical lore. The practicing clinician is invited, and encouraged, to read this text and all reports of potential treatments with a critical and judicious eye. However, until we have established further efficacy data, the adage, "Absence of proof is not proof of absence" may need to be our guiding principle.

TREATMENT CANDIDACY

Candidacy for rehabilitation efforts will be guided by the presenting etiol-ogy of the dysphagic physiology, as well as the cognition, motivation, and support systems presented by and offered to the patient. Thus each pa-tient presents a unique clinical picture and treatment planning cannot be easily generalized. Many patients with neurodegenerative disorders are not appropriate rehabilitative candidates. The focus of intervention in this population will focus heavily on compensation and ongoing, intermittent diagnostic evaluation. Certainly, in some diagnoses, such as myasthenia gravis, rehabilitative efforts are not only inappropriate, but may be contraindicated because concentrated exercises may deplete the neuro-logical reserve and exacerbate symptoms. Energy conservation and care-fully timed compensatory programs will be the rule in these populations. Parkinson's disease is considered neurodegenerative in nature. However, for patients in whom the progression of the disease is slow, the window for muscle strengthening may be opened.

In all neurologic diagnoses, cognitive deficits may certainly hinder rehabilitative efforts. Many of the techniques to be described below require sequencing of motor events and conceptualization of a rather abstract process. Thus, patients with significant cognitive or communica-tion deficits may be unable to benefit fully from this type of intervention and may require compensation as a sole management course. However, the importance of oral intake to the social, medical, and emotional well-being of the patient should entreat us to give every patient the opportu-nity to participate in rehabilitation that is carefully planned and clearly instructed. If the opportunity yields no rewards, then compensation as lifelong management will be the indicated method for ensuring optimal function and quality of life. Creativity by the clinician is required in teaching and facilitating execution of these maneuvers in order to maximize rehabilitative potential.

CHARACTERISTICS OF NEUROMUSCULAR DEFICITS

In general, neuromuscular deficits can be classified into three categories of physiologic impairment: muscle spasticity or hyperfunction, muscular weakness or hypofunction, and muscle dyscoordination or apraxia. All muscle tissue at rest demonstrates a characteristic elasticity, or tone. This inherent tone maintains joint flexibility, but establishes slight resistance to enforce some stability. Hypertonic muscle tissue however is dysfunctional and impedes coordinated, smooth movements. It can be classified by either spasticity or rigidity. Spasticity is typically symptomatic of patients with upper motor neuron lesions involving the pyramidal system and is characterized by increased tone that is variable within an individual muscle and across muscles. Thus, movement may be imprecise and difficult to initiate but without limitation of range of motion. Rigidity, on the other hand, is typical of patients with lesions of the extrapyramidal system, such as Parkinson's disease. This disorder is characterized by consistent muscle tension across muscles, which greatly inhibits range of motion.

Hypotonicity or flaccidity of musculature is characteristic of patients with cranial nerve lesions or cortical stroke and typically presents unilaterally. As weakness is the cardinal feature, this type of neuromuscular disorder is considered to respond to muscle-strengthening exercises.

Finally, dyscoordination of muscle contraction results from improper sequencing or timing of muscle contraction, or from deficits of motor programming. Considered to emerge as a result of central nervous system injury, the deficits of motor programming may present as the clinical picture of apraxia. Certainly, oral apraxia is well reported. Verbal, or speech, apraxia is less clearly documented. To date, little documentation has emerged describing a presentation of swallowing apraxia; however, it could seem likely given the nature of the disorder (Robbins, 1988; Tuch, 1965;).

A hierarchy of rehabilitative effort will address increased muscular tone as a prerequisite to other motor tasks. By decreasing tone in the initial stages of intervention, the myogenic substrates are normalized to allow for improved motor learning in other areas. Discussion of the following rehabilitative exercises will thus target the myogenic features of hyperfunction, hypofunction, and dyscoordination associated with each physiologic swallowing deficit, when appropriate or substantiated.

REHABILITATIVE EXERCISES

Physiologic Abnormality: Oral Motor Inefficiency

Oral motor inefficiency in the patient with dysphagia may result in a variety of dysphagic symptoms secondary to limitations of strength, range of motion and/or flexibility. Clinical presentation may include both anterior and posterior loss of control of the bolus with premature spillage of the bolus into the pharynx, incomplete development of a cohesive bolus, decreased effectiveness of mastication, inability for lingual sweep and postswallow residual in buccal, sublingual, or general oral cavities. Dysphagic symptoms may, but do not always, coexist with speech production impairment (Martin & Corlew, 1990).

Although used extensively in speech pathology interventions across dysphagic and nondysphagic disorders, the efficacy of oral motor exercises on oral function is obscure. It is an interesting phenomena in the profession of speech language pathology that so much of our work across the discipline involves the oral mechanism, yet we have few supportive data for intervention efforts. This is true for dysphagia management as well as dysarthria management. The issue of efficacy is compounded in swallowing management. It is fairly well accepted that the neurologic pathways for speech and swallowing differ, despite the shared anatomic structures for production. We can identify no empirical evidence that volitional rote exercises will have a subsequent effect on the highly programmed motor response required in the oral phase of swallowing. Nonetheless, and perhaps rightly so, clinicians have developed a variety of methods for oral intervention with patients who are neurologically impaired. Although these authors do not heavily utilize these practices, an overview of some of these techniques will be provided in the interest of thoroughness, as well as to foster discussion and clinical investigation. The interested reader is directed to other readings for greater detail in oral motor intervention (Dworkin, 1991; Ylvisaker & Logemann, 1986; Ylvisaker & Weinstein, 1989).

Primary Physiologic Target: Reduced Labial Closure

Increased and decreased labial tone may lead to difficult removing a bolus from a utensil or an inability to maintain the bolus within the oral cavity after it is accepted. Increased tone may as well inhibit bolus acceptance altogether in the case of abnormal reflexes. Generally, these exercises are thought to improve oral motor function with the effect of improving bolus control and inhibition of anterior oral leakage.

Patient Instruction. Tasks to improve hypertonicity of the lips may consist of slow, progressive stretching exercises in an effort to relieve the spasm or hyperfunction. Using a gloved finger, the clinician provides firm directed pressure to the outer lip in both lateral and superior/inferior directions. For labial hypofunction, exercises may include pursing, retracting, and relaxing the lips either in rote range of motion tasks, or against resistance. The use of a candy, funnel-shaped "rocket pop" that increases in diameter, may be used to encourage progressive lip closure. Functionally, strengthening of lip closure may be addressed by providing the patient with a button or lifesaver on a string with the instruction to maintain the disc within the oral cavity against pressure using only lip closure. An even more functional task to address coordination and strengthening of labial closure consists of using a strip of moistened gauze. The patient is instructed to pull the gauze into the oral cavity without the assistance of hands or tongue. The patient stabilizes the end of the gauze between his or her teeth and uses lip protrusion and retraction to slowly pull the gauze inward.

Contraindication. No contraindications are identified for the tasks themselves. Use of lifesavers, buttons, and other hard objects should be externally anchored in a patient with impaired lingual control to inhibit accidental swallowing.

Example of Possible Short-Term Clinical Objectives. During oral ingestion of one level teaspoon of pudding, the patient will fully clear the bolus from the spoon with no more than trace residual on 90% of trials.

Primary Physiologic Target: Reduced Lingual Control

Lingual weakness or dyscoordination is not uncommonly observed in neurologic injury and can result in significant functional impairment necessitating a compensated diet. Efficient tongue control moves the bolus between the teeth for mastication, collects the bolus from the buccal and sublingual cavities to inhibit postswallow oral residual, and effectively manipulates the food into a cohesive bolus for transfer. Deficits of lingual control, in addition to compromising the efficiency of this process, can lead to unintentional premature spillage of the bolus into the oral pharyngeal aperture and increase the potential for preswallow aspiration. Thus poor lingual control can effect not only nutritional but pulmonary stability.

The following exercises are designed to enhance bolus manipulation, mastication, and control for efficient anterior to posterior transfer.

Patient Instruction. As with hyperfunctional labial function, increased tone of the lingual musculature may respond to gentle stretching techniques to inhibit spasticity. These should be done cautiously using a gloved hand and a gauze pad to grasp the tongue tip. In addition, monitoring of submental, and thus sublingual, musculature using surface electromyographic (SEMG) biofeedback technology (refer to Chapter 4) may also allow the patient to gain greater volitional control and thus inhibit increased tone. For lingual hypofunction, exercises may consist of protruding, elevating, retracting, and lateralizing the tongue. General instructions would focus on repetition of these movements for limited periods of time with relaxation between contractions. A component of work-against-resistance can be added. Patient is instructed to complete range of motion exercises in all planes of movement against a firm source of resistance, such as a tongue blade. Resistance is then progressively increased to accommodate increased strength of movement. Commercially available devices such as the Iowa Oral Pressure Instrument (IOPI) or the Kay Elemetrics oral pressure tranducers may also facilitate the increase of intraoral pressure and increase lingual strength.

Exercises to improve functional flexibility of movement differ somewhat, and ultimately, may be of greater benefit to the patient. Several methods may address this goal. The activity described above wherein the patient pulls gauze into the oral cavity can be advanced further to address lingual flexibility and coordination. As the patient pulls the entire gauze into the mouth (with the exception of a small tail secured outside for safety), he or she utilizes oral lingual movements to simulate oral manipulation of a bolus. The patient is to simulate oral mastication with emphasis on rotary jaw movement and inhibition of buccal stasis, and then uses lingual movement to form a cohesive bolus. When the gauze texture is mastered, a more difficult task would be a length of household string. For patients with difficulty maintaining the bolus in the anterior oral cavity and thus at risk of premature leakage into the pharynx prior to volitional transfer, a similar activity would use small hard candy that is secured on a string. The candy is placed far into the posterior oral cavity, or in regions of the mouth that are otherwise poorly accessible to lingual sweep. The patient is instructed to retrieve the candy and move it to within a more accessible region of the oral cavity.

Contraindication. As with labial exercises, no contraindications are identified for the tasks themselves. Use of lifesavers, buttons, and other hard objects should be externally anchored in a patient with severely impaired lingual control to inhibit accidental swallowing. As with any exercise, patients with neurodegenerative disease are poor candidates for strengthening exercises, which may be contraindicated based on the nature of the disorder.

Example of Possible Short-Term Clinical Objectives.

1. Patient will masticate and manipulate one-fourth of a shortbread cookie into a cohesive bolus prior to oral pharyngeal transfer, with no sublingual or buccal residual.
2. Patient will demonstrate no radiographic evidence of premature spillage secondary to poor oral control during ingestion of any texture.

Primary Physiologic Target: Decreased Palatal Elevation

Reduced velopharyngeal closure certainly can have deleterious effects on speech production. The effects on swallowing are less clear. Although nasal regurgitation is occasionally seen in cases of severe pharyngeal phase dysphagia, the physiologic abnormality leading to this symptom appears more often to be related to dyscoordination of pharyngeal stripping rather than velopharyngeal closure directly. However, poor palatal closure may produce functional deficits in oral intake methods by reducing intraoral pressure for sucking or straw drinking. As with other oral exercises, data to support the efficacy of palatal strengthening exercises are scant and carryover to functional activity is even less well documented. Very functional tasks to facilitate velopharyngeal closure during oral intake may be the most direct route to intervention.

Patient Instruction. Straw-sucking tasks may encourage velopharyngeal closure as a functional outcome. Task difficulty may be graded by increasing the texture presented (liquid, yogurt, pudding) and decreasing the diameter of the straw (large bore straw used in barium swallows, large commercially available straw such as that dispensed at McDonald's, small commercially available straw, coffee stirrer). For patients who are unable to tolerate oral intake because of aspiration risk, the activity can be completed by aborting the task just as bolus reaches the lips.

Contraindication. None documented.

Example of Possible Short-Term Clinical Objectives. Patient will ingest 4 ounces of thin liquid using straw sips.

Physiologic Abnormality: Delayed Pharyngeal Swallow

A delayed pharyngeal swallow occurs when the patient volitionally or responsively transfers the bolus posteriorly out of the oral cavity and a synergistic pharyngeal response fails to occur in a timely manner. This represents a deficit of the neurosensory system in which inadequate sensory feedback mechanisms fail to communicate the oncoming bolus. As addressed in earlier sections, it is crucial that this deficit be distinguished diagnostically from premature spillage secondary to poor oral control, a neuromuscular deficit. Although the radiographic image is similar, the management is quite different for each disorder.

Of the variety of physiologic deficits that can occur subsequent to neurologic disease, delayed pharyngeal swallow is perhaps the most prevalent. Unfortunately, it is likely the deficit that we have the least to offer in term of rehabilitation. There is no behavioral intervention identified that will change the physiology of onset of responsive swallow on a long-term, permanent basis.

In Chapter 6, thermal stimulation, or thermal gustatory stimulation, is presented as a compensatory technique for delayed pharyngeal swallow. This is its rightful context based on available research, which will be reviewed. There is inadequate evidence to support the use of thermal stimulation as a rehabilitative modality with the goal of long-term physiologic shift to more timely onset of swallow. Unfortunately, we have little else to offer in terms of rehabilitation of this physiologic deficit.

Physiologic Abnormality: Reduced Strength and Coordination of Pharyngeal Contraction, Laryngeal Excursion

Impaired pharyngeal phase swallowing is common in neurologic disease, more often in patients with right cortical stroke and brain stem injury. The physiologic abnormalities that can occur in the pharynx and the subsequent symptoms are many. Abnormal physiology can include:

▶ Reduced palatal closure
▶ Inadequate base of tongue to posterior pharyngeal wall approximation
▶ Decreased laryngeal excursion (elevation and/or anterior movement)
▶ Reduced pharyngeal stripping
▶ Inadequate epiglottic deflection with ineffective airway protection

Symptoms can include bolus passing into the nose upon attempted swallowing, residual throughout the pharynx, slow movement of the bolus through the pharynx, and penetration or aspiration. As previously discussed, the symptoms are not the target of rehabilitative intervention; rather the underlying physiology is addressed. Most of the maneuvers that we use toward this end are targeted primarily toward a specific feature but may have secondary effects on other physiologic characteristics.

Primary Physiologic Target: Decreased Laryngeal Elevation and Reduced Pharyngeal Contraction

Treatment: Modified Valsalva (Effortful) Swallow. The modified Valsalva swallow, or effortful swallow, was initially introduced by Kahrilas and colleagues (Kahrilas, Logemann, Lin, and Ergun, 1991; Kahrilas, Logemann, Lin, Ergun, & Facchini, 1993; Kahrilas, Logemann, & Gibbons, 1992; Logemann & Kahrilas, 1990). This treatment is generally targeted toward patients with decreased laryngeal elevation and pharyngeal contraction in which the primary radiographic findings are postswallow vallecular and pyriform sinus residual with presence or potential for aspiration. There may be additional effects of the maneuver on base of tongue to posterior pharyngeal wall approximation. The effect of this treatment is not well documented. First presented as a compensatory mechanism, clinical practice suggests that this treatment, when repeated over time, may facilitate improved function of the suprahyoid and pharyngeal musculature, thus improving laryngeal excursion and pharyngeal contraction. Additionally, repetitive effortful swallows may facilitate base of tongue to posterior pharyngeal wall approximation.

Patient Instruction. Execution of this maneuver is relatively simple. The patient is instructed to sit comfortably in a chair with both feet firmly on the floor. He or she is instructed to swallow "hard" with increased effort as he or she executes a swallow. The patient may respond to the cue to "swallow a ping-pong ball" or similar analogy to effect increased effort. Repetitive dry swallows are considered by many to be very difficult to execute. If the patient is allowed liquid intake, small sips of water to moisten the oral mucosa may be helpful. For those patients in which oral intake is contraindicated, a single squirt with a spritzer bottle may be a safe alternative.

Contraindications. Although no identified data document adverse effects, it may be wise when working with patients with underlying unstable, cardiac conditions to obtain specific physician clearance before participation in a treatment protocol using this and other Valsalva-type maneuvers. Among the perpetuated clinical lore, there is concern for use of Valsalva-type maneuvers secondary to increased vascular pressure. In the absence of negating data, caution may be prudent.

Examples of Possible Short-Term Clinical Objectives.

1. After 10 treatment sessions using repetitive modified Valsalva swallows, the patient will tolerate mechanical soft diet with a maximum of two swallows per bolus to clear subjectively and no clinical indication of postswallow residual (appropriate only if the patient has radiographically confirmed accurate pharyngeal sensation).
2. The patient will independently complete a home program consisting of one modified Valsalva swallow approximately every 30 seconds for 15 minutes with rest periods as needed.

Primary Physiologic Target: Decreased Base of Tongue to Posterior Pharyngeal Wall Approximation with Subsequent Diminished Positive Pressure on the Bolus; Decreased Strength of Pharyngeal Swallow

Treatment: Masako Maneuver. Clinicians who have worked with patients who are status post base-of-tongue resection have likely observed a spontaneous increase in posterior pharyngeal wall excursion to compensate for the resected base of tongue. Fujiu, Logemann and Pauloski (1995) have documented this tendency. Based on this documented observation, Fujiu and Logemann (1996) investigated the effects of a maneuver designed to mimic tongue resection on the swallowing of individuals with nonresected anatomy. The derived maneuver, referred to as *the Masako maneuver* or *tongue holding maneuver,* involves anterior stabilization of the tongue during volitional swallowing. Ten normal subjects with no history of oral pharyngeal resection were evaluated radiographically for the effects of this maneuver on a variety of temporal measures and radiographic observations. Although many parameters of swallowing were not affected, there was a statistically significant increase in anterior bulging of the posterior pharyngeal wall as a function of the maneuver. Thus, anterior stabilization of the tongue is observed to result in greater recruitment of the pharyngeal constrictors as a compensation.

To date, no research has been published that documents the long-term effects of repetitive execution of the maneuver. It is speculated that with the positive short-term effects of the maneuver on intact anatomy and the observation of long-term changes in resected individuals, this technique may offer promise as a rehabilitative exercise to strengthen pharyngeal contraction.

Patient Instruction. As with an effortful swallow, a patient is instructed to sit comfortably in a chair with both feet firmly on the floor. He or she is directed to place the tongue anteriorly between the upper and lower central incisors and swallow with the tongue anchored in this position. Thus base-of-tongue movement is inhibited and posterior pharyngeal wall movement is facilitated. As well, it may be beneficial to pair this maneuver with a valsalva swallow by instructing the patient to swallow "hard" with increased effort as he or she executes the swallow. It may be difficult for some patients to execute a swallow under these conditions. During the teaching process, gently holding the tongue tip with gauze anteriorly may inhibit the natural tendency to retract the tongue during swallowing. For the comfort of the patient, this practice should be discontinued as soon as the learning process is completed or it is determined that the patient will not be successful in using this exercise. As with the modified Valsalva swallow, repetitive swallowing to execute the maneuver may require intermittent moistening of the oral mucosa.

Contraindications. Use of this maneuver is contraindicated with a bolus. Fujiu and Logemann (1996) documented reduced emptying of the valleculae with post-swallow residual as well as latency in onset of swallow when subjects used this technique. Thus, airway protection may be significantly compromised. Because of this, the Masako maneuver should be considered a rehabilitative maneuver only, with no role in compensation. As with the modified valsalva swallow, or effortful swallow, precautions should be taken when applying the technique to the treatment plan of a patient with unstable cardiac function.

Examples of Possible Short-Term Clinical Objectives.

1. After 10 treatment sessions utilizing repetitive Masako maneuvers, the patient will tolerate a pureed diet with a maximum of four swallows per bolus to clear the bolus subjectively, with no clinical indication of postswallow residual (appropriate only if the patient has radiographically confirmed accurate pharyngeal sensation).
2. The patient will independently complete a home program consisting of one Masako maneuver approximately every 30 seconds for 15 minutes with rest periods as needed.

Physiologic Abnormality: Inadequate Laryngeal Valving and Airway Protection

There is occasional debate between experienced dysphagia clinicians and some otolaryngologists regarding the impact of vocal fold paresis on swallowing function. Some tend to believe vocal adduction disorders by definition imply a swallowing disorder and aspiration risk. However, clinicians have observed innumerable cases in which vocal adduction was impaired without associated dysphagia. The prevailing clinical belief holds that if pharyngeal swallowing is efficient and the higher levels of airway protection are patent (epiglottic deflection, supraglottic closure), then laryngeal closure is not inherently required. Ekberg (1986) radiographically evaluated 22 patients with paresis of the recurrent laryngeal nerve. Of this group of patients, 86% demonstrated defective closure of the laryngeal vestibule. However, 14% demonstrated normal pharyngeal swallowing in the presence of impaired vocal fold closure. It would appear from these data that recurrent laryngeal nerve impairment may result in both specific laryngeal and more diffuse supraglottic deficits, but that laryngeal closure at the glottis is not necessarily a prerequisite for safe oral pharyngeal swallow.

This finding was confirmed and elaborated on by Wilson, Pryde, White, Maher, and Maran, (1995). Pharyngeal swallowing was studied using pharyngoesophageal manometry and videolaryngoscopy in a group of 27 patients who exhibited impaired vocal fold motion. Although 15 of the 27 patients demonstrated symptomatic dysphagia, there was no significant difference in the groups in pharyngoesophageal pressure dynamics or measures of pharyngeal peristalsis. The authors conclude that vagus nerve involvement may influence laryngeal and pharyngeal swallowing mechanisms, but that impaired laryngeal kinetics do not specifically contribute to dysphagic symptomatology.

In patients with impaired supraglottic swallowing, vocal adduction is critical to maintain the airway and protect the pulmonary system (Ardran & Kemp, 1952; Rontal, Rontal, Morse, & Brown, 1976; Woo, Van Hasselt, & Chan, 1992). Thus, a swallowing rehabilitation program for patients with impaired vocal fold closure should include exercises to address laryngeal function.

Treatment: Vocal Adduction Exercises. As a therapeutic response for vocal fold paresis, adduction exercises serve to increase vocal fold adduction by increasing movement of a paralyzed fold or facilitating overadduction of the functioning fold for compensation of the paralyzed fold. These techniques are utilized to improve vocal fold adduction for phonatory production and airway protection.

Patient Instruction. Several techniques are used for increased vocal adduction:

▶ Patient is instructed to link fingers at the chest or on the seat of a straight-back chair and pull or push with effort during production of sustained phonation.

▶ Patient is instructed to utilize coughing, grunting, and laughing to increase effort of glottic closure and improve vocal fold adduction.

▶ Increased effort during vocal adduction may be combined with execution of supraglottic swallowing strategy to facilitate improved airway protection.

Contraindications. As is the case any time that vocal function treatment is initiated, it is important to identify the source of the deficit with a referral to otolaryngology as indicated. May be contraindicated for patient with unstable cardiac conditions secondary to increased vascular pressure.

Examples of Possible Short-Term Clinical Objectives. The patient will sustain breath hold with no air escape for 30 seconds on 90% of trials.

Physiologic Abnormality: Reduced Opening of the Upper Esophageal Sphincter

The following two maneuvers are designed for patients with decreased laryngeal elevation and pharyngeal contraction, or those with hyperfunction of the cricopharyngeal sphincter. Primary radiographic findings may include postswallow vallecular greater than pyriform sinus residual with the presence or potential for post-swallow aspiration, and forced, segmented transfer of the bolus through the cricopharyngeal sphincter.

Treatment: Mendelsohn Maneuver. The initial documented report of Mendelsohn maneuver as an intervention was presented by Logemann and Kahrilas (1990). This article provided a case report of the recovery course of a 45-year-old patient with medullary stroke. Selected compensatory and rehabilitative interventions were provided over the course of 60 months. Response to interventions was measured via a variety of temporal and descriptive characteristics, including oropharyngeal swallow efficiency. Oropharyngeal swallow efficiency is defined by the authors as the percent of bolus swallowed divided by the duration of the oropharyngeal transit time in seconds. Although some improvement was observed in oropharyngeal swallow efficiency using postural changes and supraglottic swallow, use of the Mendelsohn maneuver increased this measure greater than twofold, to a level approximating normal.

Given the positive clinical effects of the maneuver, Kahrilas, Logemann, Krugler, and Flanagan (1991) evaluated the physiologic effects of this maneuver via concurrent videofluoroscopic and manometric procedures in eight healthy volunteers. Research data suggest that the technique results in prolonged opening, but not increased diameter, of the upper esophageal sphincter (UES). This prolongation of UES opening allows greater time for the tail or the bolus to pass into the cervical esophagus. In addition, the maneuver was noted to significantly increase maximal hyoid superior displacement, as well as laryngeal elevation, although anterior displacement of both structures did not appear to be influenced by the maneuver. Thus it is evident that although pharyngeal phase swallowing is generally considered to be a highly programmed motor response, direct intervention allows for manipulation of this response to facilitate swallowing.

As with the Valsalva or effortful swallow, the Mendesohn maneuver was initially described as a compensatory technique. However, clinical experience suggests that repetition of this exercise provides long-term effects on the opening of the upper esophageal sphincter, as a result of progressive and prolonged manipulation. This particular intervention is clinically observed to be remarkably effective in a very short period of time in patients with sometimes severe pharyngeal phase deficits. Crary (1995) and Huckabee and Cannito (1998) have presented data in which patients with chronic dysphagia secondary to brain stem injury recovered functional swallowing physiology to the point of return to full oral intake following a short-term treatment regime focused heavily on this exercise.

Indeed, it is not uncommon for patients with severe dysphagia to report improved secretion management within days of initiating a treatment regime utilizing this maneuver. Bartolome and Neumann (1993) likewise reported on effects of treatment in which the Mendelsohn maneuver was heavily used to rehabilitate upper esophageal sphincter deficits.

Each of these studies used the Mendelsohn maneuver in conjunction with other rehabilitative maneuvers, compensatory techniques, and treatment modalities. Thus, reported patient recovery could be attributed to many independent management strategies or to a combination of interventions. However, these data provide support for the clinical observation of the effect of the maneuver.

Unfortunately, this maneuver can be extremely difficult for patients to master. It requires fairly astute cognitive skills to process, sequence, and recall the maneuver, as well as tremendous muscular control to interrupt a swallow in progress and considerable effort to sustain maximal swallowing elevation. Thus, it is a typical assumption that the majority of patients will be unable to benefit from the technique. As with all of our rehabilitative efforts, this technique will challenge not just the patient. The clinician providing intervention services will be equally challenged to structure the learning environment and maximize feedback modalities to give each patient ample opportunity to benefit from the technique. Several biofeedback modalities, including surface electromyography (SEMG), electroglottography (EGG), tactile, visual, and acoustic feedback may foster mastery of the skill. These techniques are covered in more detail in a Chapters 4 and 5. If instrumental techniques are not available to the clinician, simple line drawings may provide the patient with some feedback. Derived from SEMG tracings of swallowing, the clinician can draw a representation of the maneuver on paper with a flat line signifying the resting position of the thyroid, an abrupt elevation of the line signifying rise of the thyroid cartilage, an elevated flat line representing sustained elevation and an abrupt fall of the line representing return to resting posture.

Given the difficulty of the maneuver, it is somewhat presumptive to assess the effects of the maneuver radiographically in neurologic patients who have not been previously instructed in the task. Although radiographic confirmation of effect would be optimal, it is likely rare in this population. Despite our best efforts at rapidly teaching the technique in the fluoroscopy suit, it is probably infrequently evaluated fairly in the context of the videofluoroscopic exam. Thus, elimination of the technique as a potential intervention based on a single trial after teaching may be premature.

Patient Instruction. As with the modified Valsalva swallow, patients are instructed to sit comfortably in a chair with their feet firmly planted on the floor. Initially they are guided to palpate their thyroid notch (or Adam's apple) during execution of a normal swallow and are educated regarding the excursion of the larynx during the swallow. They are then instructed to initiate a swallow and when they feel the peak of thyroid elevation, they are to hold this contraction for several seconds prior to terminating the swallow with release of laryngeal elevation and pharyngeal relaxation. Descriptive phrases such as, "Swallow long and strong" or "Stretch out the swallow" may be of benefit to some patients. Imaging exercises, such as visualization of swallowing a bolus of marshmallow cream or peanut butter may also be of use. As before, palpation may be helpful to teach and gain mastery of this strategy. Additional feedback to the patient may come in the form of visualization in a mirror, instrumental biofeedback, or acoustic feedback via cervical auscultation. These techniques are discussed further in Chapters 4 and 5.

Contraindication. The Mendelsohn maneuver was initially described as a compensatory mechanism, thus to be applied with ingestion of a bolus. Although not empirically confirmed, clinical observation suggests, however, that using this technique with a bolus may actually increase aspiration risk in patients who are neurologically impaired. Swallowing is an exquisitely coordinated process. Execution of this maneuver is not only adapting the strength, but the temporal characteristics of swallowing. In normal subjects, as utilized in the Kahrilas and Logemann study (1991), there is no reported increase in aspiration. However, in a neurologically compromised system, it appears clinically that some patients are unable to compensate for the shift in the temporal components of swallowing, thus aspiration risk may be increased. It is therefore suggested that the Mendelsohn maneuver be used as a rehabilitative exercise, not as a compensatory maneuver. And again, as with the effortful swallow described earlier, caution should be used in applying this exercise to patients with underlying unstable, cardiac conditions.

Examples of Possible Short-Term Clinical Objectives.

1. The patient will maintain laryngeal elevation for 3 seconds during execution of Mendelsohn maneuver on 90% of trials during the treatment session as measured by thyroid palpation and the intraswallow apneic period.
2. After 10 treatment sessions focusing on repetition of the Mendelsohn maneuver, the patient will ingest one level teaspoon of a puree without clinical signs of aspiration and will expectorate less than 1 cc after two dry swallows. (*Note:* This is appropriate for patients with radiographically confirmed reflexive cough and ability to clear the pharynx fully with pharyngeal expectoration.)
3. Following 15 minutes of repetitive Mendelsohn maneuvers the patient will tolerate mechanical soft diet with no more than three swallows per bolus required to clear the bolus from the pharynx subjectively on 90% of trials. (*Note:* This is appropriate only for patients with accurate pharyngeal sensation observed radiographically.)

Treatment: Head-Lifting Maneuver. This is the newest technique in our arsenal of interventions for dysphagia, developed by Shaker and colleagues (1997). These studies demonstrated that a very simple technique of head lifting resulted in facilitation of UES opening compared with a placebo exercise. Two groups of normal elders were evaluated for the duration and extent of cricopharyngeal sphincter opening prior to an exercise regime focused on one of two maneuvers. The therapeutic maneuver consisted of execution of an isotonic-isometric head-lifting exercise which was performed in supine position three times daily, consisting of three 1-minute sustained lifts, followed by 30 brief repetitions. The placebo maneuver consisted of fist clenching executed on the same schedule. Following 6 months, the subjects were reevaluated and the subjects in the sham group were then reassigned to the therapeutic exercise. As expected, no change in swallowing physiology was observed subsequent to participation in the placebo group. However, subsequent to participation in the treatment condition, subjects demonstrated significantly increased laryngeal excursion, increased width and duration of UES opening, and decreased intrabolus pressure, suggestive of decreased resistance at level of the cricopharyngeal sphincter.

Two additional studies further documented the effect of this exercise on the biomechanics of swallowing through the use of electrophysiologic techniques. Jurell (1996) demonstrated electromyographic evidence of fatigue in the muscles of the submental region, suggesting increased work by the mylohyoid and geniohyoid muscle groups during execution of the head lifting maneuver. Alfonzo, Ferdjallah, Shaker, and Wertsch (1998) demonstrated increased EMG amplitude of the supra- and infra-hyoid muscle groups during execution of the technique.

This is a remarkable development in its simplicity. For those patients with deficits associated with upper esophageal sphincter opening who are cognitively unable to perform the Mendelsohn maneuver, this technique offers another option for long-term change in physiology. As the technique is not an adaptation of the pharyngeal swallow and involves no complicated sequencing of motoric behavior, it can be executed by many patients. Although some degree of strength and stamina is required, adaptations such as decreasing intensity of rehabilitation efforts or allowing a pillow behind the head can ease the patient into the maneuver.

Patient Instruction. This is presented entirely as a rehabilitative technique and thus is not completed with food. The patient is instructed very simply to lie down in bed without a pillow and slowly lift the head off of the bed before sustaining this posture for up to 10 seconds. This is repeated three times. Another adaptation consists of requiring the patients to lift the head up briefly and then relax for up to 30 repetitions. As mentioned, adaptations in the intensity or number of repetitions can be made to accommodate less able patients. Tactile cues may also be useful. A quarter or small mirror can be placed immediately below the sternal notch with instructions to the patients to bring the chin to the chest until they feel the item or can see themselves in the mirror. A simple switch can be placed on the chest with compression turning on a light during execution of the maneuver. As well, one patient responded well to the use of adhesive Velcro dots placed on the chin and the chest.

Contraindications. No documented contraindications have been documented related to the execution of this exercise. It would appear logical that the maneuver should not be completed with a bolus because of increased risk of aspiration in the supine posture. Patients with cervical spine injury should be cleared by the physician before proceeding.

Examples of Possible Short-Term Clinical Objectives.

1. The patient will recall and implement head-lifting exercise three times daily as prescribed with minimal reminders.
2. After 4 weeks of treatment focusing on the head-lifting maneuver, the patient will expectorate less than 1 cc of pudding after two dry swallows of a 5 cc bolus. (*Note:* This is appropriate for patients with radiographically confirmed ability to clear the pharynx fully with pharyngeal expectoration.)
3. After 4 weeks of treatment focusing on the head-lifting maneuver, the patient will ingest a mechanical soft diet with no indication of postswallow aspiration secondary to pyriform sinus residual. (*Note:* This is appropriate only for patients with reflexive cough observed radiographically.)

Physiologic Abnormality: Decreased Sensory Feedback

Swallowing is the product of a fine integration between sensory input with motor output. Thus, efficient swallowing requires intact sensory and motor systems and rehabilitation may need to address both issues. Perlman, Luschei, and Dumond (1989) suggest that greater muscular effort may be required for swallowing than for other functions of the oral pharyngeal structures. Thus, the best treatment for swallowing may be swallowing. The rehabilitation exercises available to the patient with dysphagia primarily address the motor components of swallowing. Most of these exercises consist of adaptations of pharyngeal swallowing that are executed repetitively and with great effort over time. They are designed to increase the strength of the oral pharyngeal musculature associated with swallowing. However, the component of sensory input is absent unless a bolus is paired with execution of the maneuvers, which may be contraindicated in some situations because of the overriding risk of aspiration imposed by the maneuver itself.

The decisions to begin oral feeding as a component of the treatment plan are highly individualized to the patient. These decisions will be influenced by the patients' overall physical and pulmonary stability, cognition, swallowing physiology and airway protection mechanisms. The patient, family, and referring physician should be involved in the decision to begin oral feeding. Certainly, the safest route would be to continue nonoral status until aspiration risk is minimized or absent. However, delaying oral feeding until swallowing is improved to the point of a negligible aspiration risk may result in no functional recovery in swallowing because of the paucity of sensory feedback to the swallowing mechanism. At some point in the rehabilitation process, particularly for the patient with chronic dysphagia, the risks of long-term nonoral feeding to the physical and emotional well-being of the patient may be greater than the risk of aspiration. In this situation, the patient may balance the risks and benefits of oral feeding and elect to initiate therapeutic feedings in the presence of significant aspiration. *Clearly this decision should be made by the patient and family, rather than the clinician,* after adequate information is provided to facilitate an informed decision.

If patients elect to begin oral feedings under these conditions, precautions should be taken to minimize the existing, known risks. Patients should be realistically counseled regarding the aspiration risk and potential outcomes of aspiration. As well, they should be educated in the signs and symptoms of developing pulmonary symptomotology and should take an active role in minimizing these risks and assuring pulmonary safety.

Treatment: Neurosensory Stimulation.

Patient Instruction.   If the patient elects to initiate therapeutic feeding, the initial goal of oral intake may not be actually to ingest the bolus, rather to accept the neurosensory feedback provided. The patient may be instructed to swallow a bolus and then immediately expectorate pharyngeal residual. In cases where physiology results in post-swallow aspiration of residual, this technique may provide the benefits of swallowing while inhibiting aspiration risk by prompt expectoration. Swallowing compensatory mechanisms, as outlined in Chapter 6, should be rigorously utilized. As well, general precautions should be implemented. The patient should ingest PO only in upright position and should remain upright and active for a period of at least 30 minutes following PO trials. Temperature should be monitored at the same time daily and the pulmonary sounds should be checked frequently. Short-term progress may be measured by the amount of expectorate produced, in the event that the patient has radiographically confirmed ability for pharyngeal expectoration.

If the patient elects not to pursue oral feeding because of the risk of aspiration, an alternative technique may provide some sensory feedback but with no aspiration risk. A latex finger mitt can be partly filled with sherbet or cold yogurt and tied at the open end. After securely tying the knotted end to a string, this pseudobolus can be placed in the oral cavity for the patient to "swallow on." In doing so, the weight, temperature and malleable form of the bolus provide sensory input to the neurologic system. The pseudobolus can be adapted to provide more or less sensory feedback as needed, by adjusting the amount of food substance. Care should be taken to secure the end of the pseudobolus firmly with a string external to the oral cavity to prevent accidental ingestion. Double gloving may be beneficial to minimize the risk of tears and leakage.

Contraindications. Aspiration risk should be thoroughly discussed with the patient and family. A patient with poor airway protection and clearance mechanisms may be rejected for therapeutic feeding by the speech pathologist if the risk of pulmonary failure is judged to be too great.

Potential Goals. After ingestion of 10 cc of pudding, the patient will expectorate less than 5 cc after two swallows.

SUMMARY

To summarize this chapter on rehabilitation, three points are made:

1. Our current state-of-the-art practices in dysphagia do not have the scientific support needed to prognosticate swallowing recovery accurately. In a group of 10 patients with chronic dysphagia secondary to brain stem injury reported by Huckabee and Cannito (1998), 7 had been advised by well-meaning health care workers (speech pathologists and physicians) that they would never eat again. However, 5 of those 7 and 8 of the entire group of 10 returned to full oral feeding at a mean time post onset of 27 months. Thus, if rehabilitation practices fail, another trial of rehabilitation at a later date or a referral to another clinician may be appropriate.
2. Rehabilitation practices can be difficult for the patient with dysphagia to master, particularly in the neurogenic population where cognitive deficits are not uncommon. Clearly some patients will not be able to benefit from rehabilitation because of this. However, as clinicians, we need to work diligently and creatively to assist the patient in overcoming the barriers of cognition and language. Use of multimodality feedback, from the very simple palpation to the more complex instrumental techniques, should be included as a component of rehabilitation. Clinicians should be resourceful and inventive in facilitating the execution of a rehabilitation program. Although initial failed attempts at successful teaching of swallowing maneuvers may be daunting, rehabilitation attempts should continue until all efforts have been exhausted and it is clear that the patient is not an appropriate candidate.
3. Eating is a favorite pastime in this country with the preponderance of holidays and family celebrations centered around the dinner table. Thus, in addition to the medical complications, the social implications of dysphagia are tremendous. It is not uncommon in the clinical practice of dysphagia to encounter patients who would rather eat than talk, and elect for a surgical procedure that separates the trachea from the alimentary system, thus permanently sacrificing the potential for speech.

The patient highlighted late in Chapter 13, has very articulately shared her experiences of being dysphagic and recovering from dysphagia. When writing about her experiences immediately after surgery, she expresses "Since I equated living with the ability to swallow, I thought I was just marking time until I died." She further describes the social isolation of her disorder. "It was embarrassing. At theaters, restaurants, and other public places, people with forbidding glares would move away from us after hearing me 'clear' (my secretions). Strangers did not know that I couldn't swallow." On removal of her feeding tube and return to a near-normal diet, she celebrated her recovery with a trip to Europe. She states, "Mostly swallowing is, oh, so wonderful a gift, I will never take it for granted again!"

CHAPTER

4

Biofeedback Modalities

The next two chapters will outline the role of biofeedback modalities as an adjunct to swallowing rehabilitation. The mastery of swallowing rehabilitation techniques can provide a difficult challenge to the patient and clinician. Use of instrumental feedback modalities can greatly facilitate the process and allow for significant progress in the rehabilitation program. This chapter addresses primarily the theoretical and technical underpinnings of surface electromyography biofeedback. Chapter 5 addresses the use of several other techniques, including ultrasound, endoscopy, auscultation, and oximetry.

INTRODUCTION: WHEN TRADITIONAL SWALLOWING TREATMENT FAILS

VB is a 72-year-old farmer with dysphagia subsequent to supraglottic laryngectomy. When asked about his experiences with swallowing treatment, he provided a valuable insight to his clinician.

It's like trying to find your way to the refrigerator at your in-laws' house, at night, without turning on the lights. I just can't see what I'm supposed to be doing.

These very simple words well illustrate one of the major hurdles of successful dysphagia rehabilitation.

In other realms of physical medicine and rehabilitation, such as physical or occupational therapy, muscle retraining is generally a very visible process. A patient contracts the biceps and the arm flexes; the greater strength to the contraction, the greater the movement observed. In this process, the patient and clinician receive direct feedback of the adjustment in motor behavior. Swallowing treatment is a complex and typically very abstract process. We are asking patients, frequently geriatric and/or brain injured, to execute often complex tasks using muscle groups that have previously operated only under automatic response. Execution of these tasks is not clearly observable to the naked eye, and as such, success or failure is extremely difficult to measure. We expect execution of these tasks as well in patients with neurologic deficits in whom proprioceptive and kinesthetic feedback systems may be compromised. In addition, literature suggests that clinical swallowing examination, in this case as a measure of progress in treatment, is not highly reliable for identifying aspiration and specifics of pharyngeal swallowing physiology (Horner & Massey, 1988; Horner, Riski, Lathrop & Chase, 1988; Splaingard, Hutchins, Sultan, & Chaundhuri, 1988). Thus, the techniques for dysphagia rehabilitation are abstract, clinical measurement is imprecise, and treatment is largely clinician dependent. Given this, both the patient and clinician may become frustrated and abandon rehabilitative efforts prematurely. The techniques may be theoretically sound, but if the clinician cannot adequately teach and the patient cannot adequately learn, they are without clinical value. The task of the therapist working with dysphagia is to find ways to maximize teaching and reinforcement. Compensatory maneuvers may be facilitated through a variety of environmental controls such as strategic location of the meal to assure positioning or cue cards to remind the patient of swallowing techniques. Rehabilitative maneuvers are perhaps more difficult to reinforce.

DEFINITIONS

In earlier chapters, we have discussed the need for the clinician to be creative and persistent in identifying alternative modalities that will enhance the ability of the rehabilitative candidate to benefit from treatment. These modalities can collectively be referred to as "biofeedback techniques." John Basmajian, MD, is considered by many to be the elder statesman of modern-day electromyographic biofeedback. He defines biofeedback as:

> The technique of using equipment (usually electronic) to reveal to human beings some of their internal physiological events, normal and abnormal, in the form of visual and auditory signals, in order to teach them to manipulate these otherwise involuntary or unfelt events by manipulating the displayed signals.

Another definition is provided by Kasman (1994), who clarifies that biofeedback provides "instantaneous, performance-contingent feedback regarding the function of a physiological or psychophysiological system. It is an extension of the patients or clinicians senses." This perspective seems particularly applicable to swallowing rehabilitation. In patients with neurogenic dysphagia who may have impaired proprioception and sensation, the information provided through some biofeedback modality may augment their own impaired sensory system. To the clinician working with these patients, some forms of biofeedback may provide a much-needed quantitative measure to support the clinician's qualitative judgment.

When we address rehabilitation of swallowing, biofeedback modalities, regardless of the source, serve to bring a largely automatic function, to a higher level of awareness so the patient can directly address it. Biofeedback makes the abstract concrete. A 68-year-old male with dysphagia subsequent to left lateral medullary infarct summarized the importance of providing some form of biofeedback in swallowing treatment as follows:

> It gives you a target to shoot at, and most people need that in life. You can't have a general theory and expect someone to react to it. You have to have something that you can see, feel, and hear that gives you direction. This way you can relate to it.

> In other words, when you see you have a good swallow, you know what it feels like. Without this equipment, this feeling of your Adam's apple, that doesn't do me any good at all. If I have a target, I'll work for it, and I think most people are the same way. You can see progress and determine what was good and what was bad.

Biofeedback modalities, from the very simplest form to the most complex, contribute an alternate system of proprioception, thus accentuating the patient's or clinician's awareness of one aspect of swallowing behavior. By yielding a visible or auditory representation of some component of the swallowing response, a window into rehabilitative efforts is opened, allowing the patient and the clinician a means of confronting this largely inaccessible physiologic function and enhancing access to volitional motor control.

HOW BIOFEEDBACK MODALITIES FACILITATE THE LEARNING PROCESS

In the psychology literature there has been considerable discussion regarding the role of biofeedback in motor learning, highlighting both pros and cons of external feedback. Rubow (1984) identifies two models of learning that represent conceptually different approaches to the rehabilitative process: operant conditioning and the cybernetic model of learning. He elaborates that a critical issue in discriminating between these two models and their appropriate applications to treatment is the relative importance assigned to reinforcement and dynamic feedback.

The *operant conditioning model* implies that learning and behavioral adaptation occur as a consequence of reinforcement or punishment that is provided in temporal association with a given task. This model of learning suggests that reinforcement is effective if it is provided within a few seconds of a desired response. Thus, the operant conditioning model of learning would typically represent a clinician-guided treatment in which the patient's rehabilitative behavior is followed by initially consistent, albeit delayed, feedback provided by the clinician. The consistency of the feedback is progressively withdrawn as the patient assumes greater independence in the learning process.

The *cybernetic model* of learning, however, relies in concept on a continuous, closed-loop learning process. This model requires that continuous and immediate reinforcement regarding performance is the key to perceptual-motor learning. The cybernetic model thus reflects the immediacy of instrumental feedback in that the feedback is continuously integrated into the patients ongoing motor control processes. Rubow summarizes that feedback in accordance with the cybernetic model is important in the early stages of rehabilitation, while the role of reinforcement, via operant conditioning, increases in later stages.

Wolf (1994) outlines two stages of motor learning, the acquisition and transfer phases, which correlate well with the cybernetic models and operant conditioning models, respectively, as described earlier and outlined in Table 4–1. In his review of motor learning theory, he acknowledges data that suggest that normal learning and retention are enhanced with periodic rather than continuous reinforcement. However, he questions the validity of these data when applied to the initial motor relearning process

Table 4–1. Summary of Aspects of Motor Learning Theories

	Biofeedback-Assisted Treatment	Traditional Treatment
Learning Phase	Acquisition of motor skills	Transfer of motor skills
Feedback Type	Continuous	Consistent but not continuous
Feedback Proximity to Motor Behavior	Immediate	Delayed

Sources: Adapted from R. Rubow (1984), "Role of biofeedback, reinforcement, and compliance on training and transfer in biofeedback based rehabilitation of motor speech disorders." In M. McNeil, J. Rosenbek, & A. Aronson (Eds.), *The dysarthrias: Physiology, acoustics, perception, and management* (pp. 207–209). San Diego: College Hill Press; and S. L. Wolf (1979), "EMG biofeedback applications in rehabilitation." *Physiotherapy Canada, 31,* 65–72.

in patients with neurologically based disorders. He suggests that the feedback signal in the initial phases of treatment may serve as substitute for the patient's inadequate proprioceptive signals, which in normal settings are instantaneous and consistent, and that these exteroceptive signals ultimately engage the internal sensorimotor networks. Thus, the acquisition phase of relearning a motor skill requires continuous reinforcement, whereas the transfer phase begins upon engagement of the internal sensorimotor networks, thus requiring less immediate or continuous external feedback. The success of rehabilitative programs, when following this model, is considered to be secondary to a relearned appreciation of internal cues, as well as potential "recalibration" of the proprioceptive system (Wolf, 1979). The use of biofeedback modalities is considered a temporary adjunct to treatment with the inherent goal of internalization of the feedback signal and extinction of the need for external feedback.

Given this theoretical support for biofeedback, consideration can be paid to the various modalities that can potentially be applied to swallowing rehabilitation. Five modalities are formally reviewed.

1. Surface electromyography
2. Acoustic: cervical auscultation
3. Endoscopy
4. Ultrasonography
5. Pulse oximetry

Franklin Delano Roosevelt once said, "Take a method and try it. If it fails, admit it frankly and try another. But by all means, try something!"

Techniques for swallowing rehabilitation may be theoretically sound and physiologically beneficial, but if the complexity of the task exceeds the cognitive power of the patient, they are of little functional use. It is the responsibility of the clinician, or swallowing coach, to work diligently and creatively to assist the patient in overcoming the barriers of impaired cognition and language, whenever feasible. Use of multimodality feedback should be regularly included as a component of rehabilitation. The clinician however is challenged to go beyond what is offered in these chapters and develop new modalities. From a basic paper-and-pencil sketch of hyoid movement to more complex beeps, whistles, and images, external feedback will only enhance the rehabilitative process and may offer the chance for recovery to the patient with cognitive deficits. The following two chapters outline options for biofeedback monitoring and are offered with the challenge to "Try Something!"

SURFACE ELECTROMYOGRAPHY

History of Surface EMG as a Biofeedback Modality

Perhaps the biofeedback modality that is receiving the greatest clinical and research attention is surface electromyography (SEMG). The use of SEMG as a biofeedback modality has its origins as early at the late 1920s, with documentation of early clinical attempts at using primitive electromyographic signals to facilitate relaxation therapy for so-called "psychoneurotic" patients (Jacobson, 1933). Several key studies followed that provide a foundation for the clinical applications of electromygraphy (EMG) biofeedback that we use today.

Adrian and Bonk (1929), in a study of normal subjects, determined that the electrical responses in individual muscles provided an accurate reflection of the actual functional activity of the muscle; that is, there is a direct linear correlation between the EMG tracing and muscle force. Reliable measurements of functional activity are prerequisite for clinical usefulness. Two other studies provided early documentation of the subject's ability to control consciously the biofeedback tracing. Smith (1934) and Lindsley (1935) in a series of similar studies documented that subjects could exert conscious control on even smallest motor unit potential and, at rest, demonstrated no inherent muscular tension. In addition, they documented that normal subjects could achieve complete relaxation as demonstrated by no measurable motor response with little difficulty.

Clinical SEMG biofeedback has been extensively evaluated in other realms of physical medicine and rehabilitation with numerous studies demonstrating clinical efficacy for a variety of neuromuscular disorders. Wolf (1994) documents over 300 clinical studies addressing the efficacy of biofeedback in physical rehabilitation of neuromuscular disorders, not including associated disorders of pain. The discipline of speech language pathology, although encompassing rehabilitation of motor deficits associated with speech, voice, and swallowing, has yet to extensively evaluate this modality. Cooper and Perlman (1997) devote a detailed chapter to summarize the neurophysiology and technology of electromyography, including subcutaneous, as a diagnostic tool. In addition, Carman and Ryan (1989) provide an overview for clinical uses of SEMG biofeedback in speech pathology. The reader is referred to these chapters and others for further information. However, substantiation of therapeutic applications has received little attention.

Clinical Application

A string of case studies has begun to emerge regarding the use of SEMG biofeedback in swallowing treatment. The first such paper was presented by Drazier (1986). In this paper, she outlines the use of biofeedback in the treatment of dysarthria and dysphagia; however, little detail is provided regarding specific treatment methods or evaluation of progress. A more detailed account was provided by Bryant (1991), who presented a description of the use of SEMG biofeedback in the treatment of a patient with oral pharyngeal carcinoma. This patient, a 40-year-old female with severe dysphagia secondary to resection and radiation was able to discontinue tube feedings and return to a near-normal diet after 10 weeks of treatment. Subsequent to this report, Crary (1995) described the treatment course of six patients with chronic dysphagia secondary to brain stem infarct treated with SEMG biofeedback. Of these six patients, with a mean time post onset of 18.8 months (5 to 54), five were able to return to oral feedings with discontinuation of tube feedings. Crary and Baldwin further investigated patterns of swallowing dysfunction as measured by SEMG (Crary & Baldwin, 1997).

Several other unpublished projects have addressed the technical aspects and clinical efficacy of SEMG in swallowing treatment. In 1995, at the Dysphagia Research Association Meeting, Huckabee, Garcia, and Barofsky presented SEMG norms at rest and at maximal amplitude during the swallow as measured from six different sites around the head and neck. Although not dissimilar to a technical paper by Gupta, Reddy, and Canilang (1996), this study used commercially available devices that would be typical in clinical use. Not surprisingly, the standard deviation from the mean peak amplitude during swallowing of both liquid and secretions was significant, for some sites even greater than the mean itself. However, for electrode placement sites most commonly used to measure amplitude of the muscles directly involved in the pharyngeal swallow, the standard deviation from the mean was relatively smaller (Huckabee, Garcia, & Barofsky, 1995). This study provides a strong caution that SEMG amplitudes, although useful as a clinical biofeedback tool, are not appropriate for providing diagnostic information or comparing across subjects. As no meaningful mean amplitude values have been determined, it would not be feasible to determine what is considered "normal" SEMG amplitude. Although there is some promise that evaluation of the waveform shape will provide clinically useful information (Crary, 1995; Crary and Baldwin, 1997) not enough information is available to consider this more than clinical judgment.

Evidence of the physiologic correlation of the SEMG signal was provided by Sonies, Gottlieb, Solomon, Mathews, and Huckabee (1996) at the Annual Meeting of the Dysphagia Research Society. Using simultaneous ultrasound imaging and SEMG measurements, a very high correlation (R = .99) was noted between peak EMG amplitude and maximal hyoid elevation during all bolus consistencies. This suggests that the peak EMG waveform indicates maximum submental muscle contraction and maximal hyolaryngeal elevation.

Clinical applications have been evaluated by several groups. At the American Speech-Language-Hearing Association Annual Convention in 1994, Bednarek, Tucker, and Conlin offered data which suggested that normal subjects were able to utilize the SEMG tracing to increase muscular contraction during some swallowing maneuvers (1994). Berman, Boczko, and Licht, at the 1995 American Speech-Language-Hearing Association Annual convention, reported on their experiences in using SEMG biofeedback with mostly geriatric individuals with dysphagia in a chronic care facility, noting both successes and failures in treatment with this difficult population. Particular difficulty was noted in the very practical aspect of electrode placement.

Huckabee, Cannito, and Kahane, at the 1996 American Speech-Language-Hearing Association Convention, reported on 10 patients with dysphagia secondary to brain stem injury who participated in a 1-week accelerated swallowing treatment program with SEMG monitoring. Of these 10 patients, with a mean time post onset of 26 months, 8 eventually returned to full oral feeding with removal of feeding tube. All maintained oral feeding with the exception of 2, both of whom suffered further neurologic injury unrelated to their swallowing disorder. When pairing these data with the earlier data set of Crary and Baldwin (1996) using similar methods and treatment, 13 out of 16 patients with chronic dysphagia secondary to brain stem injury returned to oral intake following intensive treatment with SEMG biofeedback monitoring.

The Neurophysiologic Origins of the SEMG Tracing

An understanding of the origin of an electromyographic signal demands a rudimentary knowledge of motor unit physiology. The neurophysiology of swallowing is a complex process that is discussed in its very basic form in this presentation. As this is considered to be anything but a full disquisition on the topic, the reader is strongly encouraged to seek out other references for further study.

As food, liquid, or secretions collect within the oral cavity, surface and deep sensory receptors of the tongue and oral mucosa respond to the bolus and trigger excitation of sensory fibers. The neurosensory signal is projected via afferent fibers along cranial nerves V, VII, IX, and X to their respective nuclei. Sensory information regarding the attributes of the incoming bolus is ultimately received, either directly or indirectly, in the nucleus tractus solitarius within the medulla.

The nucleus tractus solitarius within the medulla is considered the primary sensory-processing center for peripheral information that influences swallowing. This nucleus recognizes the nature of the incoming bolus and, in conjunction with surrounding interneurons, prepares a "blueprint" for effective swallowing of that particular bolus. The neurologic signal for initiation of muscular contraction in swallowing originates in the nucleus ambiguous of the brain stem, which receives information from the nucleus ambiguus. As the sensory stimulus to elicit a swallow reaches this "medullary swallowing center" and a response is generated, the neurologic signal is transmitted distally from the medulla to the designated groups of muscle fibers via a "motor unit."

This motor unit is comprised of the nerve cell body localized in the brain stem, the long axon extending the length of the motor nerve, as well as the terminal branches and muscles fibers supplied by these branches. In general, the greater the number of muscle fibers stimulated by each motor unit, the coarser the motor response. For example, each motor unit extending into the gastrocnemius muscle of the posterior leg excites up to 2,000 muscle fibers. Reciprocally, a small number of muscle fibers stimulated by each motor unit results in a more refined motor response, as in the case of the human larynx, which contains between two and three muscle fibers per motor unit. As large groups of muscle fibers respond to their designated motor units, there is collective shortening of the muscle fibers resulting in contraction of the larger muscle group. Strength of contraction is regulated both by number of muscle fibers responding to the motor unit, number of motor units requiring a response, and timing, or frequency, of motor unit firing.

The electrical output measured by electromyography initiates in the cell body during firing of a motor unit. The resting state of a nerve cell presents with higher concentrations of negatively charged ions inside the cell with higher concentrations of positively charged ions outside the cell. This configuration of chemicals results in a polarized cell membrane (i.e., negative inside and positive outside). This balance of electrical energy is called a resting potential. When the neuron is stimulated by an incoming excitatory signal, the balance of ionic charges is offset, resulting in depolarization of the cell membrane. This shift in ionic concentration, or movement of positively and negatively charged ions, results in generation of a motor unit action potential, which travels down the long axon to terminate at the neuromuscular junction.

As the excitatory potential reaches the neuromuscular junction, the neurotransmitter acetylcholine is dumped into the synaptic cleft, which then binds to receptor sites and through a series of chemical changes results in eventual contraction of the targeted muscle. Electrodes used in electromyography are sensitive to the presence and degree of electrical current in the underlying muscle. These electrodes measure the amount of electricity produced within a targeted muscle. In its original form this electricity is measured as an EMG signal in a raw form, which may provide information in diagnostic procedures, but which has limited value in rehabilitative efforts. For purposes of biofeedback, several transformations occur to the produce a more responsive, comprehensible signal for patient use. The original raw EMG tracing is characterized by a positive and negative waveform around a neutral baseline. This tracing is rectified, thus deleting the negative representation of the signal. The tracing is then averaged and amplified to produce a smooth representation of a motor response. In SEMG biofeedback assisted treatment, this tracing represents amplitude, or strength, on the vertical axis and timing of contraction on the horizontal axis (See Figure 4–1.)

The Technique of Electromyographic Biofeedback

Electromyography is a method of measuring myoelectric impulses initiated in the cell body during firing of a motor unit. For diagnostic purposes, specificity requires hooked wire or other needle electrodes inserted directly into target muscles. For purposes of clinical biofeedback, surface electrodes adhere to the skin surface overlying the target muscle or muscle group. As discussed in the preceding section, in its very simplest form, SEMG biofeedback may consist of a raw electromyographic signal. However, most commercially available SEMG biofeedback devices provide several transformations which produce a more responsive, comprehensible signal for patient use. The ultimate signal produced by the device provides the patient with a continuous line tracing that represents both timing and

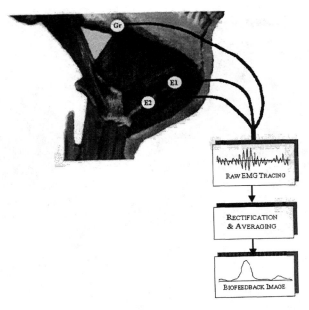

Figure 4–1. Submental muscle anatomy to Raw SEMG tracing to SEMG biofeedback tracing. The process of rectification and averaging produces a more "user-friendly" signal for patient interpretation.

amplitude, or strength. Most devices are dual or multichanneled, allowing for measurement of multiple muscle sites to observe and retrain agonist/antagonist muscle groups (See Figure 4–2). Rubow (1984) provides a detailed summary of many of the parameters available on commercially biofeedback equipment and is a suggested reading for any clinician venturing into this area.

Complications are inherent in the application of this technology for both evaluation and treatment. Electromyography is an inexact procedure using sensitive equipment. Many external factors have the potential of interfering with adequate measurement even in a carefully controlled clinical setting. There are three basic principles for electrode placement (See Figure 4–3).

1. First, electrodes should be placed over the "belly" of the targeted muscle, not the insertion points.
2. Second, electrodes will measure as deep as the active and reference electrodes are spaced apart. Thus, if monitoring of lingual movement is

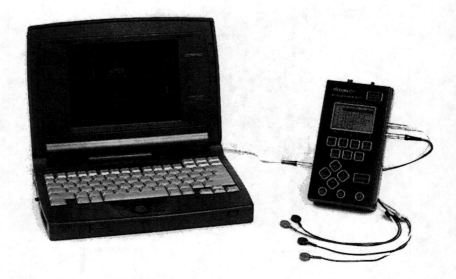

Figure 4–2. Portable SEMG biofeedback Device with electrode leads. (Photo courtesy of Verimed Intl., Ft. Lauderdale, FL.)

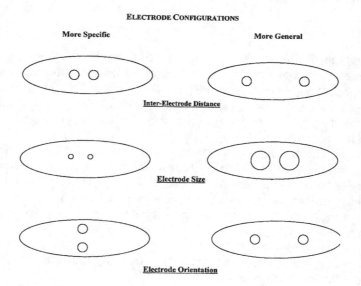

Figure 4–3. Principles of electrode configuration for recording electrodes (active and referent).

targeted, optimal electrode placement may be farther apart in order to pick up lingual activity. Conversely, if lingual movement is distracting, closer electrodes placement may minimize artifact.
3. Finally, the smaller the electrode, the more specific the measurement. Conversely, the larger the electrode recording surface, the more activity will be measured, thus losing specificity.

Despite the best underlying theory, the options for commercially available electrode sizes are limited and the muscles around the head and neck that would be measured in swallowing rehabilitation are small and overlapping. Thus, surface electrode placement is a highly inferential process. At best, one can only assume the targeted muscle group to be measured. This is particularly true in regions of the head and neck where the muscle tissue itself is frequently small in both depth and width and a complex mantle of overlying muscle is required to produce the intricacies of swallowing. Because of this, it is important to recognize the limitations of SEMG. Although these complications do not preclude the knowledgeable use of this modality, they caution careful interpretation of findings. Although the biofeedback tracing may provide the patient and clinician with valuable insights for enhanced motor learning, *SEMG should not be considered a diagnostic tool.* As previously discussed, our understanding of normal surface electromyographic data is limited. This is compounded by the limitations on accurate, repeatable measurements using surface electrodes.

Electrode placement for SEMG biofeedback will vary depending on the goals of treatment. Unfortunately, because of the density of tissue in and around the neck region and the overlying muscle, there is no feasible way to measure myoelectric activity from the pharyngeal constrictor muscles. Thus, SEMG biofeedback will not provide the clinician or patient with direct feedback about the strength of pharyngeal contraction. However, swallowing is a synergistic response with coordinated contraction of multiple muscle groups. Given this, measurement of the muscles that contribute to laryngeal excursion provides direct feedback about the function of only those muscle groups, but the clinician may be able to infer information about the function of the pharynx.

A commonly used placement for most patients is a submental method, with the active and reference electrodes placed in line between the spine of the mandible and the superior edge of the palpable thyroid cartilage. The ground electrode is then placed over the mandible or lateral to the two recording electrodes if triode patch electrodes are used. Using this placement, one receives myoelectric feedback from the collective suprahyoid muscles that are associated with laryngeal excursion, as well as some feedback from the floor of mouth and lingual musculature. Although movement of the tongue can produce artifact that needs to be clinically discriminated from swallowing behavior, for many patients intervention may be targeted toward minimizing or facilitating this tongue movement, thus observation of this behavior is important. If rehabilitation is not addressing lingual components and the patient is distracted by the artifact, placement of the electrodes approximately over the lateral lamina of the thyroid cartilage is likely to provide information about the function of the strap muscles, which also contribute to laryngeal excursion. Alternative electrode placements may include monitoring of the masseters or sternocleidomastoids to target relaxation and eliminate overall tension. Again, electrode placement is dependent on the goals of intervention and the knowledge of muscle anatomy.

Treatment Protocol

Traditional physical rehabilitation of neuromuscular deficits tends to be addressed within three areas of focus: muscle relaxation/inhibition in cases of hyperfunction or spasticity, coordination/patterning of the muscle response to address poor coordination of agonist/antagonist muscle groups, and muscle recruitment to address weakness or paresis. Although swallowing is a finely orchestrated process requiring viability and integration of multiple physiologic motor and sensory systems, at its most fundamental level, it is a motor task. Thus, through biofeedback monitoring, one clear component of swallowing can be directly, and measurably, addressed. It should be clear that SEMG treatment goals are a means to an end; that is, safe swallowing behavior. Traditional swallowing treatments and compensations are integral components of a well-rounded treatment protocol for efficacious service delivery. Standing alone, an achieved SEMG objective holds little information; however, when paired appropriately with a functional swallowing goal, this information is quite valuable as a relative measure of progress.

Initial Teaching

Substantial initial teaching is critical to the success of treatment using this modality, particularly for patients with cognitive deficits. Prior to placing electrodes, it is important to discuss with the patient and the caretaker, if appropriate, the nature of the swallowing disorder and the treatment plan outlined. When introducing SEMG biofeedback, a full explanation of motor potentials and myoelectric activity will likely exceed the interest and cognition of most patients. It is important to explain to the patient that the device that will be used to facilitate treatment is a way of measuring the electrical activity of muscles used in swallowing. This information is then displayed on a computer screen so the patient can learn what those muscles are doing as he or she executes swallowing maneuvers.

As a means of ensuring that the patient understands this very basic concept, it is usually helpful to place electrodes first on the forearm, and then ask the patient to clinch his or her fist and observe the change in the feedback tracing. Using this method initially allows the patient to learn the technique of biofeedback using muscles that are easily observable, and thus the method is more concrete. Next, the electrodes are placed submentally and the patient is not asked to swallow, but to open and close the mouth. With a small movement, there should be a relatively small amplitude excursion of the feedback tracing; with a larger movement, the tracing should demonstrate a greater amplitude excursion. If it is needed for patients with cognitive deficits, a mirror can be used to provide visual feedback and enhance learning. This exercise allows the patient to begin relating to degrees of movement and the relative effects on the feedback tracing. Finally, the patient is asked to swallow and observe the effect of the swallow on the SEMG tracing.

It is important during initial teaching as well as throughout the course of therapy that the patient be encouraged to interpret the SEMG tracing and associate that tracing with what he or she feels proprioceptively. For this purpose, the availability of a "freeze frame" option is essential. It is important, after each screen sweep, to hold that image and asked the patient to describe his or her motor events as related to the biofeedback tracing.

Education and understanding are key to successful rehabilitation. As an important initiation to treatment and as an ongoing review, it is important that patients have some understanding of the nature of their swallowing disorder, within the constraints of their cognitive ability. Viewing a videofluoroscopic examination with the patient is important. Although the patient may not grasp the intricacies of the image, most patients are able to appreciate the differences in a normal versus their impaired study.

Muscle Relaxation and Inhibition

CK is a 58-year-old male, 1 year status post brain stem infarct with a severe to profound swallowing disorder. He had previously attempted and failed traditional swallowing treatment attempts. Interestingly, when monitoring his submental musculature at rest, the patient was unable to demonstrate relaxation of the suprahyoid musculature for greater than 3 consecutive seconds. He was observed at rest to demonstrate an SEMG reading spread erratically within a very broad range of 35 mv range. With focused attention, after nine sessions, he was able to maintain a baseline rest average within a range of ± 5 mv for a maximum of 10 seconds prior to again,

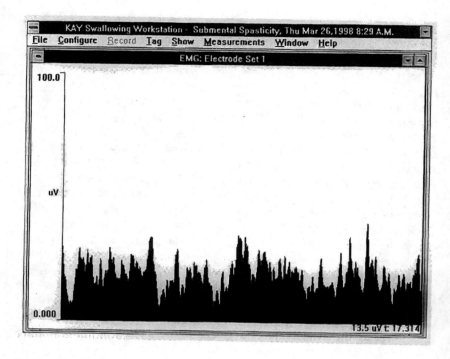

Figure 4–4. SEMG tracing characteristic of submental muscle hyperfunction as described in the case study of Patient CK. (Tracing courtesy of Kay Elemetrics, Lincoln Park, NJ.)

experiencing atypical, nonvolitional contractions. This apparent hyperfunction was not correlated with the presence of the speech deficit of spastic dysarthria, although a mild spastic hemiplegia was evident in the right upper extremity. At the conclusion of 1 week of treatment attempts, CK elected to terminate treatment efforts (see Figure 4–4).

Swallowing rehabilitation requires that a patient develop conscious control over a generally automatic process. One of the basic functions of a muscle is relaxation or rest. Early research by Smith in 1934 indicated that nonimpaired individuals should be able, with minimal training, to completely inhibit a measurable muscle response. Although swallowing requires a programmed muscle contraction it may be useful initially to evaluate the patient's ability to monitor muscle function at rest. The case of CK above raises interesting issues regarding swallowing function that would not be apparent without the benefit of SEMG monitoring. Is there a subgroup of individuals with dysphagia that can be characterized as demonstrating spastic features, so that treatment attempts will be futile without first addressing this abnormal muscle function?

Physical and occupational therapists know very well that a spastic muscle is not likely to perform a functional motor activity effectively. A goal of their rehabilitative efforts, then, may initially be to inhibit this spastic response, thus freeing the muscle group to function under volitional control. Although this issue has not been addressed in the dysphagia literature, clinical practice using SEMG biofeedback suggests that this may be a contributing feature in the dysphagic symptoms of some patients. Other populations that may demonstrate atypically increased SEMG amplitude at rest include patients with spastic cerebral palsy or those with psychogenic, or functional, dysphagia.

Therapeutic instruction for this type of disorder focuses on differential contraction and relaxation of the targeted muscle group with visual feedback of the relative degree of muscle tension provided via the biofeedback tracing. Although the focus of this goal is not on swallowing, the patient should be instructed to swallow as necessary to manage secretions. Clinically, in some patients who have achieved a degree of success with this treatment activity, transiently increased amplitude may reflect inadequate secretion clearance. It would appear that increased pharyngeal secretions result in "posturing" of the pharynx to inhibit aspiration, thus resulting in increased muscle contraction.

Coordination and Patterning of Muscle Response

SJ is a 66-year-old male with a 4-year history of Parkinson's disease. Although he was maintaining nutrition on an oral diet, he was experiencing significant weight loss associated with progressively increasing time required to eat. These symptoms appeared to be due to abnormal tongue pumping and pharyngeal tremor that are characteristic of the dysphagia of Parkinson's disease. When his swallowing was monitored with a SEMG biofeedback tracing, SJ demonstrated an ability to relax submental musculature at rest. However, during attempts to elicit a pharyngeal swallow, either with or without a bolus, he demonstrated multiple peaks of amplitude prior to onset of the swallow that were well correlated with tongue pumping and swallowing gesture behaviors. This pattern was pointed out to the patient, with the treatment goal of extinguishing this nonpurposeful movement. With practice, SJ was able to limit extraneous movement to one preswallow gesture for exaggerated bolus transfer, with associated decreased time required for ingestion of adequate PO and eventual weight gain (see Figure 4–5).

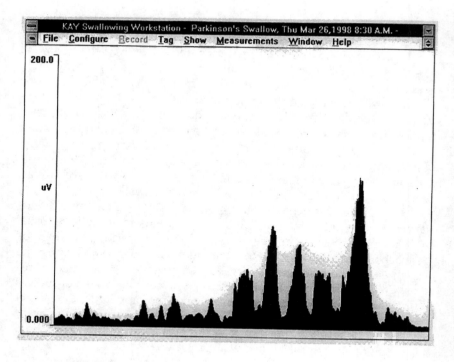

Figure 4–5. SEMG tracing characteristic of a patient with Parkinson's disease as described in the case study of patient SJ. Note the series of peaks of increased amplitude prior to onset of swallowing consistent with extraneous lingual movement. (Tracing courtesy of Kay Elemetrics, Lincoln Park, NJ.)

During normal swallowing behavior, we all demonstrate some variation in patterns of muscular contraction. Rarely do we demonstrate a clean pattern of complete relaxation followed by sharp contraction representing execution of the swallow and followed immediately by complete relaxation. These variations are not, however, of great enough magnitude to impact the efficiency of deglutition. Crary identifies in his study of six patients with brain stem infarct four distinct swallowing patterns, which he correlates with degree of swallowing coordination (Crary, 1995). Clearly, in patients with diseases such as Parkinson's disease, brain stem infarct, and psychogenic dysphagia, these patterns of muscular contraction may be so pronounced as to be intrusive to the effectiveness of swallowing. In this case, rehabilitative efforts may focus on reinforcement and mastery of a more efficient swallowing pattern as described above in the case of SJ.

Muscle Recruitment

SR is a 51-year-old female, 28 months status post excision of a right foramen magnum meningioma. Intraoperatively, she hemorrhaged into her tumor site. She received traditional swallowing treatment for 18 months without significant change in swallowing behavior. A videofluoroscopy completed 3 weeks prior to a SEMG-assisted treatment program revealed profound pharyngeal phase dysphagia characterized by absent swallow on approximately 70% of attempts. Despite the guarded prognosis, SR elected to attempt treatment. By the end of nine treatment sessions, she demonstrated persisting severe dysphagia but with remarkable gains in the coordination of swallowing components. She was started on a puree diet and continued progress in swallowing through traditional treatment. Her feeding tube was removed 5 months following her SEMG-assisted swallowing treatment. At that time, the patient was tolerating a near-normal diet with no pulmonary symptoms and a needed weight gain of approximately 20 pounds.

A patient with weakened or dyscoordinated pharyngeal swallowing from neurological injury or resection/radiation secondary to carcinoma may experience a variety of dysphagic complications. The traditional exercises of modified Valsalva (or effortful) swallow, Mendelsohn maneuver, the newly described Masako, or tongue holding, maneuver are described in detail in Chapter 3 of this text. These can be highly effective maneuvers if they are executed correctly. For execution of the modified Valsalva maneuver, the patient is instructed to "swallow hard," with the presupposition that repetitive execution with increasing effort will produce overall stronger pharyngeal contraction. However, subjective estimates of strength of the swallow or relative degree of laryngeal excursion are difficult to assess by observation or palpation. The Mendelsohn maneuver requires an abstract alteration in the way we swallow. The patient is instructed to initiate a normal swallow, but when the larynx is at its highest point of excursion, the patient is to sustain this maximal contraction volitionally. This maneuver is clinically thought not only to strengthen the pharyngeal swallow but enhance opening of the sphincter muscle that separates the pharynx from the esophagus. Because of the complexity of the maneuver and the required alteration of an automatic process, many patients are not able to master the technique and thus do not reap the benefits. Both of these traditional swallowing treatment exercises can be greatly enhanced via SEMG monitoring (see Figure 4–6).

The patient described above would, by many accounts, be considered to present chronic, perhaps hopeless, dysphagia. Certainly, the extent of her injury and time since onset would tend toward a poorer prognosis.

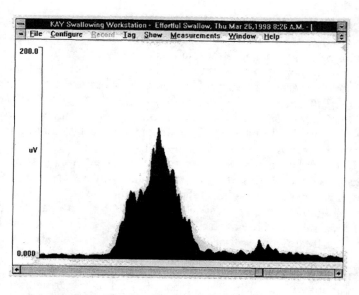

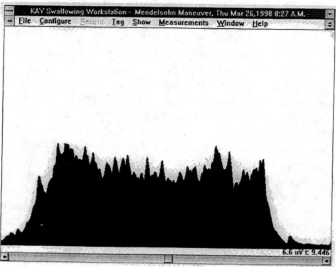

Figure 4–6. Target SEMG tracings during execution of therapeutic maneuvers. (a) The top tracing is characteristic of an effortful swallow with a high amplitude peak of short duration. (b) The lower tracing represents execution of a Mendelsohn maneuver. The initial onset peak amplitude is associated with peak laryngeal excursion, while the sustained amplitude is representative of prolonged laryngeal excursion. (Tracing courtesy of Kay Elemetrics, Lincoln Park, NJ.)

She illustrates, however, our lack of knowledge regarding accurate prognostication and perhaps our underestimation of the effects of rehabilitation. In this case, once she was able to accurately master several swallowing exercises, SR demonstrated not only increased strength of the pharyngeal swallow, but also remarkably increased coordination of the swallow response. This raises another interesting, but as yet, unanswered question. What exactly are we affecting through our rehabilitative efforts? If execution of these exercises were only to strengthen the swallowing musculature, why then, do we not see as a result only a stronger, poorly coordinated swallow? Can we in some ways reprogram a swallowing response, thus not only affecting strength but, as well, coordination and elicitation of a pharyngeal swallow? These questions are yet unanswered in the swallowing literature, but as improved swallowing rehabilitation modalities yield better results, we are gaining more insights into the issues related to swallowing treatment.

Home Programming

The ultimate goal of SEMG biofeedback monitoring in any rehabilitative program is for the patient ultimately to internalize the biofeedback signal, thus maximizing carryover to alternate environments and eventually eliminating the need for direct rehabilitation. The initial steps toward this goal are introduction to rehabilitative exercises and direct intervention in the clinical setting. The logical next step is the establishment of a program to facilitate carryover of the learned behavior to alternate environments. This process initially may be well facilitated by the use of a portable SEMG biofeedback device. An optimal home program for many patients will consist of five to six brief (5 to 10 minutes) sessions daily, addressing the goals from direct treatment in the home environment. For patients who can tolerate at least a limited oral diet, these sessions may be structured to precede snacks and meals. It has been the experience of this clinician that if the patient completes an initial intensive training program with SEMG biofeedback, rental of a portable device is rarely required. As described by a patient who used this equipment, "The images you worked at my building are permanently etched on my mind."

Treatment Candidacy

Not all patient groups will benefit from the inclusion of SEMG biofeedback monitoring in dysphagia rehabilitation, just as not all patients will benefit from dysphagia intervention in its traditional form. Certainly, some disorders such as severe bilateral brain stem infarct or amyotrophic lateral sclerosis may not be responsive to any rehabilitative attempts. Traditional treatment practices for presumably treatable etiologies are difficult to comprehend and implement in many cognitively disordered, as well as intact, patients. However, utilization of an additional feedback system in the form of SEMG is thought to "widen the net" of reasonable candidates for treatment. Biofeedback monitoring facilitates an awareness of muscle contraction associated with swallowing and depicts performance of strategies. This enables many patients who otherwise could not grasp treatment concepts to participate successfully in a therapy program.

Contraindications

SEMG biofeedback monitoring is a noninvasive treatment technique. There are only a few situations that warrant precautions. The nature of the treatment tends to be a very intensive form of traditional swallowing treatment and requires considerable effort by the patient. As such, patients with unstable cardiac conditions may be unable to tolerate the intensive, Valsalva-type maneuvers required for treatment. In addition, recent surgical patients or patients undergoing radiation therapy, may be contraindicated secondary to the delicacy of fresh surgical incisions or the friability of irradiated tissue. In these patient populations, SEMG biofeedback-assisted treatment is not absolutely contraindicated, but should be approved by the referring physician with specific written orders. Also, clinical experience has identified that some patients may develop transient hoarseness as a result of the maximal effort at glottic closure during repetitive swallowing maneuvers. Although this is not a specific effect of biofeedback-assisted treatment, it may be more apparent with the increased intensity of intervention using this modality.

Equipment Availability

For swallowing rehabilitation purposes, the minimal requirement is a continuous waveform of an integrated and rectified signal. The equipment used in swallowing rehabilitation is no different from that used by our colleagues in physical and occupational therapy. Thus, in rehabilitation facilities with multidisciplinary services, equipment can be shared among departments. There are other devices especially designed for use in swallowing rehabilitation that provide similar information (Hageman & Crow, 1996; Reddy, Gupta, Simcox, Motta, & Coppenger, 1997; Sukthankar, Reddy, Canilang, Stephenson, & Thomas, 1994). Pizeoelectric transducers or electroglottography may provide a very similar waveform representing hyoid movement. Regardless of the instrumentation, it is important for the clinician to understand the variable source of the signal and the associated artifact.

SUMMARY

Several primary points should be gleaned from this chapter:

1. Although subcutaneous electromyography has diagnostic value, SEMG biofeedback cannot be considered a component of diagnostic evaluation given the variability of the signal and the lack of specificity. However, it can be a very valuable clinical adjunct to swallowing rehabilitation.
2. Electrode placement is dependent on the targeted therapeutic task and clinician knowledge of muscular anatomy. Several principles of electrode placement are outlined with the warning that SEMG electrode placement is nonspecific.
3. After full evaluation of swallowing physiology, development of a treatment plan including SEMG biofeedback monitoring may focus on the components of muscle relaxation and inhibition, coordination and patterning of a motor response, or muscle recruitment.
4. Biofeedback monitoring may not facilitate treatment in all patients, but it is considered to "widen the net" of those patients who are treatment candidates by providing additional visual and auditory cues.

SEMG biofeedback is not the only type of feedback system that can augment treatment. Chapter 5 outlines several additional sources of exteroceptive feedback that the clinician may find useful.

FOOD FOR THOUGHT

Delayed pharyngeal swallow is likely one of the most common deficits of pharyngeal swallowing in the neurogenic population. Unfortunately, it is also the one deficit for which we have little to offer in terms of rehabilitation. Part of the difficulty in addressing this disorder is the transient and elusive nature—there are currently very few reliable clinical and noninvasive ways to measure a delayed swallow or to visualize the deficit for intervention. Would SEMG, acoustic, endoscopic, or even ultrasonic biofeedback

(continued)

FOOD FOR THOUGHT *(continued)*

provide an option for observing and thus modifying this deficit? If the patient were able to visualize the differential transfer of the bolus into the pharynx followed by onset of laryngeal excursion immediately and consistently, would he or she ultimately be able to gain volitional control over this deficit? Using the compensatory technique of 3- second prep as a repetitive exercise, rather than a compensation, could the more prompt volitional swallow eventually become habituated, thus rehabilitating this difficult swallowing deficit?

Endoscopic evaluation allows for a clear view of the events associated with delayed onset of swallow. Martin, Logemann, Shaker, and Dodds (1993) and others have used SEMG to mark the onset of swallowing during research trials which investigate of the onset of swallowing within the respiratory cycle. She refers to two components of the swallowing EMG signal. One of these, EMG1, may well refer to base-of-tongue movement for bolus propulsion into the pharynx, while the other, EMG2, may refer to actual onset of laryngeal excursion. Currently, the clinical biofeedback instrumentation that is commercially available does not appear to sample the electromyographic data at a fast enough rate to visualize these two components. However, future development may allow this discrimination. In reference to cervical auscultation, the oft-reported sound of swallowing is described as a double clunk followed by a swoosh. Although we currently are unsure what physiologic events this relates to, McKaig (1995) has reported some correlation between the interclunk distance and delayed pharyngeal swallow as viewed radiographically. As well, the acoustic waveform, as can be measured through an easily accessible computerized sound card, presents two distinct waveforms. Do these two signals correlate with bolus transfer and onset of swallow, respectively? If so, could they be visualized and perhaps amenable to treatment as just described?

5

Other Biofeedback Modalities: Endoscopy, Ultrasound, Auscultation, and Oximetry

A biofeedback device must provide visualization of some component of swallowing. Given this, traditional diagnostic techniques may provide valuable information to the patient and clinician when adapted for therapeutic purposes. This chapter describes the application of several clinical and diagnostic techniques to the rehabilitation process. A brief overview of the technique and equipment is provided, followed by a description of how the technique could be applied to the therapeutic process.

ENDOSCOPY

The use of fiberoptic endoscopy in the field of dysphagia is relatively new. Initially, otolaryngologists developed the procedure as a way to assess laryngeal pathology and physiology. Langmore first described its use as an instrumental tool in diagnosing pharyngeal dysphagia in 1988. She described a procedure called FEES®, Fiberoptic Endoscopic Evaluation of Swallowing, which involves inserting a flexible fiberoptic endoscope into the hypopharynx, via the nares, to obtain information regarding the presence and pathophysiology of pharyngeal dysphagia.

More recently, a new endoscopic test to evaluate sensory capacity in the supraglottic larynx and pharynx has been described by Aviv and colleagues (1993). This test requires a special endoscope (Pentax Precision Instrument Corp, Orangeburg, NJ) that can deliver a brief pulse of air to the pharynx and supraglottic larynx. The air pulse is precisely controlled in amplitude (strength). By delivering variations in air pulse strength to subjects, information can be gained regarding sensory thresholds in their larynx. Aviv suggests that sensory testing, using this special endoscope, may be a useful addition to FEES. This evaluation is known as FEEST, Fiberoptic Endoscopic Evaluation of Swallowing with Sensory Testing (Aviv, Martin, Keen, Debell, & Blitzer, 1993; Aviv et al., 1998).

The importance of sensory discrimination in these areas may be important, since it is suggested that decreased sensation or anesthesia in these structures could cause severe dysphagia and increased frequency of aspiration (Aviv et al., 1996). It is known that both motor and sensory deficits occur after a patient sustains a stroke (Mohr, 1986) and, therefore, it is hypothesized that the larynx and pharynx would not be spared. In addition, studies have reported decreased oral cavity sensation with increasing age (Aviv, Hecht, Weinberg, Dalton, & Urken, 1992; Aviv et al., 1994; Calhoun, Gibson, Hartley, Minton, & Hokanson, 1992). However, the role that sensory deficits of the pharynx or larynx play in the development of dysphagia and aspiration is not known.

FOOD FOR THOUGHT:

In a recent publication, Langmore (1998) raises several significant questions for clinicians to ponder regarding how sensory deficits may influence dysphagia management. For example, what would constitute appropriate intervention for a patient with sensory loss and dysphagia? What is the best management for a patient with sensory loss who does not aspirate or exhibit a high risk of aspiration during instrumental testing? More research and discussion are clearly needed to answer these important questions.

FEES®: The Procedure

FEES® involves the insertion of a flexible fiberoptic endoscope into the hypopharynx via the nares. The placement of the endoscope is high in the hypopharynx, and allows a direct view of the larynx and pharyngeal structures.

Initially, a careful assessment is conducted regarding the anatomy of the laryngeal and pharyngeal structures, presence of oral secretions, sensation, and functional physiology for swallowing. Direct assessment of the physiology (function) of the anatomic structures occurs first, and the information gained from this assessment is then applied to swallowing physiology. It includes voluntary and involuntary movements, such as vocal cord adduction during breath hold, and laryngeal/pharyngeal movements during phonation. In addition, spontaneous and voluntary dry swallows and laryngeal activity during respiration are observed.

The swallowing examination involves the presentation of controlled amounts of food and liquid to the patient to swallow. All material is dyed with green food coloring for contrast. Varying consistencies and amounts may be presented, depending on the patient's status and the objectives of the particular exam. If desired, drops of green food coloring can be placed in the mouth to mix with saliva and assess the management of secretions as they fall to the pharynx. The examination is videotaped to optimize clinical use and interpretation. For more information regarding the use of endoscopy as a diagnostic tool in swallowing, see Langmore and McCulloch (1997).

Equipment

A flexible fiberoptic endoscope and portable light source, coupled with a chip camera, videotape recorder, and monitor system, allow real-time viewing of pharyngeal and laryngeal structures during swallowing. This allows the procedure to be recorded for review and interpretation later. This is important since the pharyngeal swallow occurs rapidly and much information could be missed if videotape review were not possible. The equipment is placed on a cart that can be rolled to a patient.

Endoscopy as Biofeedback Modality

Endoscopy has many valuable uses as a biofeedback tool (Table 5–1). It allows patients to observe their laryngeal and pharyngeal anatomy in real time, and its response to voluntary and involuntary movements. Clinicians can visually point out various anatomical structures and explain the

Table 5–1. Uses of endoscopy as a biofeedback tool.

Increase understanding of swallowing disorder

Increase understanding of surgical reconstruction

Increase sensory awareness of residue

Observe effect of diet modifications (consistency, bolus amount, taste, temperature, placement; adaptive equipment)

Train/observe effect of chin tuck

Train/observe effect of head rotation

Train/observe effect of head tilt

Train/observe effect of head extension

Train/observe effect of vocal cord adduction

Train/observe effect of velopharyngeal closure

Train/observe effect of supraglottic and super-supraglottic maneuver

functional impairments of swallowing physiology seen. This is especially useful in patients who have had surgical reconstruction. Denk and Kaider (1997) report that videoendoscopic biofeedback significantly increased the chance of therapeutic success in patients following head and neck surgery, when compared to conventional swallowing therapy alone. Anecdotally, patients typically demonstrate rapid understanding of their disorder, since the monitor allows a graphic display of their anatomy and functional physiology. This is especially important in patients with apparent decreased sensation, who are often unaware of residue or secretions in their pharynx or larynx.

Endoscopy can be useful in providing continuous, immediate feedback regarding the training and effect of various compensatory and rehabilitative techniques used in treatment. For example, patients can readily see the effect of a head rotation or chin tuck and how these postures influence bolus transfer and clearance. Figure 5–1 portrays head rotation and chin tuck. Views such as these can rapidly show a patient the rationale for a certain treatment recommendation, and most important, how to use it correctly. It is hoped that the patient can then develop an internal guideline system that will help him or her in using these techniques independently.

Endoscopy is an exceptional biofeedback tool to help a patient learn how to voluntarily protect the airway. Vocal cord adduction does not always occur with normal breath-holding, even in normals (Langmore & McCulloch, 1997; Martin, Logemann, Shaker, & Dodds, 1993). Patients can readily see the adequacy of their vocal cord adduction during breath-holding, and effectively learn how to voluntarily protect their airway during swallowing. Figure 5–2 portrays endoscopic views of both normal and tight breath-holding. Seeing such images may improve a patient's learning of a complicated maneuver.

The abstract nature of a patient's swallowing disorder, and the rationale, effect, and training of treatment recommendations may be more easily understood by using FEES as a biofeedback tool. As patients are able to understand what is wrong and what they can do to "fix" it, it is hoped that their recovery may be quicker and more complete.

Patient Candidacy

Not all patients with dysphagia are appropriate candidates for endoscopy. Careful screening of a patient's medical history and current status must occur, prior to accepting a patient for endoscopy. This will greatly minimize the risk of an adverse reaction.

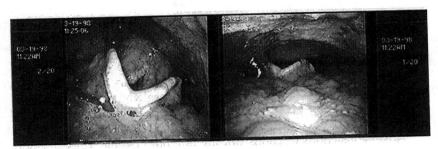

Figure 5–1. Endoscopic view of head rotation (left)and chin tuck (right). (Courtesy of Nicholas Tsaclas, Pentax Precision Instrument Corporation, Orangeburg, NJ.)

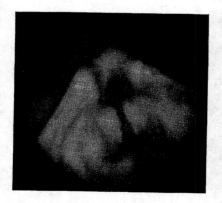 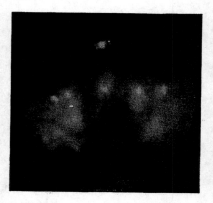

Figure 5–2. Endoscopic view of normal breath-holding (left) and tight breath-holding (right). (Reprinted with permission of Singular Publishing Group, Inc.)

Contraindications for endoscopy are patients with a history of bleeding disorders, epistaxis (severe nosebleeds), acute cardiac problems which predispose the patient to bradycardia, movement disorders (dyskinesia), and/or extreme agitation or combative behavior. If a topical anesthetic or nasal decongestant (vasoconstrictor) is used in the nasal mucosa to increase patient comfort prior to inserting the endoscope, patients should be evaluated for a history of allergic reactions or contraindications due to present medical status or current medications.

The routine use of a topical anesthetic or vasoconstrictor to increase patient comfort during insertion of the endoscope has recently been questioned. Leder, Ross, Briskin, and Sasaki (1997) conducted a prospective, double-blind, randomized study on the use of a topical anesthetic, over-the-counter vasoconstrictor, and a nasal placebo (designed to have both a medicinal taste and smell) on patient comfort levels during transnasal endoscopy. Similar patient comfort levels were reported given all three variables, and no significant differences were found. In addition, patient comfort levels were found to have no significant differences even when nothing was administered to the nasal mucosa prior to endoscopy. It was concluded by the authors that no treatment is necessary prior to inserting an endoscope comfortably into the nasal mucosa when the procedure is performed by a trained endoscopist, such as a speech-language pathologist or physician.

Adverse reactions to endoscopy are rare but possible. These include nosebleed, fainting, laryngospasm, allergic reaction to the topical anesthetic, and/or a possible stinging sensation or sneezing if a nasal decongestant (vasoconstrictor) is used. Aspiration pneumonia is also possible if food or liquid is introduced, since it may be aspirated. However, endoscopy does not require the introduction of any food or liquid if it would appear unsafe, or when used as a biofeedback tool to practice voluntary vocal cord adduction, for example.

Clinician Training and Competence

Prior to performing FEES independently, it is generally agreed that clinicians must receive specialized training, in addition to what is normally received in graduate school. They must be able to demonstrate both the technical and clinical skills necessary to insert an endoscope safely, conduct the exam, and interpret the results. These skills are typically gained only after extensive training and supervision. Since no specific guidelines for training are currently available, clinicians are encouraged to attend workshops and develop mentoring relationships with otolaryngologists and/or speech-language pathologists who are trained to perform FEES.

ULTRASOUND

Ultrasound imaging is a noninvasive technique that uses high-frequency sounds waves to visualize the movement of soft tissue structures during functional activity. This type of biologic imaging for the assessment of swallowing was developed and refined in the 1980s through the efforts of Sonies, Shawker, and others at the National Institutes of Health (Sonies, Baum, & Shawker, 1984; Shawker, Sonies, Hall, & Baum, 1984; Shawker, Sonies, Stone, & Baum, 1983). The diagnostic uses of ultrasonic imaging are outlined extensively in other readings and thus are not addressed in this chapter.

The Procedure

Through the work of Sonies, Shawker, and others, several features of swallowing can be visualized using selective placements and orientations of the transducer. The density of the hyoid bone produces a black triangular shadow in the ultrasound image and thus can be tracked easily during swallowing to track laryngeal excursion and timing of the oropharyngeal swallow (Cordaro & Sonies, 1993; Sonies, Parent, Morrish, & Baum, 1988). The air-tissue interface on the lingual surface appears as a darkened line outlining the tongue surface. With the transducer in the midline sagittal plane, information would be provided about bolus control in reference to anterior to posterior transit and premature spillage. With the tranducer in the coronal plane, the lateral tongue surfaces are visualized and thus can provide information about symmetry of bolus control. An inspection of the timing between tongue movement and hyoid elevation will provide a clinical picture of timing of the onset of swallow after bolus transfer (Sonies et al., 1988). More recent work by Miller and Watkin (1997) highlights the use of ultrasound to view the movement of the lateral pharyngeal walls during swallowing as a relative indication of pharyngeal constriction.

Equipment

A linear transducer placed submentally in the coronal, saggital, or transverse planes emits high-frequency sound impulses (2 to 10 MHz) into the structures of the oral and hypopharyngeal cavity. As these ultrasonic impulses pass through the soft tissue structures, they are reflected back to the transducer, with the brightness of the measured response proportionate to the reflective properties of the intervening tissue. Highly reflective tissues such as fibrous tissue appears bright, while liquid reflects little sound and thus appears very dark. Bone and air-filled spaces reflect no sound, and will thus appear black. These gradations in reflected energy collectively reproduce an image of the oral and hypopharyngeal structures. Figures 5–3, 5–4, and 5–5, provided courtesy of Dr. Barbara Sonies, show sagittal and coronal views of a normal tongue and a coronal view of lingual asymmetry. More recent advances have used color flow doppler ultrasound to evaluate bloodflow during lingual muscle contraction (Miller & Watkin, 1996). Although, ultrasound may be considered costly in respect to its benefits to swallowing diagnosis and rehabilitation, it may be found in other departments of a major medical center.

Ultrasound as Biofeedback Modality

The clinical use of ultrasound as a biofeedback modality to enhance swallowing rehabilitation has been sparsely documented and procedures have yet to be fully developed, but it is discussed in two references (Shawker & Sonies, 1985; Shawker et al., 1984). Since ultrasound is noninvasive and can be repeated without risk or significant cost, aspects of swallowing that can be visualized using this tool can be monitored by the clinician and patient during therapeutic tasks.

Other modalities do not provide an image of the lingual surface or shape. Using ultrasound imaging, patients with oral phase deficits and subsequent bolus control deficits may reap significant benefits. For patients with anterior leakage or posterior spillage into the pharynx, visualization of tongue tip or tongue base elevation using midline sagittal positioning may allow the patient to produce a tighter intraoral seal and inhibit these

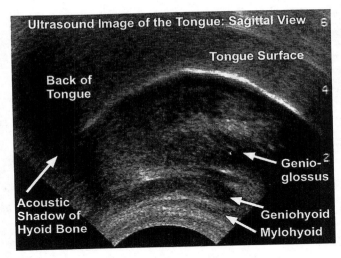

Figure 5–3. Sagittal view of the tongue at rest with the tip on the right side and the back of tongue on the left. The tongue surface is the top curved white line with the major lingual muscle, genioglossus, depicted by arrow. The floor of the mouth muscles (geniohyoid and mylohyoid) are seen below the tongue. The dark triangular acoustic shadow cast by the hyoid bone radiates from the lower left of the ultrasound scan.

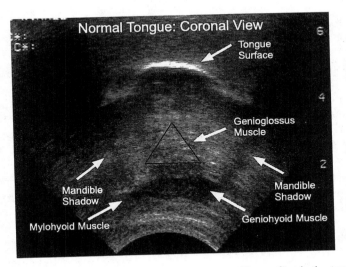

Figure 5–4. Coronal view of the tongue blade at rest. The surface is the top curved line. The triangular area is the bundling of the genioglossus muscle. The floor of the mouth muscles are seen below the tongue. Because the image is taken from a submental location, the mandible casts a shadow on either side of the tongue.

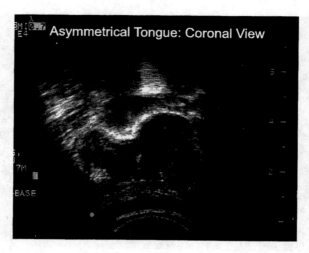

Figure 5–5. Coronal view of an abnormal, asymmetric tongue blade at rest. Note that the tongue surface, the indented white line, is snakelike and the tongue surface is larger on the right side.

adverse dysphagic symptoms. For patients with asymmetry of lingual movement from unilateral stroke, for example, modeling the tongue surface shape with the transducer in the coronal plane may allow the patient to gain greater bolus control. Extent of laryngeal excursion both during swallowing and during therapeutic tasks such as the Mendelsohn maneuver can likewise be visualized and subsequently manipulated. With the transducer placed over the vocal folds during phonatory exercises, vocal fold adduction can be visualized as a technique to address glottic closure in the patient who is at aspiration risk secondary to poor airway protection at the glottic level. Glottic closure during execution of a supraglottic swallow will be more difficult to visualize because of the movement of the vocal folds out of the transducer range during swallowing.

As with other biofeedback modalities, patient education regarding the technique and interpretation of the ultrasound image will be prerequisite to clinical use as a biofeedback tool. The ultrasound image for some patients may be difficult to interpret because of the sometimes grainy nature and indistinct borders. However, ultrasound provides a direct image of structural components, unlike SEMG and auscultation; thus, it may be more easily understood by patients with cognitive impairment. Certainly, the biofeedback benefits of ultrasound can be maximized by a skilled clinician with precise transducer placement leading to an optimally clear image.

CERVICAL AUSCULTATION

Cervical auscultation is a relatively new technique that is receiving considerable research attention. In summary, cervical auscultation can be defined as listening to the sounds of swallowing with a stethoscope at or around the level of the laryngopharyngeal junction to gain information about pharyngeal swallowing.

The Procedure

This technique has been the focus of significant recent research in an attempt to define the physiologic correlates of the acoustic signal, determine the optimal recording techniques and establish its role as a clinical diagnostic tool (Boiron, Rouleau, & Metman, 1997; Chicero & Murdoch, 1998; Hamlet, Nelson, & Patterson, 1990; Smith, Hamlet & Johns, 1990; Takahashi, Groher, & Michi, 1994; Zenner, Losinski, & Mills, 1995). To date, there is little consensus regarding the physiologic correlates of the perceived sounds of swallowing, thus clinical application as a diagnostic tool is hindered. The reader is directed elsewhere for specifics regarding clinical diagnostic use. Application of this technique as a biofeedback modality is similarly affected by lack of information; however, the goals of its use as a therapeutic tool are significantly less complex and not as dependent on absolute knowledge of what is perceived. Thus, for many patients in the early stages of rehabilitation, auditory feedback of the acoustic signal associated with swallowing can provide valuable information to guide the learning process.

Equipment

Listening with a stethoscope can typically provide auditory input to only one listener; thus, an adapted device can be created to project the acoustic signal through a loudspeaker. Doing so makes the information available to the patient and clinician for discussion and critique. An inexpensive amplified speaker serves as the output for a small lapel microphone that is connected via flexible plastic tubing to the housing of a stethoscope bell (see Figure 5–6). As the signal is adequately amplified with the speaker and microphone, the membrane of the stethoscope bell can be removed because it can create additional noise when it is placed over the skin surface. With the loudspeaker set at an appropriate level, the stethoscope is placed over the lamina of the thyroid cartilage to monitor the acoustic signal associated with swallowing.

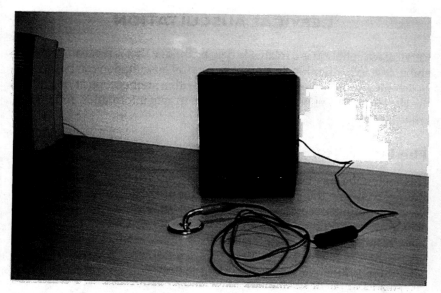

Figure 5–6. An inexpensive biofeedback device for cervical auscultation can be easily made using material available at an electronics store. An inexpensive speaker, lapel microphone, and stethoscope bell can be combined to allow the patient and clinician to monitor the acoustics of swallowing.

Auscultation as a Biofeedback Modality

As a biofeedback modality, cervical auscultation can facilitate correct execution of a Mendelsohn maneuver. As discussed in prior chapters, execution of a Mendelsohn maneuver requires sustaining laryngeal excursion during the swallow, or prolonging the swallow. Unfortunately, many patients demonstrate difficulty with the sequencing of swallowing and sustained contraction. Thus, they may be observed to execute the swallow and, after the return of the thyroid to resting posture, maintain contraction primarily of the tongue. Or conversely, they may contract musculature of the oropharynx and only execute a swallow on release of the contraction. Either way, the effect of the technique may be lost, as the sustained muscle contraction does not occur synergistically with the height of laryngeal excursion and cricopharyngeal sphincter opening. Acoustic feedback may be used to monitor the release of tracheal air during execution of an attempted Mendelsohn maneuver. Inherent in the correct completion of the exercise is a period of intraswallow apnea. Except in cases where vocal fold pathology inhibits glottic closure, there should be no air escape during execution of this technique, as would be consistent with intraswallow apnea. As with any rehabilitative method, some patients appear to benefit from this type of information while others are merely puzzled by it.

Further applications of cervical auscultation as a biofeedback modality may emerge as we gain greater insights into the nature of the acoustic signal. If the clinical correlates of auscultation are further developed for diagnostic purposes, the same information could be used to support and encourage rehabilitation practices.

FOOD FOR THOUGHT:

Using cervical auscultation as a biofeedback modality in rehabilitation reveals enormous variability in the sounds of swallowing both between and within patients. Some cognitively intact patients report great benefit in monitoring the acoustic signal and claim that they can judge the relative strength and efficiency of the swallow by the acoustic feedback. "That sounded like a good one." Indeed, subjective clinical impressions tend to support this, with the perception of a "cleaner" or "crisper" acoustic signal developing as rehabilitation progresses. Is there anything to this? So far we have no data to support such an observation; however, we are yet in the early stages of evaluating this technique.

PULSE OXIMETRY

Pulse oximetry has recently received attention as a possible tool in the management of neurogenic dysphagia (Rogers, Msall, & Shucard, 1993; Sellars, Dunnet, & Carter, 1998; Zaidi, Smith, King, Park, O'Neill, & Connolly, 1995). Pulse oximetry is a noninvasive, continuous visual measure of arterial blood oxygenation that can detect changes in oxygenation levels within 20 seconds (New, 1985). It also provides continuous pulse rate (Figure 5–7). Arterial blood saturation is measured as a percentage of hemoglobin filled with oxygen, with 100% as the maximum reading possible. This provides a measure of how well oxygen is being transported within the blood. Readings between 95 and 100% are considered normal, while anything below 90% may be life threatening (Carroll, 1997).

It is hypothesized that arterial blood oxygenation, as determined by pulse oximetry, may dramatically drop because of aspiration of foods or

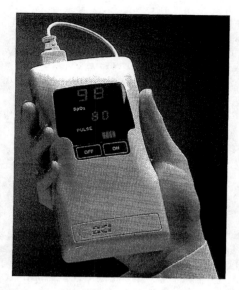

Figure 5–7. Pulse oximeter.(Reprinted with permission of BCI International.)

liquids. A significant drop in level is considered a variation of 4% (Sulllivan, 1985). Therefore, pulse oximetry may provide biofeedback of the presence but not the nature of aspiration, without traditional instrumental examination, such as videofluoroscopy or FEES. Since pulse oximetry requires little patient cooperation, provides objective measures, and is portable to a patient, it may be a valuable tool in the management of dysphagia if this hypothesis is proven correct.

The Procedure

Pulse oximetry involves the placement of a visual light sensor probe over a finger usually, but it also may be placed over a toe, earlobe, or ear pinna. The sensor has a light source and a light detector. As explained by Carroll (1997), the light source emits red and infrared light in alternating bursts over the vascular bed where the probe is placed. The red light is absorbed by the unoxygenated hemoglobin while the infrared light is absorbed by the oxyhemoglobin. The light detector then measures how much light is absorbed by each hemoglobin as it passes through the finger, toe, or earlobe/pinna (Figure 5–8). This information is calculated by a microprocessor in the oximeter into an average of the ratios of red light to infrared light, and presented as a percentage reading. Good arterial blood flow is necessary to get a reliable reading (Carroll, 1997).

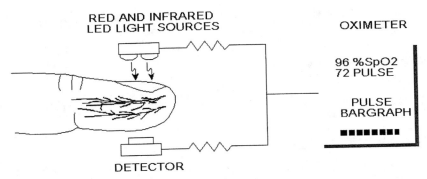

Figure 5–8. Theory of pulse oximeter operation. (Reprinted by permission of BCI International.)

Pulse oximetry has proven to be quite accurate and reliable in a variety of settings, but there are several artifacts that need to be controlled (Alexander, Teller, & Gross, 1989; Bowes, Corke, & Hulka, 1989; Cote, Goldstein, Cote, Hoaglin, & Ryan, 1988; Kagle, Alexander, Berko, Gruffre, & Gross, 1987; Tremper & Barker, 1989). The following factors, agents, or situations may affect the readings and limit the precision, performance, and application of pulse oximetry (Carroll, 1997):

Motion artifact. The probe must remain motionless during all readings. May need to move the probe to the ear to prevent motion artifact due to Parkinsonism tremors, or other movement disorders.

Abnormal hemoglobins. Pulse oximeters cannot tell the difference between hemoglobin that has bonded with oxygen or carbon monoxide. Therefore, both conditions would provide high readings, and provide a falsely elevated reading for patients with carbon monoxide poisoning. This may commonly be seen in patients who are smokers, since carbon monoxide is often elevated in their blood. This condition is called carboxyhemoglobin.

Exposure of the probe to high ambient light. Sunshine or artificial light can skew readings, since pulse oximetry relies on the measurement of light emitted through arterial blood. Covering the sensor with a washcloth or any opaque material will eliminate this artifact.

Decreased circulation. If a patient has a weak or absent peripheral pulse, inaccurate readings will occur. Patients at highest risk for low blood perfusion rates are those with hypotension, hypovolemia, and hypothermia. Those with cardiac problems that lead to weak perfusion may also have poor readings. Warming the extremity or placing the probe on the earlobe may be helpful. The earlobe is least affected by poor peripheral blood perfusion. Comparing the pulse rate reading on the oximeter against palpated pulse or apical heart rate can provide a way to check whether the device is picking up arterial pulsation and providing reliable readings.

Nail polish, false fingernails, or fungus. Since light needs to pass through a vascular bed, anything that may impede this passage may alter the reading. Use of an earlobe or pinna, or taping the sensor sideways on the finger rather than the nailbed, may eliminate this artifact.

Mechanical problems with the device. Low battery readings or equipment malfunction can always occur with any mechanical device. Check the pulse readings against apical heart rate periodically, and examine the device carefully occasionally for malfunction. Test it on your own finger as well for a normal reading and matching pulse rate. Check the signal strength indicator frequently during use since lower signal levels may provide unreliable readings.

Equipment

The only equipment necessary is a pulse oximeter in good working condition. These devices are small, battery-operated devices, with adapters to plug into electricity available. Some devices can store the recordings to be downloaded into a computer later (Sellars et al., 1998). They also may provide a continuous paper reading, in addition to the reading provided on the device.

Pulse Oximetry as a Biofeedback Modality

It has been suggested that pulse oximetry may be a useful, noninvasive tool to monitor cardiopulmonary stress during oral eating with patients who exhibit dysphagia (Rogers et al., 1993). These authors reported significant, acquired hypoxemia that occurred only during oral feedings in two patients with chronic dysphagia. Other unpublished reports (Iskowitz, 1997) state that a correlation has been shown between oxygen desaturation and documented aspiration, as determined by simultaneous modified barium swallow studies and pulse oximetry.

If pulse oximetry were shown to reliably demonstrate an effect of aspiration, its application in clinical assessment and intervention would be greatly beneficial. Patients could possibly be classified into high- and low-risk aspiration groups, and the objective data would be helpful in determining the need for further instrumental studies (Iskowitz, 1997). Based on the information gathered in an instrumental diagnostic study, patients possibly could use pulse oximetry to monitor the effectiveness of intervention strategies continuously as they eat. This would be very beneficial during initial oral feeding trials with a patient known to aspirate, and as an aid to monitor the effect of fatigue over the course of a meal.

However, convincing data to support the use of pulse oximetry in this manner have not yet been reported. Sellars and colleagues (1998) were unable to find a clear-cut relationship between aspiration and a significant change in arterial oxygenation in six dysphagic subjects, using videofluoroscopy and pulse oximetry simultaneously. They did find some support that respiratory status may change during oral feedings, but the mechanisms responsible for these alterations are still illusive.

The relationship of respiration, oral feeding, and aspiration to arterial oxygenation levels is complex and not well-understood. Given the variety of artifacts that may influence readings, as well as the complexities involved in the relationship of aspiration and respiration, further research is needed with both normals and individuals with dysphagia before the value of pulse oximetry as a management tool for dysphagia can be evaluated. As with all of the biofeedback techniques described in this chapter, pulse oximetry is not intended to replace traditional diagnostic or intervention procedures. Clinicians are cautioned to continue with their standardized methods of diagnosis and rely on their clinical skills to manage dysphagia. While new technology is exciting and perhaps beneficial to our plethora of tests and tools, it is important not to abandon our past practices without careful scrutiny.

SUMMARY

Rehabilitative efforts in their current state will challenge not just the patient. The clinician providing intervention services will be equally challenged to structure the learning environment and maximize feedback modalities to give each patient ample opportunity to benefit from the rehabilitative techniques. Several biofeedback modalities, including SEMG, ultrasound, endoscopy, tactile, visual and acoustic feedback may foster mastery of the skill.

Again, the clinician is encouraged not to stop with these suggestions. Taking the advice of Roosevelt in the last chapter, if one treatment approach fails, try another. A vivid imagination and sharp problem-solving skills are required of clinicians in this area, particularly those with little funds for instrumentation. The use of a paper-and-pencil drawing may well suffice to enhance understanding of rehabilitative maneuvers. Using thyroid palpation as a guide, the clinician may ask the patient to draw a line that represents perceived relative strength of the pharyngeal swallow. Collaboration with colleagues in biomedical engineering or occupational therapy may yield a variety of inexpensive tools that can effectively augment treatment.

As clinicians involved in the provision of services to patients with a variety of handicapping conditions, it behooves us to listen carefully to our patients and let their words motivate us to discover innovative therapies or alternative applications of well-known treatment modalities. Biofeedback modalities provide great potential for the enhancement of clinical rehabilitation of the patient with dysphagia. Bryant (1991) and Crary (1995) have documented case studies of patients with chronic dysphagia successfully treated with SEMG biofeedback, even after failing traditional treatment. Clinical experience suggests benefit from other biofeedback modalities as well. Regardless of the modality, the concept is quite simple. As described by one patient, "It gives you a target to shoot at." Biofeedback monitoring provides a clear window into a difficult and abstract treatment process, affording both patient and clinician a visual or auditory representation of the swallow, and, in some cases, concrete short-term objectives and clear measurement of one aspect of patient progress.

6

Compensatory Interventions for Dysphagia

This chapter provides a definition and tutorial on compensatory management of dysphagia. Categories of compensatory techniques are provided, followed by discussion of specific techniques in conjunction with the physiologic deficits that they are typically applied toward. Instructions for the techniques, coaching techniques, and examples of short-term objectives are included.

The focus of this chapter is to provide the reader with a tutorial on defining and implementing compensatory techniques in the management of the patient with dysphagia. As a prerequisite to this discussion, however, several fundamental principles should be reiterated from earlier chapters. First, effective management of any oral pharyngeal swallowing impairment relies on accurate diagnosis and individualization of the treatment plan to the specific physiology. This applies to compensation and rehabilitation and is crucial to the success of the intervention program. Second, a "cookbook approach" to dysphagia management is inappropriate and may be contraindicated. As an example, chin tuck posturing is widely applied as a technique to inhibit preswallow aspiration in patients with delayed pharyngeal swallow. However, in a small percentage of patients, prescription of a chin tuck posture may actually facilitate, rather than inhibit, aspiration (Ekberg, 1986). Thus, therapeutic maneuvers, including compensatory mechanisms which have an immediate effect on bolus propulsion, should be evaluated thoroughly prior to application. The information gleaned from the diagnostic evaluation is used to select specific techniques to address physiologic abnormalities. These techniques in turn address the goals of minimizing aspiration risk and nutritional compromise and maximizing quality of life. Treatment planning in all aspects is an ongoing problem solving process of weighing risks, benefits, patient wishes, and underlying physiology.

DIFFERENTIATION OF COMPENSATION AND REHABILITATION

The goals for intervention can be addressed by the speech language pathologist via two routes: compensation and rehabilitation. It is important to distinguish between these two categories as separate modalities. Those patients who are not candidates for rehabilitative management may be prognostically at a disadvantage by virtue of the severity or etiology of the underlying disorder. The optimal treatment plan in this case will utilize compensatory maneuvers as a sole interventional approach to enhance quality of life and nutritional support and to inhibit aspiration risk. For those patients who are appropriate for rehabilitation, it is important that we address both compensation in the short-term, and treatment in the long term.

Compensatory strategies have been defined earlier in this text as those maneuvers that provide an *immediate but typically transient* effect on the efficiency or safety of swallowing. As a rule, if the strategy is not consistently executed, swallowing will return to the prior dysfunctional status. Compensatory strategies do not change the physiology of swallowing; that is, there is no cumulative effect on the underlying physiology, but they may allow a person to be successful in eating orally. Compensatory strategies do exactly what their name says; they *compensate* for disordered swallowing physiology. They change the flow and gravitational direction of a bolus to allow for safe passage into the stomach. They must be used with every swallow, or safety for oral eating will not be maintained. Depending on the compensatory strategy, the patients themselves must be rigorous in following the technique or the caregivers must assure compliance with the strategies.

Management practices that focus on compensation are considered to be, by nature, only either short term or sporadic. A trial period of training the compensatory strategy, with a follow-up reevaluation, is a reasonable way to assess the acceptance, benefits, and understanding of the treatment plan. Direct feeding of a patient for every meal is not necessary. Once the patient and/or caregivers are able to demonstrate competency in following the compensatory strategy, the clinician withdraws from direct intervention but can be available for ongoing consultation when necessary. Reimbursement for long-term intervention is typically not supported. In the case of patients with neurodegenerative disease processes, the patient may be followed for a long period of time, but with only intermittent short-term treatment visits to adapt the compensatory plan to the changing needs of the patient.

CATEGORIZATION FOR COMPENSATORY MECHANISMS

Compensatory strategies may be categorized into five areas:

▶ Postural strategies
▶ Bolus control techniques
▶ Volitional airway protection strategies
▶ Diet modifications
▶ Prosthetic devices

A brief overview is provided of the categorization of compensatory maneuvers. However, given the importance of physiology in defining the components of the treatment plan, the specific techniques that are available for compensation are presented in detail not by technique, but by the physiological deficit that they are primarily intended to address.

Postural strategies can be considered from two aspects:

▶ Body posturing to support self-feeding and swallowing
▶ Pharyngeal posturing to facilitate bolus transfer during the swallow

Both of these are valuable compensations. It is important to evaluate a patient's ability to achieve normal head/neck posture prior to implementing pharyngeal posturing techniques; that is, to sit upright, with normal chin flexion. This critical posture is frequently difficult for many institutionalized patients and thus may become a prerequisite goal to oral intake. As adequate body positioning is not physiology specific, but provides a foundation for all interventional efforts, it is addressed independently at the conclusion of this chapter.

Examples of pharyngeal posturing strategies include:

▶ Chin tuck posturing
▶ Head rotation
▶ Head tilt
▶ Side lying
▶ Neck extension

Pharyngeal posturing strategies have been reported to eliminate aspiration in 75 to 80% of patients with dysphagia (Horner, Massey, Riski, Lathrop, & Chase, 1988; Logemann, 1989a, 1989b, 1993a; Logemann, Kahrilas, Kobara, & Vakil, 1989b; Logemann, Rademaker, Pauloski, & Kahrilas, 1994; Rasley et al., 1993; Shanahan, Logemann, Rademaker, Pauloski, & Kahrilas, 1993; Welch, Logemann, Rademaker, & Kahrilas, 1993). These postures involve certain head and/or neck movements that redirect the flow of the bolus in specific ways to compensate for identified physiologic problems.

Another approach to compensation is through selection of what will be referred to as bolus control techniques. These are techniques that the patient completes independently or the caregiver facilitates in which the flow of the bolus is redirected not by structure but by function. Examples of this class of compensation include:

▶ 3-second prep
▶ Lingual sweep
▶ Cyclic ingestion
▶ Dry swallows
▶ Thermal gustatory stimulation
▶ Bolus placement
▶ Modification of bolus size
▶ Adaptations in the rate of intake
▶ Slurp and swallow

The successful implementation of these techniques depends heavily on the cognitive abilities of the patient or the subsequent support provided by caregivers. Environmental cues thus play a secondary role to education in the implementation of these strategies.

Volitional airway protection strategies may be utilized in patients with aspiration risk to directly address the laryngeal components of swallowing.

▶ Supraglottic swallow
▶ Super-supraglottic swallow
▶ Pharyngeal expectoration
▶ Vocal quality checks

By virtue of the nature of these techniques, the patient must be a fairly cognizant participant in the interventional process for these to be successful. Although verbal cuing can be used to facilitate recall, caregiver intervention cannot directly assure execution of the tasks.

Diet modification, or adaptation of the texture of food and liquid consistencies in a diet should be the last option in a treatment regimen, according to Logemann (1993b), since diet modifications often are quite difficult for patients and caregivers to accept and implement. In many clinical settings, however, texture modifications and the avoidance of certain foods or liquids are often the first treatment recommendations. The complications of imprecise terminology and the complexities of diet modification have been discussed at length in Chapter 9 . Thus, this chapter does not attempt to define diet levels or readdress texture issues. However, intervention usually focuses around adaptations in two areas:

▶ Liquid modifications
▶ Solid modifications

Recommendations in dysphagia intervention should address both of these areas. As discussed, modified diets are routinely used in many long-term care facilities. Although no figures are available in other settings, the prevalence is high. Diet modification as a compensatory strategy in dysphagia management is arguably the most widely used treatment strategy employed, despite being recommended as a last resort.

Prosthetic devices, by their narrowest definition, are not widely used in swallowing management, particularly in the neurogenic population. However, a broader definition of the term may include:

▶ Palatal lifts
▶ Tracheostomy valves

The application of these devices may alter the underlying structural substrates for swallowing and thus affect physiology significantly. However, if they are not used consistently, they are considered to have no cumulative, or rehabilitative, effect on swallowing physiology. For this reason, they are regarded as compensatory in nature.

COMPENSATORY TECHNIQUES BASED ON PHYSIOLOGY

The previous section emphasized the need to base the selection of compensatory techniques of the underlying swallowing physiology, rather than using a "cookbook" approach to management. We have attempted to outline the following compensatory techniques by virtue of the physiologic impairment that they are assumed to address. But this organization carries a precaution: All techniques should be evaluated for effectiveness. Inclusion of a technique under a given physiologic abnormality doesn't imply that that technique is always appropriate for that deficit in all patients.

Physiologic Abnormality: Oral Motor Inefficiency

Oral phase deficits can be founded in weakness or spasticity of the oral and lingual musculature or in dyscoordination of a volitional oral motor response. The resulting symptomotology that is observed radiographically can be diverse. Reduced lip and jaw closure results in poor seal around a cup, straw, or spoon and anterior leakage of the bolus from the oral cavity. Decreased or dyscoordinated lingual control and buccal tension may result in the symptoms of inefficient mastication and premature spillage of the bolus into the pharynx preceding the swallow or sublingual, buccal, or diffuse oral stasis postswallow. Reduced base of tongue to palate approximation also allows for premature spillage during mastication.

The radiographic interpretation of the symptomotology associated with premature spillage from poor oral control is frequently confused with delayed pharyngeal swallowing. This is an important distinction, as options for intervention will differ remarkably. Premature spillage from poor oral control is a motor-based deficit. Although there is significant variability in swallowing, several features may be apparent radiographically to assist the clinician in differentially diagnosing these symptoms.

1. Premature spillage may be more apparent during ingestion of heavier semisolids or solids as these textures require greater demands on oral lingual control during bolus preparation. Conversely, ingestion of liquid requires little oral manipulation and will thus be less likely to manifest this symptom, but will be more reflective of delayed pharyngeal swallow as there is less tactile information for neurosensory stimulation.
2. Evaluate the position of the base of tongue during oral preparation. If the tongue is flaccid and not in close approximation to the palate, this may suggest premature spillage from poor oral control as a physiologic

deficit. In the case of delayed swallow the base of tongue should maintain soft contact with the palate, unless there are coexisting oral motor deficits.
3. Observe the bolus as it enters the pharyngeal cavity. Patients with poor oral control will more likely spill the contrast into the pharyngeal cavity in small pieces as opposed to the more cohesive bolus seen with delayed pharyngeal swallow in the absence of poor oral control.

Differential diagnosis between the motorically based premature spillage and the sensory based delayed swallow is important and is reflected in subsequent suggestions for compensatory management.

Postural Strategies: Chin Tuck Posturing

Supporting Research/Description of Technique. Chin tuck posturing is a widely used and very beneficial technique for neurogenic patients. It is most commonly recommended for patients who demonstrate the physiologic deficit of delayed pharyngeal swallow. Thus, the bulk of the discussion on the topic is included on page 109. In some patients with premature spillage secondary to oral motor control of the bolus, this technique may inhibit premature transfer by gravitational pull anteriorly.

Patient Instruction. Patients contain the bolus anteriorly with chin tuck posturing until they are ready to swallow, then lift their head, transfer the bolus, and swallow in a coordinated effort. Care should be taken to keep the cervical spine upright and bring the chin down to the chest, rather than moving the head and neck forward as a combined unit (i.e., "birdnecking").

Coaching Tips. Refer to the coaching tips suggested on page 111 under delayed pharyngeal swallow.

Contraindications. In many patients with poor oral control, the technique complicates the oral phase deficit by encouraging anterior leakage and requiring the patient to work against anterior gravity to pull the bolus over the base of tongue. Thus applications for premature spillage from poor oral control are limited.

Example Goal. The patient will recall and implement chin tuck posturing with no evidence of anterior leakage on 90% of solid boluses with minimal verbal cues.

Postural Strategies: Neck Extension

Supporting Research/Description of Technique. The posture of leaning the head back employs the effects of gravity to propel a bolus into the pharynx and is primarily used when oral motor deficits inhibit efficient anterior to posterior transfer of a bolus into the pharynx. Head back posture appears to be beneficial primarily for those patients who suffer from difficulty in oral transit to the pharynx, as seen in patients with early bulbar amyotrophic lateral sclerosis (ALS) or oral cancer. The degree of extension must be carefully assessed for these patients to ascertain the degree necessary for beneficial oral transit, without increasing aspiration risk. It is important that a prompt, efficient swallow response be initiated when the bolus is propelled by gravity into the pharynx to elicit a safe swallow. As always, careful evaluation is needed to determine the effects of this maneuver on an individual patient.

Patient Instruction. Execution of head back posturing is simple and direct. Prior to oral intake of the bolus, the patients are instructed take a breath and hold it. They then bring the chin up and with residual lingual movement, allow gravity to transfer the bolus into the pharyngeal region. Environmental cues may consist of written reminders or, if patients are not unreasonably distracted, placing patients and their meals underneath and just in front of an elevated television set, thus encouraging them to look up to watch the program while they eat.

Coaching Tips. As with all compensatory techniques, success of the maneuver is dependent on consistent execution. Environmental cues for this technique are limited. Fortunately, patient populations that might benefit from this technique are those patients who are less likely to have concomitant cognitive impairment. Verbal instruction and cuing are suggested for those with cognitive deficits.

Contraindications. This posture can decrease a patient's ability to close the laryngeal vestibule effectively (Ekberg, 1986), and therefore, it should be recommended only after careful assessment using an instrumental evaluation. As well, it has been reported that head extension significantly decreases the ability of the UES to relax, in direct relation to the degree of extension. Using manometry, Castell, Castell, Schultz, and Georgeson (1993) found that upper esophageal sphincter (UES) relaxation began after the onset of pharyngeal contraction, and that termination of the relaxation occurred prior to the completion of the pharyngeal contraction, when the head was in extension. Incomplete UES relaxation was also noted during the pharyngeal contraction. It was concluded that the dramatic changes seen in UES and pharyngeal pressure dynamics would lead to significant difficulties in bolus transfer during eating.

Neck extension in patients with neurogenic dysphagia may increase aspiration risk, particularly in patients with concomitant delayed onset of pharyngeal swallow. Because of potentially increased risk, it is important for a clinician to recognize that this posture is unwittingly used by caregivers in institutionalized settings with patients who suffer from neurogenic dysphagia. The reasons for placing this type of patient in head extension to eat are unintentional but many. Patients often have poor body and neck control to maintain an upright sitting position and require supported seating, with geri-chairs. They frequently cannot feed themselves. Poor oral control and impaired cognitive functioning are also commonly observed with these patients. Therefore, head back, with or without the entire body being reclined, is a natural posture for many dependent patients. It does increase bolus transit into the pharynx and, thereby, increase feeding speed and intake for caregivers, but this "efficiency" may be paid for by increased risk.

Example Goals.

1. Patient will recall and implement neck extension posturing on 90% of puree trials with no verbal cues.
2. Using neck extension posturing paired with liquid wash, the patient will demonstrate minimal oral residual on 90% of mechanical soft PO trials.

Bolus Control Techniques: Lingual Sweep

Supporting Research/Description of Technique. Perhaps the most practical and "normalized" technique is one that most individuals without deficit perform regularly during mealtime. Lingual sweep can be described as actively using the tongue to clear residual from oral cavities and redirect to tongue blade for development of a bolus. A cued or volitional lingual sweep is particularly useful when decreased oral sensitivity is associated with weakness and the patient is unaware of residual

Patient Instruction. Very simply, in the absence of spontaneous compensation, the patient is cued to use tongue purposefully to sweep the entire oral cavity, particularly areas of weakness, to collect residual bolus. The patient should repeat the technique throughout meal as indicated to inhibit development of residual. In cases where lingual movement restricts search of certain regions, finger sweep may be substituted.

Coaching Tips. Lingual sweep may be facilitated in some patients with the use of a mirror placed on the meal tray to provide visual feedback to the patient. For those facilitating the feeding of the dependent patient, care should be taken to wear a glove and move quickly if using a finger sweep!

Contraindications. There are no suspected or known contraindications.

Example Goal. The patient will fully clear oral residual in the left buccal cavity with spontaneous lingual sweep after every third bolus with minimal cues.

Bolus Control Techniques: Cyclic Ingestion

Supporting Research/Description of Technique. The technique of cyclic ingestion may be indicated for patients with bolus manipulation deficits, particularly those for whom postswallow oral residual is the subsequent symptom. The patient is very simply instructed to alternate intake of liquids with solids, using the increased flow rate of the fluid to wash out the oral cavity of residual that is unable to be manipulated successfully via lingual searching. For patients with adequate base of tongue elevation who are able to inhibit preswallow spillage of the bolus into the pharynx, cyclic ingestion can be paired with "swishing" to clear oral recesses further that are not normally within the flow of the fluid. Certainly, this technique, as others, should be carefully evaluated. Patients that are at risk of aspiration of liquids may not be able to benefit from this technique.

Patient Instruction. The patient is given liquids with all meals and instructed to alternate liquid and solid intake throughout the meal, either in one-to-one ratio or as indicated by diagnostic examination

Coaching Tips. This technique relies heavily on the patient's recall of the task. Written reminders on the dinner tray may facilitate recall.

Contraindications. This technique cannot be used with patients on a liquid-restricted diet. In a limited number of patients, the subsequent liquid bolus may bypass the residual in the valleculae as opposed to washing it out and will then present potential for aspiration; thus, the strategy should be evaluated diagnostically.

Example Goal. The patient will recall and implement cyclic ingestion pattern of intake during meals with no verbal cues and no evidence of postswallow aspiration of residual.

Bolus Control Techniques: Dry Swallows

Supporting Research/Description of Technique. Dry swallow is used for several physiologic deficits that result in postswallow residual somewhere within the aerodigestive tract. In particular dry swallow can be used to clear oral residual secondary to oral motor impairment, pharyngeal residual secondary to weakness or dyscoordination, or pyriform sinus residual secondary to UES dysfunction. The technique may also be used in cases of intact pharyngeal phase swallowing when oral residual falls postswallow into the pharynx in inadequate quantity to elicit a pharyngeal swallow. In principle, repetition of the swallow without a new bolus serves to aid in clearing postswallow residual.

Patient Instruction. The patient is instructed to dry swallow after every bolus swallow or to swallow each bolus two, three or four times as indicated by the diagnostic examination.

Coaching Tips. Decreasing rate of intake may facilitate this strategy. This can be promoted by requiring patient to put down the spoon, fork, or cup between bites. For a few patients, placement of an empty bowl on the meal tray with instructions to take a bite from that bowl may also cue recall of the strategy.

Contraindications. No documented contraindications are associated with this technique.

Example Goal. The patient will recall and implement dry swallows after bolus swallows with minimal verbal cues on 90% of bolus swallows.

Bolus Control Techniques: Bolus Placement

Supporting Research/Description of Technique. When techniques to redirect the bolus within the oral cavity via muscular or gravitational forces fail, techniques may be employed to alter the intake of the bolus to serve the same end. Bolus placement techniques are heavily used with oral cancer patients who have undergone lingual resection. Neurogenic patients with unilateral paresis of the oral musculature or oral desensitivity may benefit from these techniques as well. Very simply, bolus placement techniques position the bolus at the onset of the oral phase in a location that is either more sensate or more available for manipulation by the weakened oral musculature. For patients who are unable to search for a bolus because of limitations of weakness or cognition, this technique may facilitate oral intake.

Patient Instruction. In a patient with unilateral lingual hemiparesis, the bolus is purposefully placed on the side of the oral cavity where the residual lingual movement is better able to move the bolus within the oral cavity. Placement can be accomplished with a spoon or fork, or with specialized feeding devices, such as glossectomy spoon or syringe if needed.

Coaching Tips. Verbal and written instructions near the patient during a meal may facilitate recall of the technique. A mirror placed on the tray may facilitate accurate placement.

Contraindications. Care should be taken in patients with cognitive deficits when using devices for bolus placement. Respect for the patient's wishes regarding oral intake should be a priority. If the goal of syringe or glossectomy spoon feeding is to overcome oral weakness, these devices are likely appropriate. If the goal is to inject the bolus in an unaccepting patient, the clinician should seriously consider the ethical issues associated with such actions.

Example Goal. The patient will demonstrate minimal oral residual throughout the meal using bolus placement technique to the right buccal cavity during ingestion of solids.

Bolus Control Techniques: Modification of Bolus Size/Adaptations in the Rate of Intake

Supporting Research/Description of Technique. Bolus size and rate of intake can be critical factors in influencing the efficiency of the oral components of swallowing. Unfortunately in this area, patient physiology is so variable that no hard and fast rules, or even general tendencies, can be clearly identified. In some patients with significant oral motor impairment, smaller boluses may allow for greater control and less scatter to oral recesses. The result is more efficient manipulation and a more cohesive bolus. However, other patients, because of decreased oral sensitivity as the primary physiologic abnormality underlying inefficient oral control, may function much better with a larger more substantial bolus. With a heavier bolus and more variable texture, the patient's sensory system is better stimulated, thus facilitating greater oral awareness and more efficient oral control. The clinical sensorimotor exam and diagnostic assessment will guide the clinician in the appropriate route for the individual patient.

The rate of intake may also influence oral efficiency. In general, slowing the rate of intake may allow for greater oral efficiency by giving the patient who is neurologically impaired more time to manage the bolus. This may be particularly the case for patients with cognitive deficits that do not attend well to food preparation and pause in the process of oral ingestion. Patients with head injury or right cortical stroke tend may have oral motor impairments that are exacerbated by tachyphagia, or rapid ingestion. Thus, external controls may be required to slow the rate of intake. Patients with neurodegenerative disease or chronic obstructive pulmonary disease may demonstrate significant fatigue during oral intake, thus requiring control of the length of the meal or the rate of intake during the meal.

Patient Instruction. If the patient has adequate cognition to control the rate and quantity of intake independently, instructions are provided for the size of bolus and rate of ingestion that has been determined to maximize swallowing efficiency. Otherwise, interventions such as those that follow may be useful.

Coaching Tips. There are several techniques that can be used to facilitate slowed or controlled intake. To slow the rate or limit the quantity of liquid intake in patients with cognitive impairment, patients can take all liquids from a lidded travel mug. If the size of the hole is too large to limit flow adequately, the top can be taken off and a small piece of duct tape used to half cover the hole from the inside. Straw sips, unless otherwise contraindicated, may also slow rate of liquid ingestion, particularly if using a straw of narrow diameter. To slow the rate of solid or semisolid intake, the patient can be cued always to put spoon or fork down between bites, or to insert volitional dry swallow. A small wrist weight may provide adequate tactile information and increased effort to slow rate of intake. To limit the quantity of solid intake, use of a small spoon bowl will decrease the amount. Another option would be to have the center of a standard dining room spoon bowl removed by a metal shop. With the edges adequately smoothed, this allows a significant portion of the bolus (for puree) to fall through the spoon and only the bolus at the edges enters the patient's mouth. Portion control may also be useful; that is, providing the patient with a series of bowls only partially filled.

Contraindications. There are no suspected or identified contraindications.

Example Goal. The patient will demonstrate decreased rate of puree intake as measured by 4 ounces ingested in no less than 5 minutes.

Bolus Control Techniques: Slurp and Swallow

Supporting Research/Description of Technique. Patients demonstrating physiologically limited oral control that manifests as inefficient transfer of the bolus anterior to posterior may benefit from the slurp and swallow technique. This technique circumvents the oral phase of the swallow and rapidly transfers bolus into the pharynx. It is particularly well suited for oral pharyngeal cancer patients with partial glossectomy. In the neurogenic patient it's success is guarded and must be cautiously evaluated.

Patient Instruction. The patient is instructed to take the bolus in the oral cavity and essentially "slurp" or "suck" the bolus into the pharynx, using aerodynamic pressure as opposed to lingual control to transfer the bolus. A prompt pharyngeal swallow should follow.

Contraindications. As discussed, this technique is frequently not appropriate for neurologically impaired patients. As the bolus enters the pharynx during deep inspiration, the technique may significantly increase aspiration risk in patients with inadequate airway protection or pharyngeal phase impairment. Thus the benefits of oral transfer may be outweighed by the increased aspiration risk in patients who are neurologically "slow."

Example Goal. Using slurp and swallow technique during ingestion of puree, patient will demonstrate marginal oral residual and no clinical indication of aspiration.

Diet Modification

Modification of food and liquid is discussed at length in Chapter 9, regarding nutritional aspects of dysphagia management. As a compensatory technique, diet modification can be used with oral phase impairment of any etiology when mastication and manipulation are inadequate to prepare bolus for transfer to the pharynx. Diet modification may also be indicated for cognitively impaired patients that lack prolonged attention to prepare the bolus fully, despite adequate oral function. For treatment planning purposes, it is important to specify clearly recommendations for both solid foods and liquids.

Specificity is required as to what constitutes a restricted diet of either foods or liquids. Consultation with dietary staff will assure maintenance of caloric needs on restricted diets. The risk of malnutrition and dehydration may be increased by application of a modified diet. The reader is referred to Chapter 9 of this text for more information about indications and contraindications of modified diets.

Diet Modifications: Liquids

Supporting Research/Description of Technique. The use of thickened liquids is most often indicated when thinned liquids are aspirated prior to the initiation of the airway protection secondary to delay in onset of the pharyngeal swallow. However, thickened liquids may also be used in cases of decreased oral motor control for manipulation of thin liquid bolus. Liquids are typically thickened if it is determined by videofluoroscopy that adjustment is needed. A thickened liquid may be more easily controlled in the oral phase of the swallow. By thickening the liquid for ingestion, the rate of flow is reduced, allowing for greater control and less "splash" as the liquid enters the oral and pharyngeal cavities.

Patient Instruction. Patient should be given precise instructions as to what constitutes a thickened liquid as this is an area of terminological ambiguity among professionals and between clinician and patient. Thickened liquids may take many forms from thin nectar consistency through honey/semipuree. Degree of thickness should be determined for that patient by the diagnostic exam. Commercial products are available to thicken liquids systematically without compromising the free-water content. Liquids can also be thickened by blending with another nutritive puree texture (potatoes, applesauce, and the like).

Coaching Tips. In rehabilitation or home care settings where kitchen facilities are available, it may be helpful to evaluate the patient or caretaker preparing thickened liquids to specifications, thus assuring preparation of a safe consistency.

Contraindications. As fully discussed in the oral nutrition chapter (Chapter 9), the risk of dehydration may be significant when thickened liquids are introduced into the diet. Risks of aspiration vs dehydration should be evaluated. Care should be taken to remove liquid restrictions as soon as possible.

Example Goal. During ingestion of thickened liquids, patient will demonstrate clinical indication of aspiration on less than 1% of swallows.

Diet Modification: Solids

Supporting Research/Description of Technique. Food modification generally consists of limiting the diet to specialized foods that are of a softer texture, requiring less mastication. The use of gravies and sauces that help the bolus maintain cohesiveness may be suggested, particularly for dry or particulate foods. Heavy foods that require excessive mastication, foods that break apart (rice), or mixed textures (cereal with milk, soups with vegetables) may pose a greater challenge for the patient with oral motor impairment. As well, breads may become sticky when mixed with secretions, and jello may be harder to control in oral phase.

By adjusting the texture of the oral diet, the burden of the oral phase of the swallow in preparation of the bolus for transfer is minimized. Although these adaptations may be necessary and appropriate for patient safety and nutritional adequacy, use of restricted textures in diet should be balanced with the need for oral stimulation in patients with decreased oral pharyngeal sensitivity. Thus, careless restriction of diet texture may ameliorate the immediate problem of getting food into the pharynx for swallowing but delay the overall recovery of the patient. Thoughtful planning of the diet may allow the patients a softer, more manageable texture at some meals while challenging the patients with firmer and more varied textures at other meals. Although this poses definite challenges for direct care and dietary workers, it may offer the best solution for the patient.

Patient Instruction. Clear instructions are required for the patient and caregiver, particularly if the patient is homebound and thus does not have meals provided. Examples of specific well-tolerated foods should be given to minimize ambiguity.

Coaching Tips. As discussed in the chapter on oral nutrition, compliance may be an issue with some patients on a restricted diet. Definition and discussion with the patient of a clear plan to work off of the restricted diet may increase cooperation. Developing a diet log, in which the patient charts the nature and quantity of foods consumed, may be helpful to evaluate both compliance and nutrition and to provide the patient with a sense of progress toward an end goal of normalizing diet levels.

Contraindications. These issues are discussed fully in the oral nutrition chapter (Chapter 9). Care should be taken that a significantly altered diet does not result in a reduced appetite and thus compromise patient nutrition.

Example Goal. Patient will comply with mechanical soft diet recommendations as demonstrated by evaluation of a diet log.

Prosthetic Devices: Palatal Prostheses

Supporting Research/Description of Technique. The use of palatal prosthetics in the management of neurogenic dysphagia is a highly specialized area that is not well developed or well documented. There is little in the literature regarding prosthetic placement and the few existing reports are applicable to oral pharyngeal carcinoma with little objective documentation.

For the patient with neurogenic dysphagia, palatal prosthetics to improve oral control of the bolus are generally of two types:

▶ A palatal lift raises the soft palate to facilitate improved velopharyngeal closure
▶ Palatal augmentation or reshaping prothetics are designed to provide a lowered, contoured palatal surface for the tongue to approximate during oral bolus manipulation. Thus, for patients with significant and long-term deficits secondary to unilateral or bilateral lingual weakness the palate is lowered and "fit" to allow lingual compression on the palate.

The oromaxillofacial prosthodontist, the patient, and the speech language pathologist generally design palatal prostheses through a combined evaluation.

Patient Instruction. After the prosthesis is developed, it is important for the patient to learn correct placement of the device and advise the prosthodontist or speech-language pathologists of any discomfort that may indicate a poor fit to the existing oral cavity. In addition, meticulous oral hygiene is very important to minimize growth of oral bacteria and decrease pulmonary risks.

Example Goal. The patient will demonstrate minimal oral residual with palatal prosthesis in place for all meals.

Physiologic Abnormality: Delayed Pharyngeal Swallow

A delayed pharyngeal swallow occurs when the patient volitionally or responsively transfers the bolus posteriorly out of the oral cavity and a synergistic pharyngeal response fails to occur in a timely manner. This represents a deficit of the neurosensory system in which inadequate sensory feedback mechanisms fail to communicate the oncoming bolus. As addressed in earlier sections, it is crucial that this deficit be distinguished diagnostically from premature spillage secondary to poor oral control, which is a deficit of the neuromotor system. Although the radiographic image can be similar and the deficits may coexist, the management is quite different for each disorder.

Postural Strategies: Chin Tuck Posturing

Supporting Research/Description of Technique. The use of chin tuck posturing, also called chin flexion or chin down, is a common postural strategy because of its ease in implementation, its effect on bolus direction, and the protection it affords the airway. It was first introduced as a compensatory strategy by Logemann (1983) to treat observed delays in triggering the pharyngeal swallow, poor tongue control, reduced tongue base retraction, and/or reduced closure of the laryngeal entrance and vocal cords during a swallow, as assessed by videofluoroscopy. Many patients exhibit one or more of these physiologic impairments, and so it is not surprising that this posture is frequently assessed during instrumental examination and subsequently recommended for treatment. The symptoms observed during an instrumental examination are pre-swallow pooling in the valleculae and/or aspiration during a swallow.

Chin tuck has been observed to be beneficial in reducing aspiration during videofluoroscopy, and a variety of hypotheses have been suggested for its success. Chin tuck (1) widens the vallecular space to prevent the bolus from entering the airway, (2) narrows the airway entrance, (3) pushes the tongue base backward toward the pharyngeal wall, and (4) puts the epiglottis in a more protective position. Subsequent research to test these hypotheses using videofluoroscopy and manometry has been conducted by several researchers (Castell et al., 1993; Shanahan et al., 1993; Welch et al., 1993). The changes in the pharynx that occur with chin tuck are a posterior shift of the anterior pharyngeal structures. These serve to change several important dimensions in the pharynx. Welch and others (1993) reported that it narrows the distance from the epiglottis to the pharyngeal wall and widens the angle of the epiglottis to the anterior tracheal wall. This posterior shift of structures also serves to narrow the entrance to the larynx, and places the tongue base in a more posterior position. However, chin tuck has been found to have no significant effect on two important pharyngeal pressures, UES relaxation or the coordination between pharyngeal contraction for a swallow and UES relaxation. Overall, the greatest effect of chin tuck has been reported to be improved airway protection and tongue base retraction.

Although the benefits of chin tuck may be substantial for some patients, it appears that many dimensional changes in the pharynx are not uniform and individual differences may be observed (Shanahan et al., 1993). For example, it has been shown that not everyone will enlarge the vallecular space when using a chin tuck, epiglottic distance to the pharyngeal wall will either increase or decrease, and the distance to the airway entrance decreases in some people, but not significantly so. Shanahan et al. (1993) found differences in airway entrance distance between two groups of elderly, one slightly younger group (mean age 61.1 years ± 4.8 years) versus an older group (mean age 74.3 years ± 2.3 years). Since the larynx descends with age, it has been hypothesized that chin tuck was not as successful in eliminating aspiration with the older group because they did not exert as much direct posterior pressure on the thyroid notch into the anterior tracheal wall when they performed a chin tuck.

The differences in pharyngeal dimensions noted in the literature may be partially due to the different conditions under which chin tuck was studied (video prints of postures unrelated to actual swallows versus videofluoroscopy of neurologically impaired patients recovering from dysphagia). In any event, it is clear that an instrumental examination must be performed prior to prescribing a chin tuck posture for a patient with delayed pharyngeal swallow, poor tongue base retraction or tongue control, and/or poor laryngeal closure during a swallow. Because of the lowering of the larynx within the pharynx with aging, this is particularly important with our older patients.

Patient Instruction. Execution of chin tuck posturing is simple and direct—the patient is instructed to tuck the chin to the chest during swallowing, while maintaining an upright and straight cervical spine. Care should be taken to keep the cervical spine upright and bring the chin down to the chest, rather than moving the head and neck forward as a combined unit (i.e., "bird-necking"). Many patients are able to implement this simple one-step command, even if they have coexisting severe aphasia or poor comprehension. Chin tuck can be easily demonstrated, verbally and tactically cued, and usually is well accepted by patients.

Coaching Tips. Recall and implementation of chin tuck posturing may be enhanced using several environmental controls. Placing the food tray in a position that is low and close will encourage the patient to look down at the food. This technique often aids correct placement, and it does not bring attention to itself as an abnormal posture. Chin tuck posturing for liquid intake can be facilitated through straw drinking, if not otherwise contraindicated, with the cup held at the abdomen and the patient bending down to the straw rather than bringing the straw up to the patient. Straw drinking can further be used by securing the cup button to the table using a velcro patch. Although this encourages a more "bird-necking" posture, it may be a better option than fully upright head position. This positioning can also be passively introduced in patients who tolerate a tactile cue from a caregiver.

Other options for tactile cuing include a pillow or rolled towel behind the head or an adapted soft cervical collar, with a cut-out half-moon located in the optimal chin location and the cut out portion placed behind the neck to provide sensory feedback. Cloth tape can be used to seal the cut edges and assure placement of the cut-out portion. As described for other techniques, the use of a collar does not inhibit volitional movement by the patient, but serves to provide tactile feedback and supports the desired posture as the more comfortable position for the patient.

Contraindications. Shanahan et al. (1993) found that patients who were observed to have material enter the pyriform sinus prior to swallow response were more likely to aspirate those contents despite a chin tuck. Since the larynx and pharynx elevate significantly during a swallow (approximately 2 cm), this movement shortens and narrows the pyriform sinuses greatly, causing their contents to spill into the larynx. Therefore, the observation of spillage of material into the pyriform sinuses prior to a swallow response, as observed during an instrumental examination, may indicate that a chin tuck will not be successful in reducing aspiration. In addition, chin tuck posturing may actually increase the potential for aspiration in patients who have poor laryngeal elevation and closure (Martin-Harris & Cherney, 1996). The chin tuck posture may direct the food bolus forward, directly into the laryngeal vestibule or trachea. For patients with poor lip closure or oral control, chin tuck posture may prove problematic as most of the bolus may tend to fall out of the mouth or be poorly propelled against gravity into the pharyngeal cavity. However, for many patients who have been adequately diagnosed using an instrumental examination, chin tuck could be one of the most valuable compensatory postures a patient could employ.

Example Goal. The patient will recall and implement chin tuck posturing with no evidence of anterior leakage on 90% of solid boluses with minimal verbal cues.

Bolus Control Techniques: Three-Second Prep

Supporting Research/Description of Technique. This technique was first presented by Kagel in the late 1980s as a clinical approach to managing two physiologic deficits. Three-second prep may be useful for addressing delayed pharyngeal swallowing or, in a select number of patients, tachyphagia. The basic principle behind the technique is similar to that for supraglottic swallow in that a function that is normally considered to be reflexive in nature is compensated for by moving that task into the volitional realm. A volitional, conscious pause prior to transfer of the bolus may allow the patient a greater opportunity to organize execution of bolus transfer and elicitation of the swallow, insert a purposeful break in the rapid ingestion pattern of a tachyphagic patient, and allows greater time in the patient with delayed onset of swallow to elicit volitional airway protection. Use of this strategy alters the swallows from a reflexive response to a more volitionally controlled action.

Patient Instruction. After placement of the bolus in the oral cavity, the patient is instructed to count to three mentally prior to transfer of the bolus into the pharynx. On transfer, the patient is instructed to volitionally swallow.

Coaching Tips. This task requires some degree of cognitive power on the part of the patient, with the ability to follow instructions. Verbal cuing to "put the spoon down before you swallow" may facilitate recall of the technique is some patients. As well, insertion of some motor task ("blink three times before you swallow") may facilitate recall in some patients.

Contraindications. Some patients with poor oral motor control, particularly base of tongue to palate approximation, may experience premature spillage of bolus into the pharynx and thus increase preswallow aspiration risk.

Example Goal. The patient will recall and implement 3-second prep technique with no evidence of preswallow aspiration and minimal verbal cues on 90% of liquid swallows.

Bolus Control Techniques: Thermal Gustatory Stimulation

Supporting Research/Description of Technique. Rosenbek, at a 1995 presentation for the American Speech-Language-Hearing Association, commented that thermal stimulation is "done with kind-hearted rigor." This is perhaps the most widely used and misunderstood bolus control technique in our arsenal of compensations. Efficacy research related to thermal stimulation is fraught with difficulties, as is efficacy research in any area. Although we have more research in this area than in any other interventional practice, we have fewer answers. In 1975, Mansson and Sandberg evaluated dry swallowing in normal subjects, half of whom received anesthesia to the posterior oral cavity and half without. Using manometry as a measure of onset of pharyngeal response, they determined that anesthesia increased the latency of the pharyngeal response, or produced a delay in onset of the pharyngeal swallow. This study, as well as others, gives support for the importance of the mucosal receptors in swallowing onset.

Two studies have evaluated the effects of thermal stimulation in the normal, nondysphagic population. Ali, Lundl, Wallace, deCarle, and Cook (1996) radiographically evaluated 14 normal volunteers subsequent to thermal stimulation and local mucosal receptor anesthesia. They demonstrated no influence on the temporal relationships of motor events in normal swallowing and concluded that there is no support for thermal stimulation as a treatment modality for delayed swallow. Conflicting findings were identified by Kaatze-McDonald, Post, and Davis (1996). These researchers also evaluated 10 normals using a laryngograph to document timing issues of swallowing. After applying a warmed and cooled laryngeal mirror, as well as warm and cooled solutions of saline, glucose, and distilled water, the authors concluded that cold stimulation in the form of tactile input and fluid infusion facilitated more timely swallowing. No change in temporal measures of swallowing was observed when stimuli were presented at room temperature. Both of these reports, however, used normal, nondysphagic subjects on which to base their conclusions. One has to ask, what evidence do we have that would suggest that normals respond similarly to patients with dysphagia?

Several research groups have evaluated the short-term and long-term effects of thermal stimulation on onset of swallow. The initial, and perhaps landmark study of thermal stimulation was provided by Lazarra, Lazarus, and Logemann (1986). Twenty-five neurologically impaired subjects were radiographically identified with delayed pharyngeal swallow. Two swallows were radiographically recorded prior to thermal stimulation, then stimulation was applied and swallowing was reevaluated within 1.5 seconds. Thermal stimulation reportedly improved the total transit time in 23 of 25 subjects for at least one texture. This improved timing persisted across up to the three subsequent swallows. Although this may suggest thermal stimulation as an effective compensation with short-term positive effects, there is no support from this study that it has long-term benefits. As well, it is unclear what parameter actually facilitated the change: the temperature, the pressure, or perhaps even the aggravation of having something brushed against the oral cavity. Their findings are also confounded by the sequencing of thermal application. Some neurologically impaired patients are observed to require a "warm up" period of a few swallows before optimal functioning is observed. This tendency may have biased their findings.

Rosenbek and colleagues have studied the effects of thermal stimulation extensively. Rosenbek, Fishback, and Levine (1991) evaluated seven neurologically impaired patients with dysphagia who presented delayed pharyngeal swallow. Using an ABAB treatment design, the relative effects of thermal stimulation as compared to no stimulation on the underlying physiology were evaluated. Thus, stimulation was evaluated as a rehabilitative intervention, not compensation. Subjects were provided stimulation 15 to 25 trials each session, with an average of five sessions per day for 1 week duration prior to switching to control condition of no stimulation. In post treatment videofluoroscopies, two out of three judges reported that two out of seven subjects demonstrated decreased in latency of swallow as a long-term effect. However, several subjects demonstrated immediate short-term improvement in delay. It is important to note that the two subjects who responded to stimulation with decreased latency were still clearly in the acute phase, only 5 weeks post onset.

A follow-up study by Rosenbek and colleagues (1996) evaluated short-term compensatory effects. Twenty-two neurologically impaired patients with radiographically confirmed delayed pharyngeal swallow on semisolid bolus were used. To allay the critique of "warm-up" effects, the subjects were randomly assigned to received stimulation first or the control swallow first. As measured by videofluoroscopy, 15 of 22 subjects demonstrated decreased latency of onset of swallowing after thermal stimulation. However, the question persists. If there is an effect, how do we differentiate the cause between the temperature and pressure?

If we operate on the assumption that thermal stimulation is effective to facilitate swallowing we would need to know the most effective rate of application. Rosenbek and colleagues (1998) evaluated 43 neurologically impaired patients who received thermal stimulation for 2 weeks. Subjects were randomized to intensity of application ranging from 150 to 300 to 450 to 600 trials per week. Frozen ice sticks were used to obviate the argument about the temperature of the probe as it enters the oral cavity. The study demonstrated that 450 trials of thermal stimulation per day have therapeutic effects on 3-ml boluses, but not 10-ml boluses. Trials of up to 600 applications per week were likely more effective but also generally impossible to execute. Criteria for establishing the efficacy of a treatment modality depend not only on the patient effect, but also on the feasibility. A technique is of limited use if it cannot be reasonably executed.

Clinical practice suggests similar, if not improved results, through the addition of strong taste, particularly a tart lemon, applied more globally to the entire oral cavity. The use of frozen lemon glycerine swabs is one option. Another effective and less obtrusive option is the ingestion of limited amounts of lemon Italian water ice throughout the meal to facilitate oral pharyngeal awareness. This technique does not limit the thermal-gustatory stimulation to the anterior faucial arches but includes the entire oral cavity and is comfortably incorporated into the patient's diet. Recent research has supported that sour boluses may facilitate more timely swallowing. Logemann and colleagues (1995) evaluated the effects of a sour bolus on delayed pharyngeal swallow in two groups of neurologically impaired patients: those with stroke and those with other neurogenic etiology. The authors reported improvement in oral onset of the swallow in both groups of patients and a significant reduction in delayed onset of swallowing in the groups with a diagnosis of stroke. Interestingly, the group with other neurogenic etiology demonstrated decreased aspiration.

What can we conclude from this sometimes-contradictory information? It would appear that in some patients with the physiologic abnormality of delayed onset of pharyngeal swallowing, thermal application to the posterior oral cavity may facilitate a short-term decrease in the latency of response. The extent of the effect and the exact mechanism by which this occurs are, as yet, undetermined. There does not appear to be adequate evidence to support the use of thermal stimulation as a rehabilitative modality with the goal of long-term physiologic shift to more timely onset of swallow. Unfortunately, we have little else to offer in terms of rehabilitation of this physiologic deficit.

Patient Instruction. There are several methods of applying thermal (gustatory) stimulation. Introduced initially as only thermal stimulation, the patient or family member is instructed to use a chilled laryngeal mirror to stroke the anterior faucial arches vertically five to six times on each side prior to and intermittently during meals. As described in the Rosenbek et al. (1996) study, frozen ice sticks will assure continued cooling of the probe. Several adaptations have surfaced that may be of benefit but have not been fully evaluated. Frozen lemon glycerine swabs may also be used. In a series of educational programs, Kagel describes the use of lemon Italian ice as a form of thermal stimulation, thus applying the cold and tart sensory information throughout the oral cavity. Lemon ice is served with the meal with instructions to use cyclic ingestion pattern. Kagel also describes the use of Italian ice as an antecedent to the bolus, placed on the spoon ahead of the actual bolus. Some patients may respond, as well, to ingestion of iced lemonade with the meal. These final suggestions may be more easily incorporated into a mealtime environment but have not withstood the rigors of research.

Contraindications. Thermal stimulation is not suggested for patients with a hyperactive gag response. The use of lemon glycerine swabs may exacerbate dryness of the oral mucosa inpatients with xerostomia. The sugar content of lemon Italian water ice or lemonade should be considered in the care of the diabetic patient. For patients with abnormal primitive reflexes care should be taken when introducing anything into the oral cavity.

Example Goal. The patient will demonstrate more responsive pharyngeal swallow of liquids after ingestion of lemon ice on 90% of trials during a meal.

Bolus Control Techniques: Modification of Bolus Size

Supporting Research/Description of Technique. Use of modification of bolus size is more thoroughly discussed in the section on oral motor inefficiency (page 104). This technique may also be helpful for patients with delayed pharyngeal swallow in order to limit the amount of bolus that enters the supra-laryngeal region prior to initiation of airway protection. In general, application of modification of bolus size for delayed pharyngeal swallow consists of limiting the size of the bolus.

Patient Instruction. Specific instructions should be given to the patient and caregiver regarding optimal bolus size.

Coaching Tips. Observation of food preparation and consumption to evaluate understanding of instructions and compliance may be necessary. Refer to the section on oral motor inefficiency for more coaching tips.

Contraindications. Care should be taken to assure adequate oral intake in the presence of limited bolus size.

Example Goal. The patient will demonstrate no clinical indication of aspiration when ingesting puree with teaspoon bolus size.

Volitional Airway Protection: Supraglottic Swallow

Supporting Research/Description of Technique. The supraglottic swallow technique was first described by Larsen (1973). This technique provides volitional airway protection, when the patient presents either silent aspiration or a latent reflexive airway protection. The lungs are filled and the vocal folds firmly sealed through conscious effort prior to the swallow, with a volitional cough/forced expiration immediately following to clear laryngeal coating/potential aspiration. Martin, Logemann, Shaker, and Dodds (1993) provided a systematic evaluation of three breath-holding maneuvers: easy hold, inhale hold, and inhale/exhale hard hold. Maximal laryngeal valving was visualized by nasoendoscopy under the hard breath-hold condition. False vocal fold approximation and anterior arytenoid tilting that is optimal for airway protection was only observed during effortful breath hold conditions, not easy breath-holding. The authors of this study emphasize that considerable intrasubject and intratrial variation is observed in executing the tasks, thus, extensive teaching and perhaps biofeedback monitoring of vocal fold closure via endoscopy or electroglottography are indicated.

Patient Instruction. The patient is instructed to take a deep breath and hold it firmly while swallowing the bolus. On completion of the swallow, patient is instructed to expel the air in the lungs forcefully with a volitional cough, prior to inhalation. The patient then swallows and coughs a second time.

Coaching Tips. Because of the complexity of sequencing multiple components, the patient may require written instruction to recall sequence of events as this can be a difficult task for many patients to coordinate. A technique to facilitate learning of this strategy is to break the task, on first presentation, into discrete steps with mastery at each level prior to moving ahead.

1. Hold your breath (3, 5, 10 seconds progressively), then relax.
2. Hold your breath (3, 5, 10 seconds progressively), then exhale forcefully or with a cough.
3. Hold your breath, swallow, then exhale forcefully or with a cough.

Contraindications. There are no documented or suspected contraindications; however, this intervention may be very difficult for the patient with concomitant pulmonary disease or reduced pulmonary effort.

Example Goal. The patient will recall and implement supraglottic swallow technique on 95% of liquid swallows with no verbal cues.

Diet Modification: Liquids

Supporting Research/Description of Technique. The use of thickened liquids is very frequently indicated when thinned liquids are aspirated prior to the initiation of the airway protection, secondary to delay in onset of the pharyngeal swallow. Liquids are typically thickened if it is determined by videofluoroscopy that adjustment is needed. A thickened liquid may be more easily controlled in the oral phase of the swallow. By thickening the liquid for ingestion, the rate of flow is reduced, allowing for greater control and less "splash" as the liquid enters the oral and pharyngeal cavities.

Patient Instruction. Patient should be given precise instructions as to what constitutes a thickened liquid as this is an area of terminal ambiguity among professionals and between clinician and patient. Thickened liquids may take many forms from thin nectar consistency through honey/semipuree. Degree of thickness should be determined for that patient by the diagnostic exam. Commercial products are available to thicken liquids systematically without compromising the free-water content. Liquids can also be thickened by blending with another nutritive puree texture (potatoes, applesauce, and the like).

Coaching Tips. In rehabilitation or home care settings where kitchen facilities are available, it may be helpful to evaluate the patient or caretaker preparing thickened liquids to specifications, thus assuring preparation of a safe consistency.

Contraindications. As fully discussed in the oral nutrition chapter, the risk of dehydration may be significant when thickened liquids are introduced into the diet. Risks of aspiration versus dehydration should be evaluated. Care should be taken to remove liquid restrictions as soon as possible.

Example Goal. During ingestion of thickened liquids, patient will demonstrate clinical indication of aspiration on less than 1% of swallows.

Diet Modifications: Solids

Supporting Research/Description of Technique. Food modification is less frequently an appropriate option for the patient with delayed pharyngeal swallow. If the patient demonstrates adequate oral control, there should be no reason to restrict texture of solid consistency. However, delayed pharyngeal swallowing frequently coexists with poor oral control. Thus adaptations of texture may be appropriate to address the oral motor concerns as described in the previous section. Again, as is the case for all compensatory interventions, an understanding of swallowing physiology and patient needs will be required to determine appropriate diet level.

Patient Instruction. Clear instructions are required for the patient and caregiver, particularly if the patient is homebound, and thus does not have meals provided. Examples of specific well-tolerated foods should be given to minimize ambiguity.

Coaching Tips. As discussed in the chapter on oral nutrition, compliance may be an issue with some patients on a restricted diet. Definition of a clear plan to work the patient off of the restricted diet may increase cooperation. Developing a diet log, in which the patient charts the nature and quantity of foods consumed, may be helpful to evaluate both compliance and nutrition.

Contraindications. These issues are discussed fully in the oral nutrition chapter. Care should be taken that a significantly altered diet does not result in a reduced appetite and thus compromise patient nutrition.

Example Goal. The patient will comply with mechanical soft diet recommendations as demonstrated by evaluation of a diet log.

Prosthetic Devices: Tracheostomy Valves

Supporting Research/Description of Technique. The use of tracheostomy valves in the management of dysphagia is discussed more fully on page 141 under the discussion of the physiologic abnormality of inadequate laryngeal closure. The question of whether placement of a valve will decrease delay in onset of swallow is yet unanswered in the literature. Theroetically, one might expect that with the improved supralaryngeal sensation resulting from airflow directed through the upper airway, deficits in delayed onset of swallow due to poor sensation may be minimized.

Patient Instruction. Tracheostomy occlusion can occur by either a cap, which allows no airflow, or a one-way speaking valve, which allows inspiratory airflow through the tracheostomy. It is important that any management of a tracheostomized patient be completed in cooperation with other members of the health care team, particularly respiratory care and nursing. Meticulous hygiene is required to minimize the risk of infection.

Contraindications. The management and implications of tracheostomy management in speech and swallowing are complex. Although presence of a tracheostomy allows for access to the pulmonary system for suctioning, patients with tracheostomy may have fewer pulmonary reserves, thus requiring careful management.

Physiologic Abnormality: Reduced Strength and Coordination of Pharyngeal Contraction, Laryngeal Excursion

Impairment of the pharyngeal phase of the swallow can be secondary to a variety of specific physiologic abnormalities, many of which will be addressed similarly in management. Decreased base of tongue to posterior pharyngeal wall approximation results in diminished positive pressure on the bolus and subsequent vallecular residual. Reduced strength and coordination of the musculature involved in pharyngeal swallowing can result in the radiographically observed symptom of pharyngeal residual localized to the valleculae or distributed diffusely throughout the pharyngeal cavity. Decreased laryngeal excursion secondary to limited suprahyoid contraction can result in the symptoms of inadequate epiglottic deflection for upper airway protection and incomplete opening of the upper esophageal sphincter.

Postural Strategies: Chin Tuck Posturing

Supporting Research/Description of Technique. Chin tuck posturing is a widely used and very beneficial technique for neurogenic patients. It is most commonly recommended for patients who demonstrate the physiologic deficit of delayed pharyngeal swallow. Thus, the bulk of the discussion on the topic is included on page 109. Logemann (1983) suggests chin tuck posturing as an intervention to address not only delays in triggering the pharyngeal swallow, but also poor tongue control, reduced tongue base retraction, and/or reduced closure of the laryngeal entrance and vocal cords during a swallow, as assessed by videofluoroscopy. Refer to the prior discussion for a detailed description of the physiologic effects of this intervention.

Patient Instruction. The patients are instructed to bring their chin to their chest during swallowing. Care should be taken to keep the cervical spine upright and bring the chin down to the chest, rather than moving the head and neck forward as a combined unit (i.e., "bird-necking").

Coaching Tips. Refer to the coaching tips suggested on page 111 under delayed pharyngeal swallow.

Contraindications. Although chin tuck posturing may facilitate pharyngeal clearance in some cases, patients with severe postswallow pharyngeal residual may be at increased risk with this position. As described in earlier sections, chin tuck posturing may encourage aspiration risk by tilting postswallow residual toward the unprotected airway between swallows.

Example Goal. The patient will recall and implement chin tuck posturing with no evidence of anterior leakage on 90% of solid boluses with minimal verbal cues.

Postural Strategies: Head Rotation

Supporting Research/Description of Technique. Rotating, or turning, the head to the weaker, hemiparetic side of a neurologically impaired patient can direct the flow of a bolus down a potentially more sensate and stronger side of the pharynx (Logemann, 1983). The prevailing belief is that this rotation will, in effect, reduce the size of pharyngeal cavities on that side; thus, the bolus will be redirected toward the more functional side of the pharynx, promoting more efficient swallowing. Although not empirically evaluated, many clinicians have observed cases in which rotation toward the stronger side is more beneficial. As well, this technique may be of use when the patient demonstrates diffuse weakness and residual, therefore the strategy should be confirmed diagnostically. Effectiveness of the technique for pharyngeal weakness may be enhanced when paired with chin tuck posturing.

Patient Instruction. Execution of this position requires that the patient sit erect, but with the head turned 90°, or to the full extent comfortable, toward the designated shoulder. The torso should remain facing forward. Care must be taken to maintain this posture throughout the swallow. Training head rotation in patients with cognitive impairment may require more persistence. This position is an abnormal movement during eating; thus, it may require greater commitment to recall by the patient and caregivers. Frequently, patients forget to rotate their head prior to swallowing, or move out of rotation too early, thus limiting its beneficial effects. As well, it may be quite fatiguing to maintain for every swallow, and for an entire meal.

Coaching Tips. Environmental controls may enhance recall of the technique. Placing the patient's meal tray on the side of head rotation may be facilitory. Seating the patient with family, friends, television, or the rest of the dining room on the side of head rotation may be also be useful. In addition, an adapted soft cervical collar is useful for facilitating head rotation. A half-moon is cut from the lateral aspect of the collar where the chin would rest during optimal head rotation posturing. Cloth tape is used to seal the cut edges and the cut-out wedge can be placed between the collar and the patient on the opposite side of the neck. Thus, slight pressure from the cut-out wedge provides tactile cuing to the patient with cognitive impairment and the cut-out region provides a position for the chin. It is important to note, however, that use of the collar does not limit patient movement; a patient may easily move against the collar for comfort.

Contraindications. No suspected or documented contraindications are associated with this technique.

Example Goal. The patient will recall and implement head rotation technique with intermittent verbal cues on 90% of puree swallows.

Postural Strategies: Head Tilt

Supporting Research/Description of Technique. As with head rotation, tilting the head to the stronger, undamaged side of a neurologically impaired patient may also direct the bolus to the stronger, potentially more sensate oral and pharyngeal side (Logemann, 1983). The increased sensation and motor strength/coordination experienced on the undamaged side of a mouth and pharynx may provide immediate positive benefits to a patient. These benefits include improved oral control, bolus formation and propulsion with a stronger pharyngeal swallow response.

The degree of tilt necessary for benefit is hard to assess reliably and sustain with each swallow, and a return to an upright posture usually occurs during a meal, unless constant verbal cues are given. The difficulties in training and maintenance make this posture a less common approach in institutionalized settings, unless the patient already naturally reverts to this posture.

Patient Instruction. The patient is instructed to tilt the head toward the stronger, nonimpaired side during PO ingestion. However, as with all compensatory techniques, diagnostic assessment will help the clinician determine the most appropriate positioning for the patient. The technique must be executed consistently for all textures.

Coaching Tips. An adapted soft cervical collar is useful for facilitating head tilt. A half-moon is cut from the lateral aspect of the collar where the chin would rest during optimal head tilt. Cloth tape is used to seal the cut edges and the cut-out wedge can be placed between the collar and the patient on the opposite side of the neck. Thus, slight pressure from the cut-out wedge provides tactile cuing to the patient with cognitive impairment and the cut-out region provides a position for the chin. It is important to note, however, that use of the collar does not limit patient movement; a patient may easily move against the collar for comfort.

Contraindications. As briefly addressed in the preceding paragraph, if a patient benefits with head tilt toward the stronger side, but hemiparesis tends the patient toward the weaker side, head tilting technique will need to be consistently cued and corrected to inhibit greater impairment.

Example Goal. The patient will recall and implement head tilt positioning with no verbal cues on 90% of liquid swallows.

Postural Strategies: Side Lying

Supporting Research/Description of Technique. Lying down on one side has been suggested by Logemann (1996) as an effective posture to compensate for reduced pharyngeal contraction that results in diffuse residue in the pharynx. The rationale for this posture is that a lateral head/trunk position will reduce the gravitational force on any residue that is left in the pharynx after a swallow. Repeated swallows while on one side may effectively clear the residue, thereby reducing the risk of aspiration.

Patient Instruction. The patient is comfortably positioned in the lateral position in bed or in a semireclined or fully reclined chair. The meal tray is positioned in from of the patient, which in this position would likely be at the side of the chair, such that the patient is able to derive visual feedback prior to oral acceptance of the bolus. A small pillow may provide additional needed head support and comfort.

Coaching Tips. There are a variety of adaptive feeding utensils that can help with administering a bolus in side-lying posture, such as a swinging spoon. Drinking of liquids from this position is quite difficult and usually requires adaptive cups or straws to aid placement to the mouth.

Contraindications. Although this posture may be beneficial for selected patients, it may not be readily accepted by patients or caregivers. It is very difficult to self-feed a meal from a lateral position, as anyone who has tried to eat while lying down on the couch can attest. Excellent eye-hand coordination, flexibility, and patience must be present to attain this feat without spilling most of the food off a utensil, prior to placement in the mouth. Finally, there may be great resistance in many facilities to feeding patients while they lie in bed, with good reason. For institutionalized patients, the only place they could safely and comfortably lie on their side would be their own bed. Most residential facilities work hard to normalize all activities of daily living, especially eating. The social and physical rewards of being dressed, out of bed, and in a dining room to share a meal with others is a quality-of-life issue. These benefits would have to be weighed against the benefits of lying on one side to eat as a compensatory posture for dysphagia. Although this posture may have positive benefits for some patients, acceptance and compliance of this posture may be hard to attain. This posture may be accepted as a temporary treatment option, but long-term use may be rejected by some patients or caregivers.

Example Goal. Side-lying positioning will be implemented for all PO intake with no evidence of aspiration or poor oral control.

Bolus Control Techniques: Cyclic Ingestion

Supporting Research/Description of Technique. This technique is primarily utilized when the patient demonstrates pharyngeal weakness/dyscoordination or hypertonicity of the UES resulting in postswallow pharyngeal residual in valleculae and/or pyriform sinuses. However, it may have some applications as well in patients with significant oral motor issues with postswallow oral residual. In this case, liquid ingested after a solid bolus facilitates clearance of the oral cavity by serving as a liquid wash. No research has been published to date regarding effectiveness of the technique.

Patient Instruction. The patient is given liquids with all meals and instructed to alternate liquid and solid intake throughout the meal, either in one to one ratio or as indicated by diagnostic examination

Contraindications. This technique cannot be used with patients on a liquid- restricted diet. In a limited number of patients, the subsequent liquid bolus may bypass the residual in the valleculae as opposed to washing it out and will then present potential for aspiration; thus, the strategy should be evaluated diagnostically.

Example Goal. The patient will recall and implement cyclic ingestion pattern of intake during meals with no verbal cues and no evidence of postswallow aspiration of residual.

Bolus Control Techniques: Dry Swallows

Supporting Research/Description of Technique. Dry swallow is used for several physiologic deficits that result in postswallow residual somewhere within the aerodigestive tract. In particular, dry swallow can be used to clear oral residual secondary to oral motor impairment, pharyngeal residual secondary to weakness or dyscoordination, or pyriform sinus residual secondary to UES dysfunction. The technique may also be used in cases of intact pharyngeal phase swallowing when oral residual falls postswallow into the pharynx in inadequate quantity to elicit a pharyngeal swallow. In principle, repetition of the swallow without a new bolus serves to aid in clearing postswallow residual.

Patient Instruction. The patient is instructed to dry swallow after every bolus swallow or to swallow each bolus two, three or four times as indicated by the diagnostic examination.

Coaching Tips. Decreasing rate of intake may facilitate this strategy. This can be promoted by requiring patient to put down the spoon, fork, or cup between bites. For a few patients, placement of an empty bowl on the meal tray with instructions to take a bite from that bowl may also cue recall of the strategy.

Contraindications. There are no documented contraindications associated with this technique.

Example Goal. The patient will recall and implement dry swallows after bolus swallows with minimal verbal cues on 90% of bolus swallows.

Bolus Control Techniques: Modification of Bolus Size/Adaptations in the Rate of Intake

Supporting Research/Description of Technique. Bolus size and rate of intake can also influence the efficiency of the pharyngeal swallowing when neurosensory deficits result in inadequate feedback regarding bolus size or texture. Details regarding the use of these techniques are more fully outlined under the section for oral motor impairment. As before, patient physiology is so variable that no hard and fast rules, or even general tendencies, can be clearly identified. Thus, full diagnostic examination will facilitate correct prescription of optimal bolus size and rate.

Patient Instruction. If the patient has adequate cognition to control the rate and quantity of intake independently, instructions are provided for the size of bolus and rate of ingestion that has been determined to maximize swallowing efficiency. Otherwise, interventions such as those that follow may be useful.

Coaching Tips. There are several techniques that can be utilized to facilitate slowed or controlled intake. To slow the rate or limit the quantity of liquid intake in patients with cognitive impairment, patients can take all liquids from a lidded travel mug. If the size of the hole is too large to limit flow adequately, the top can be taken off and a small piece of duct tape used to half-cover the hole from the inside. Straw sips, unless otherwise contraindicated, may also slow rate of liquid ingestion, particularly if using a straw of narrow diameter. To slow the rate of solid or semisolid intake, the patient can be cued always to put spoon or fork down between bites, or to insert volitional dry swallow. A small wrist weight may provide adequate tactile information and increased effort to slow rate of intake. To limit the quantity of solid intake, use of a small spoon bowl will decrease the amount. Another option would be to take standard dining room spoons and have the center of the bowl removed by a metal shop. With the edges adequately smoothed, this allows a significant portion of the bolus (for puree) to fall through the spoon and only the bolus at the edges enters the patient's mouth. Portion control may also be useful; that is, providing the patient with a series of bowls only partially filled.

Contraindications. There are no suspected or identified contraindications.

Example Goal. The patient will demonstrate decreased rate of puree intake as measured by 4 ounces ingested in no less than 5 minutes.

Volitional Airway Protection: Super-Supraglottic Swallow

Supporting Research/Description of Technique. The super-supraglottic swallow technique has mostly been described in reference to patients with dysphagia subsequent to oral pharyngeal carcinoma. However, application of this intervention may be appropriate as well for patients with neurogenic dysphagia who demonstrate compromised airway protection and concurrent pharyngeal phase weakness. The super-supraglottic swallow consists of pairing the sequence of airway protective mechanisms in supraglottic swallow with the effort in swallowing generated by effortful or modified Valsalva swallow.

Patient Instruction. As with the supraglottic swallow technique, the patient is instructed to take a deep breath and tightly hold, then swallow "hard" or swallow with greater effort than usual. Following completion of the swallow, the patient should cough on exhale, prior to the initiation of subsequent inspiration.

Coaching Tips. See the coaching tips for supra-glottic swallow on page 139.

Contraindications. There are no suspected or documented contraindications.

Example Goal. The patient will recall and implement super-supraglottic swallow technique on 95% of solid boluses with no clinical evidence of aspiration and minimal postswallow pharyngeal expectoration.

Volitional Airway Protection: Pharyngeal expectoration

Supporting Research/Description of Technique. Pharyngeal expectoration as a compensatory technique may be particularly appropriate for the patient with impaired opening of the upper esophageal sphincter given the frequently observed symptom of postswallow pyriform sinus residual. As described more fully under airway protection strategies, pharyngeal expectoration consists of expelling residual in the pharynx through the oral cavity.

Patient Instruction. The patient is instructed to bring up secretions from the back of the throat and expectorate them into a cup, basin, or tissue.

Coaching Tips. Colloquialisms such as "truck driver's spit" or "hawking up a clam" may communicate more effectively the intent of the instruction.

Contraindications. Aside from the social implications of expectoration, there are no suspected contraindications. However, as patients progress in swallowing rehabilitation, they should be encouraged to swallow, rather than expectorate, oral pharyngeal secretions.

Example Goal. The patient will demonstrate transfer of the bolus through the UES as evidenced by decreased postswallow expectorations of residual.

Diet Modification: Liquids

Supporting Research/Description of Technique. The use of thickened liquids is most often indicated when thinned liquids are aspirated prior to the initiation of the airway protection, secondary to delay in onset of the pharyngeal swallow; thus, a more detailed description of this intervention is described on page 118. Thickened liquids may also be applied when the patient demonstrates aspiration during the swallow secondary to pharyngeal phase impairment that contributes to poor supralaryngeal airway protection. By thickening the liquid for ingestion, the rate of flow is reduced, allowing for greater control and less "splash" as the liquid enters the oral and pharyngeal cavities.

Patient Instruction. As always, clear instructions are needed in defining the texture of thickened liquids. Thickened liquids may take many forms from thin nectar consistency through honey/semipuree. Degree of thickness should be determined for that patient by the diagnostic exam. Commercial products are available to thicken liquids systematically without compromising the free-water content. Liquids can also be thickened by blending with another nutritive puree texture (potatoes, applesauce, and the like).

Coaching Tips. In rehabilitation or home care settings where kitchen facilities are available, it may be helpful to evaluate the patient or caretaker preparing thickened liquids to specifications, thus assuring preparation of a safe consistency.

Contraindications. As fully discussed in the oral nutrition chapter, the risk of dehydration may be significant when thickened liquids are introduced into the diet. Risks of aspiration versus dehydration should be evaluated. Care should be taken to remove liquid restrictions as soon as possible.

Example Goal. During ingestion of thickened liquids, patient will demonstrate clinical indication of aspiration on less than 1% of swallows.

Diet Modifications: Solids

Supporting Research/Description of Technique. Food modification may be appropriate for patients with pharyngeal phase impairment if pharyngeal weakness or dyscoordination results in inadequate propulsion of the bolus through the pharynx. If oral motor control is maintained, and the patient has adequate cognition to prepare the bolus fully prior to pharyngeal transfer, a modified diet may not be required. As in the case of oral motor inefficiency, food modification generally consists of limiting the diet to specialized foods that are of a softer texture, requiring less mastication. The use of gravies and sauces that help the bolus maintain cohesiveness may be suggested, particularly for dry or particulate foods. Heavy foods that require excessive mastication, foods that break apart (rice), or mixed textures (cereal with milk, soups with vegetables) may pose a greater challenge for the patient with oral motor impairment. As well, breads may become sticky when mixed with secretions, and jello may be harder to control in oral phase.

By adjusting the texture of the oral diet, particularly limiting sticky or dry textures, patients with pharyngeal weakness or inefficiency may be better able to propel the bolus through the pharyngeal cavities. This should result in decreased postswallow residual as a symptom of the physiologic abnormality.

Patient Instruction. Clear instructions are required for the patient and caregiver, particularly if the patient is homebound, and thus, does not have meals provided. Examples of specific well-tolerated foods should be given to minimize ambiguity.

Coaching Tips. As discussed in the chapter on oral nutrition, compliance may be an issue with some patients on a restricted diet. Definition of a clear plan to work the patient off of the restricted diet may increase cooperation. Developing a diet log, in which the patient charts the nature and quantity of foods consumed, may be helpful to evaluate both compliance and nutrition.

Contraindications. These issues are discussed fully in the oral nutrition chapter. Care should be taken that a significantly altered diet does not result in a reduced appetite and thus compromise patient nutrition.

Example Goal. The patient will comply with mechanical soft diet recommendations as demonstrated by evaluation of a diet log.

Prosthetic Devices: Tracheostomy Valves

Supporting Research/Description of Technique. The use of tracheostomy valves are discussed more fully on page 141 under the section on physiologic abnormalities associated with poor laryngeal closure. As discussed in that section, the effects of valving on swallowing are not fully clarified through the available research. In association with the abnormality of reduced pharyngeal stripping with postswallow residual, clinical practice suggests improved function with tracheostomy closure. Further research is needed in this area, as others, to substantiate these impressions.

Patient Instruction. Tracheostomy occlusion can occur by either a cap, which allows no airflow, or a one-way speaking valve, which allows inspiratory airflow through the tracheostomy. It is important that any management of a tracheostomized patient be completed in cooperation with other members of the health care team, particularly respiratory care and nursing. Meticulous hygiene is required to minimize the risk of infection.

Contraindications. The management and implications of tracheostomy management in speech and swallowing are complex. Although presence of a trach allows for access to the pulmonary system for suctioning, patients with tracheostomy may have fewer pulmonary reserves, thus requiring careful management.

Physiologic Abnormality: Reduced Opening of the Upper Esophageal Sphincter

Opening of the upper esophageal sphincter during swallowing is a complex process requiring coordination of several biomechanical processes. As a sphincteric muscle, the UES is tonically contracted; thus, bolus passage requires transient relaxation. Failure of the neurologic system to signal relaxation will result in incomplete UES opening and postswallow, primarily, pyriform sinus residual. Second, the UES has no internal mechanism by which to open itself and requires contribution of external biomechanical forces. This is provided by laryngeal excursion, which provides anterior and superior traction forces on the UES. Finally, relaxation of the UES and pharyngolaryngeal excursion must work in a coordinated fashion. A patient may demonstrate adequate laryngeal excursion as well as relaxed tone of the UES, but if these events do not work in synchrony, bolus passage will be impeded. Compensation for UES dysfunction generally focuses on facilitating biomechanical pull on the UES by increasing laryngeal exursion.

Postural Strategies: Chin Tuck Posturing

Supporting Research/Description of Technique. Chin tuck posturing is most commonly recommended for patients who demonstrate the physiologic deficit of delayed pharyngeal swallow. Thus, the bulk of the discussion on the topic is included beginning on page 109. Although chin tuck posturing may facilitate opening of the upper esophageal sphincter, this technique may also facilitate aspiration is patients with upper esophageal sphincter impairment, as cited by Shanahan et al. (1993). Thus, its application to this physiologic deficit may be significantly limited and should be very carefully evaluated.

Patient Instruction. After confirmation of safety via diagnostic procedure, the patient is instructed to bring the chin to the chest during swallowing.

Coaching Tips. Refer to the coaching tips suggested on page 111 under delayed pharyngeal swallow.

Contraindications. As cited above, this technique should only be very cautiously applied to patients with UES impairment secondary to aspiration risk.

Example Goal. The patient will recall and implement chin tuck posturing with no evidence of aspiration and clinical indication of decreased pyriform sinus residual on 90% of solid boluses with minimal verbal cues.

Postural Strategies: Head Rotation

Supporting Research/Description of Technique. The technique of head rotation is discussed in detail under the physiologic impairment of pharyngeal phase weakness/dyscoordination (page 121). Although not empirically evaluated, it also appears that this technique facilitates opening of the upper esophageal sphincter by posturally providing external pull to the sphincter. Head rotation appears to have a similar effect on UES function as chin tuck posturing but with decreased aspiration risk. For patients who are diagnosed with increased cricopharyngeal pressure as their primary problem, head rotation has been found to give great relief and is embraced as a compensatory technique. These patients are usually highly motivated, aware of and aggravated by their problem, and willing to use this technique with every swallow.

Patient Instruction. Execution of this position requires that patient sit erect, but with the head turned 90°, or to the full extent comfortable, toward the designated shoulder with the torso remaining forward.

Coaching Tips. Environmental controls may enhance recall of the technique. Placing the patient's meal tray on the side of head rotation may be facilitory. Seating the patient with family, friends, television, or the rest of the dining room on the side of head rotation may be also be useful. In addition, an adapted soft cervical collar is useful for facilitating head rotation. A half-moon is cut from the lateral aspect of the collar where the chin would rest during optimal head rotation posturing. Cloth tape is used to seal the cut edges and the cut out wedge can be placed between the collar and the patient on the opposite side of the neck. Thus slight pressure from the cut out wedge provides tactile cuing to the patient with cognitive impairment and the cut-out region provides a position for the chin. It is important to note, however, that use of the collar does not limit patient movement; a patient may easily move against the collar for comfort.

Contraindications. There are no suspected or documented contraindications associated with this technique.

Example Goal. The patient will recall and implement head rotation technique with intermittent verbal cues on 90% of puree swallows.

Bolus Control Techniques: Cyclic Ingestion

Supporting Research/Description of Technique. This technique is primarily used when the patient demonstrates pharyngeal weakness/dyscoordination or hypertonicity of the UES resulting in postswallow pharyngeal residual in the valleculae and/or pyriform sinuses. However, it may have some applications as well in patients with significant oral motor issues with postswallow oral residual. In this case, liquid ingested after a solid bolus facilitates clearance of the oral cavity by serving as a liquid wash. No research has been published to date regarding effectiveness of the technique.

Patient Instruction. The patient given liquids with all meals and instructed to alternate liquid and solid intake throughout the meal, either in one to one ratio or as indicated by diagnostic examination

Coaching Tips. This technique relies heavily on the patient's recall of the task. Written reminders on the dinner tray may facilitate recall.

Contraindications. This technique cannot be used with patients on a liquid-restricted diet. In a limited number of patients, the subsequent liquid bolus may bypass the residual in the valleculae as opposed to washing it out and will then present potential for aspiration; thus, the strategy should be evaluated diagnostically.

Example Goal. The patient will recall and implement cyclic ingestion pattern of intake during meals with no verbal cues and no evidence of postswallow aspiration of residual.

Bolus Control Techniques: Dry Swallows

Supporting Research/Description of Technique. Dry swallow is used for several physiologic deficits that result in postswallow residual somewhere within the aerodigestive tract. In particular, dry swallow can be used to clear oral residual secondary to oral motor impairment, pharyngeal residual secondary to weakness or dyscoordination, or pyriform sinus residual secondary to UES dysfunction. The technique may also be used in cases of intact pharyngeal phase swallowing when oral residual falls postswallow into the pharynx in inadequate quantity to elicit a pharyngeal swallow. In principle, repetition of the swallow without a new bolus serves to aid in clearing postswallow residual.

Patient Instruction. Patient is instructed to dry swallow after every bolus swallow or to swallow each bolus two, three or four times as indicated by the diagnostic examination.

Coaching Tips. Decreasing rate of intake may facilitate this strategy. This can be promoted by requiring patient to put down the spoon, fork, or cup between bites. For a few patients, placement of an empty bowl on the meal tray with instructions to take a bite from that bowl may also cue recall of the strategy.

Contraindications. No documented contraindications are associated with this technique.

Example Goal. The patient will recall and implement dry swallows after bolus swallows with minimal verbal cues on 90% of bolus swallows.

Bolus Control Techniques: Modification of Bolus Size/Adaptations in the Rate of Intake

Supporting Research/Description of Technique. Bolus size and rate of intake are more fully described in the section on oral motor efficiency, but bear some mention as an intervention for UES impairment. Although no research is identified to support this observation, it would appear that some patients with impairment of UES opening demonstrate improved passage of contrast into the esophagus when provided with larger bolus size. It appears as if larger bolus size provides greater superior pressure or force on the UES and facilitates opening.

Patient Instruction. If the patient has adequate cognition to control the rate and quantity of intake independently, instructions are provided for the size of bolus and rate of ingestion that has been determined to maximize swallowing efficiency. Otherwise, interventions such as those that follow may be useful.

Contraindications. The potential benefits of increased bolus size should be carefully weighed, however, with the patient's ability for airway protection. Significant postswallow pyriform sinus residual may increase aspiration risk.

Example Goal. The patient will ingest large rounded tablespoons of puree during PO trials with less than half a teaspoon of expectorated pharyngeal residual.

Volitional Airway Protection: Pharyngeal Expectoration

Supporting Research/Description of Technique. Pharyngeal expectoration as a compensatory technique may be particularly appropriate for the patient with impaired opening of the upper esophageal sphincter given the frequently observed symptom of postswallow pyriform sinus residual. As described more fully under airway protection strategies, pharyngeal expectoration consists of expelling residual in the pharynx through the oral cavity

Patient Instruction. The patient is instructed to bring up secretions from the back of the throat and expectorate them into a cup, basin, or tissue.

Coaching Tips. Colloquialisms such as "truck driver's spit" or "hawking up a clam" may communicate more effectively the intent of the instruction.

Contraindications. Aside from the social implications of expectoration, there are no suspected contraindications. However, as patients progress in swallowing rehabilitation, they should be encouraged to swallow, rather than expectorate, oral pharyngeal secretions.

Example Goal. The patient will demonstrate transfer of the bolus through the UES as evidenced by decreased postswallow expectorations of residual.

Diet Modification: Liquids

Supporting Research/Description of Technique. The use of thickened liquids is most often indicated when thinned liquids are aspirated prior to the initiation of the airway protection, secondary to delay in onset of the pharyngeal swallow. However, thickened liquids may also be used in cases of decreased oral motor control for manipulation of thin liquid bolus. Liquids are typically thickened if it is determined by videofluoroscopy that adjustment is needed. A thickened liquid may be more easily controlled in the oral phase of the swallow. By thickening the liquid for ingestion, the rate of flow is reduced, allowing for greater control and less "splash" as the liquid enters the oral and pharyngeal cavities.

Patient Instruction. The patient should be given precise instructions as to what constitutes a thickened liquid as this is an area of terminal ambiguity among professionals and between clinician and patient. Thickened liquids may take many forms from thin nectar consistency through honey/semipuree. Degree of thickness should be determined for the patient by the diagnostic exam. Commercial products are available to thicken liquids systematically without compromising the free-water content. Liquids can also be thickened by blending with another nutritive puree texture (potatoes, applesauce, and the like).

Coaching Tips. In rehabilitation or home care settings where kitchen facilities are available, it may be helpful to evaluate the patient or caretaker preparing thickened liquids to specifications, thus assuring preparation of a safe consistency.

Contraindications. As fully discussed in the oral nutrition chapter, the risk of dehydration may be significant when thickened liquids are introduced into the diet. Risks of aspiration versus dehydration should be evaluated. Care should be taken to remove liquid restrictions as soon as possible.

Example Goal. During ingestion of thickened liquids, patient will demonstrate clinical indication of aspiration on less than 1% of swallows.

Diet Modifications: Solids

Supporting Research/Description of Technique. Food modification generally consists of limiting the diet to specialized foods that are of a softer texture, requiring less mastication. This is particularly the case for patients who demonstrate oral motor inefficiency. Modification of solids for the patient with impairment in UES opening may present a greater challenge and require more critical diagnosis. For most patients with impaired opening of the UES, a softer texture is desirable, allow for greater malleability of the bolus as it passes through the restricted opening to the esophagus. In some cases, solids may need to be severely limited until improvement in UES opening is evidenced. However, clinical practice suggests that in some patients with impairment of UES opening, greater texture and weight of solid boluses provide more sensory information and thus greater responsiveness of hyolaryngeal excursion, and subsequently UES opening. Critical evaluation of multiple textures under videofluoroscopic guidance will be required.

Patient Instruction. Clear instructions are required for the patient and caregiver, particularly if the patient is homebound, and thus, does not have meals provided. Examples of specific well-tolerated foods should be given to minimize ambiguity.

Coaching Tips. As discussed in the chapter on oral nutrition, compliance may be an issue with some patients on a restricted diet. Definition of a clear plan to work the patient off of the restricted diet may increase cooperation. Developing a diet log, in which the patient charts the nature and quantity of foods consumed, may be helpful to evaluate both compliance and nutrition.

Contraindications. These issues are discussed fully in the oral nutrition chapter. Care should be taken that a significantly altered diet does not result in a reduced appetite and thus compromise patient nutrition.

Example Goal. The patient will comply with mechanical soft diet recommendations as demonstrated by evaluation of a diet log.

Physiologic Abnormality: Inadequate Laryngeal Valving and Compromised Airway Protection

Although aspiration and penetration are definitely issues associated with dysphagia, it is important to recognize that aspiration is a symptom of another physiologic deficit, not impairment in and of itself. Aspiration does not occur in the absence of some other physiologic abnormality. Thus, rehabilitation of aspiration is somewhat of a misnomer, as rehabilitative practices would focus on the underlying physiologic abnormality, not the aspiration itself. However, compensatory techniques may address aspiration or airway compromise directly as a means to minimize the risks associated with the underlying physiologic abnormality. For example, a patient may demonstrate the symptoms of aspiration postswallow, secondary to the symptom of pyriform sinus residual caused by the physiologic abnormality of decreased UES opening. Rehabilitation would address not the aspiration directly, but the impaired opening of the UES. Compensation however may address both issues: UES opening and aspiration. The physiologic etiologies resulting in aspiration are numerous and exceed the scope of a text on treatment. It is important for both rehabilitation and compensation that this underlying physiology be identified prior to implementation of a treatment plan.

Postural Strategies: Chin Tuck Posturing

Supporting Research/Description of Technique. Chin tuck posturing is most commonly recommended for patients who demonstrate aspiration secondary to the physiologic deficit of delayed pharyngeal swallow. Thus, the bulk of the discussion on the topic is included on page 109. As discussed, chin tuck has been observed to be beneficial in reducing aspiration during videofluoroscopy based on the work by several research groups (Castell et al., 1993; Shanahan et al., 1993; Welch et al., 1993). It is important to realize, however, that in conditions where chin tuck posturing is effective, the observed aspiration is a symptom of delayed or incomplete airway protection secondary to nonlaryngeal issues. Chin tuck posturing may not have direct influences on laryngeal valving.

Patient Instruction. Chin tuck posturing is executed by instructing patients to drop their chin down and in toward their chest. Care should be taken to maintain the cervical spine and avoid anterior movement of the base of skull.

Coaching Tips. Refer to the coaching tips suggested on page 111 under delayed pharyngeal swallow.

Contraindications. Chin tuck posturing in this situation is used to compensate for a primary physiologic impairment (e.g., delayed pharyngeal swallowing) that results in aspiration as a secondary symptom. Chin tuck posturing may not be effective to address aspiration secondary to a laryngeal etiology, such as poor vocal fold closure, or sensory etiology, such as absent cough reflex.

Example Goal. The patient will recall and implement chin tuck posturing with no evidence of aspiration on 90% of solid boluses with minimal verbal cues.

Bolus Control Techniques: 3-Second Prep

Supporting Research/Description of Technique. This technique is fully described under the category of delayed pharyngeal swallow (page 112) and only indirectly addresses aspiration/airway protection issues by inhibiting delayed pharyngeal swallow. However, as it has been observed to inhibit aspiration in many patients, it is covered briefly in this section. A volitional, conscious pause prior to transfer of the bolus may allow greater time in the patient with delayed onset of swallow to elicit volitional airway protection. Use of this strategy alters the swallows from a reflexive response to a more volitionally controlled action.

Patient Instruction. After placement of the bolus in the oral cavity, the patient is instructed to count to three mentally prior to transfer of the bolus into the pharynx. On transfer, the patient is instructed to swallow volitionally.

Coaching Tips. This task requires some degree of cognitive power on the part of the patient, with the ability to follow instructions. Verbal cuing to "put the spoon down before you swallow" may facilitate recall of the technique is some patients.

Contraindications. Some patients with poor oral motor control, particularly base of tongue to palate approximation, may experience premature spillage of bolus into the pharynx and thus increase preswallow aspiration risk.

Example Goal. The patient will recall and implement 3-second prep technique with no evidence of preswallow aspiration and minimal verbal cues on 90% of liquid swallows.

Volitional Airway Protection: Supraglottic Swallow

Supporting Research/Description of Technique. The supraglottic swallow technique was first described by Logemann (1984). This technique provides volitional airway protection, when the patient presents either silent aspiration or a latent reflexive airway protection. The lungs are filled and the vocal folds firmly sealed through conscious effort prior to the swallow, with a volitional cough/forced expiration immediately following to clear laryngeal coating/potential aspiration. Martin et al. (1993) provided a systematic evaluation of three breath-holding maneuvers: easy hold, inhale hold, and inhale/exhale hard hold. Maximal laryngeal valving was visualized by nasoendoscopy under the hard breath-hold condition. False vocal fold approximation and anterior arytenoid tilting that is optimal for airway protection was only observed during effortful breath-hold conditions, not easy breath-holding. The authors of this study emphasize that considerable intrasubject and intratrial variation is observed in executing the tasks; thus, extensive teaching and perhaps biofeedback monitoring of vocal fold closure via endoscopy or electroglottography are indicated.

Patient Instruction. The patient is instructed to take a deep breath and hold it firmly while swallowing the bolus. On completion of the swallow, patient is instructed to expel the air from the lungs forcefully with a volitional cough, prior to inhalation. The patient then swallows and coughs a second time.

Coaching Tips. Because of the complexity of sequencing multiple components, the patient may require written instruction to recall sequence of events, as this can be a difficult task for many patients to coordinate.

A technique to facilitate learning of this strategy is to break the task, on first presentation, into discrete steps with mastery at each level prior to moving ahead.

1. Hold your breath (3, 5, 10 seconds progressively), then relax.
2. Hold your breath (3, 5, 10 seconds progressively), then exhale forcefully or with a cough.
3. Hold your breath, swallow, then exhale forcefully or with a cough.

Contraindications. There are no documented or suspected contraindications; however, this intervention may be very difficult for the patient with concomitant pulmonary disease or reduced pulmonary effort.

Example Goal. The patient will recall and implement supraglottic swallow technique on 95% of liquid swallows with no verbal cues.

Volitional Airway Protection: Super-Supraglottic Swallow

Supporting Research/Description of Technique. The super-supraglottic swallow technique has mostly been described in reference to patients with dysphagia subsequent to oral pharyngeal carcinoma. However, application of this intervention may be appropriate as well for patients with neurogenic dysphagia who demonstrate compromised airway protection and concurrent pharyngeal phase weakness. The super-supraglottic swallow consists of pairing the sequence of airway protective mechanisms in supraglottic swallow with the effort in swallowing generated by effortful, or modified Valsalva swallow.

Patient Instruction. As with the supraglottic swallow technique, the patient is instructed to take a deep breath and tightly hold, then swallow "hard" or swallow with greater effort than usual. Following completion of the swallow, the patient should cough on exhale, prior to the initiation of subsequent inspiration.

Coaching Tips. See the coaching tips for supra-glottic swallow (page 139).

Contraindications. There are no suspected or documented contraindications.

Example Goal. The patient will recall and implement super-supraglottic swallow technique on 95% of solid boluses with no clinical evidence of aspiration and minimal postswallow pharyngeal expectoration.

Volitional Airway Protection: Pharyngeal Expectoration

Supporting Research/Description of Technique. Pharyngeal expectoration is a clinically useful technique for clearing pharyngeal residual postswallow in the presence of the physiologic abnormality of decreased pharyngeal contraction and laryngeal excursion of impaired UES opening. By inhibiting the buildup of postswallow residual, there is less likelihood for postswallowing aspiration of residual. Although not documented through empirical research, clinically this technique appears to be very useful in advancing severely impaired patients toward an oral diet.

Patient Instruction. The patient is instructed to bring up secretions from the back of the throat.

Coaching Tips. Colloquialisms such as "truck driver's spit" or "hawking up a clam" may communicate more effectively the intent of the instruction.

Contraindications. Aside from the social implications of expectoration, there are no suspected contraindications. However, as patients progress in swallowing rehabilitation, they should be encouraged to swallow, rather than expectorate, oral pharyngeal secretions.

Example Goal. The patient will demonstrate increased efficiency of pharyngeal swallow as evidenced by decreased postswallow expectorations of residual.

Volitional Airway Protection: Vocal Quality Check

Supporting Research/Description of Technique. More of a clinical assessment procedure, assessment of vocal quality bears a brief mention under techniques for swallowing compensation. Given the risks of silent aspiration, however, reliability of the technique should be confirmed radiographically.

Patient Instruction. The patient is instructed to monitor vocal quality during oral intake. Wet vocal quality, as a clinical sign of aspiration, should be promptly followed by a cough response or throat clear until the dysphonia clears. The patient may also be aware of changes in vocal resonances secondary to an increase of pharyngeal residual.

Coaching Tips. Considerable teaching may need to precede independent use of this technique by a patient. Audio recordings of vocal quality under various conditions may be used as a focus of discussion during initial teaching.

Example Goal. The patient will recognize wet vocal quality following ingestion of liquids with minimal cues and will successfully clear until vocal quality is clear.

Prosthetic Devices: Tracheostomy Valves

Supporting Research/Description of Technique. Tracheostomy in the patient with neurologic disorder is generally indicated in a patient post ventilation for treatment of pneumonia or when access to the lungs for pulmonary toilet is required in patients with pulmonary illness or aspiration. There have been a number of studies evaluating the effects of tracheostomy on swallowing (Bonano, 1970; Buckwalter & Sasaki, 1984; DeVita & Spierer-Rundback, 1990; Eibling & Gross, 1996; Nash, 1988; Sasaki, Suzki, Horiuchi & Kirchner, 1977). In summary, tracheostomy has been found to influence swallowing by:

1. Minimizing laryngeal excursion by anchoring the trachea to the overlying skin, mucosa and muscle, thus influencing airway protection and bolus propulsion
2. Compressing the anterior wall of the esophagus by the pressure of the tracheostomy tube on the shared tracheo-esophageal wall
3. Altering intra-tracheal pressure

4. Creating desensitization of the upper airway with prolonged presence of the tube secondary to the diversion of airflow away from the oropharyngeal cavity
5. Weakening vocal fold closure for airway protection

Closure of the tracheostomy tube via cap or one-way valve has been evaluated as a mechanism to improve airway protection and facilitate more efficient swallowing. In the head and neck cancer population it has been documented that occlusion of a tracheosomy will decrease the incidence of aspiration occurring with a non-occluded trach tube (Dettelbach, Gross, Mahlmann, & Eibling, 1995; Logemann, 1983; Muz, Hamlet, Mathog, & Farris, 1994; Muz, Mathog, Nelson, & Jones, 1989). However, this finding has not been as strongly supported in other populations. According to a 1997 study by Leder and colleagues, occlusion of the tracheostomy tube does not decrease aspiration risk. It is suggested, however, that the duration of occlusion may play an important role on its physiologic effects, with the possibility that "short-term" occlusion is not as adventageous as "long-term" occlusion. This research, in contrast to what is seen frequently in clinical practice, suggests the need for full evaluation of various swallowing conditions before outlining a treatment plan. Instructions for overall management of the patient with tracheostomy tube, including the weaning process, is beyond the scope of this text and the reader is referred to other more comprehensive texts (Dikeman & Kazandjian, 1995).

Patient Instruction. Tracheostomy occlusion can occur by either a cap, which allows no airflow, or a one-way speaking valve, which allows inspiratory airflow through the tracheostomy. It is important that any management of a tracheostomized patient be completed in cooperation with other members of the health care team, particularly respiratory care and nursing. Meticulous hygiene is required to minimize the risk of infection.

Contraindications. The management and implications of tracheostomy management in speech and swallowing are complex. Although presence of a tracheostomy allows for access to the pulmonary system for suctioning, patients with tracheostomy may have fewer pulmonary reserves, thus requiring careful management.

A FEW COMMENTS ABOUT POSITIONING

The unique issues and complications of managing the dependent feeder are discussed in Chapter 10. But, there exists a broad range of

skills between autonomy and dependence. Thus, as appropriate positioning can be considered a prerequisite to optimal oral intake, it is addressed
briefly in this section as well. When addressing positioning for feeding in
the neurogenic population, the necessity of maximizing multidisciplinary
efforts cannot be overstated. Colleagues in physical and occupational
therapy should be consulted and included in the treatment planning process. The importance of appropriate positioning for eating, whether the
patient eats in the dining room or in bed, is critical. Appropriate positioning improves a patient's ability to self-feed, will aid in airway protection,
and provide maximal comfort (Hotaling, 1990). Whenever possible, a patient should be sitting upright with the pelvis as far back as possible in a
solid chair, with solid arms. This will add stability and allow upper extremity movement for self-feeding. The hips should be at a 90-degree angle,
with both feet placed flat on the floor and shoulders slightly forward. The
arms of a patient should be supported on the table or arms of the chair; it
is important the affected arm of adults with hemiplegia not be allowed to
lie in the lap as they cannot use it for self-feeding in that position (Koltin
& Rosen, 1996b). The head should be upright and aligned with the trunk.
Patients should be positioned for feeding according to the following sequence: pelvis, trunk, legs, arms, and head.

Koltin and Rosen (1996b) discuss the importance of establishing and
maintaining trunk control, beginning in the pelvis, in the treatment of stroke
patients who need to relearn how to feed themselves. The embarrassment
of not being able to feed themselves in a socially appropriate way may
impact nutritional intake (Levy, 1993). They suggest that clinicians should
first understand what constitutes normal self-feeding movements and subsequently assess the abnormal movements observed in the stroke patient.
Based on these observations, a variety of treatment approaches can be introduced to meet the goals of helping the patient quickly achieve feeding
independence, control, adequate intake, and improved self-esteem.

Three common interventions to improve self-feeding skills in the
stroke patient are facilitation, motor learning, and compensation (Koltin
& Rosen, 1996c). Facilitation focuses on motor recovery by altering the
sensory motor input. This treatment is based on the theory that central
nervous system (CNS) lesions lead to abnormal movements, because the
higher cortex does not adequately inhibit these movements. It hypoth-
esizes that CNS lesions, not biomechanical factors, cause the motor deficits. It postulates that increased sensory motor input improves CNS integration and organization for correct movement patterns. The treatment
approaches associated with facilitation are the Bobath neurodevelopmental
approach (NDT) and the proprioceptive neuromuscular facilitation approach (PNF).

NDT focuses on inhibiting abnormal movements and facilitating normal ones even on the affected side, and allows for movement to take place at a normal speed. NDT attempts to normalize tone and improve the quality of movement in stroke patients so that they can learn to feed themselves and perform other functional activities. Clinicians use various techniques such as weightbearing, rotation, elongation, and positioning, to counteract or inhibit abnormal motor patterns. They use key points of control either proximally (head/neck, pelvis, shoulder girdle) or distally (wrist, fingers) to provide sensory motor input and, thereby, enhance stability in one area to allow skilled movement in another. The clinician can manually guide a patient in the desired movement, and gradually decreases the input as the patient begins to relearn the movement and actively assume control (Bobath, 1990). Some clinicians have become interested in the application of NDT adapted techniques in the treatment of dysphagia and self-feeding. The literature does not offer any reports of improved physiologic benefits of swallowing using these techniques. However, the importance of body position in directing bolus flow in dysphagia is wellknown, thus NDT may be a useful tool in establishing and enhancing normal body positioning to provide a foundation for feeding.

PNF focuses on quickening the response of neuomuscular movements using proprioception and other sensory input, such as quick stretch, manual guiding, maximal resistance, rhythmic stabilization, and slow reversals in movements to enhance coordinated reciprocal movements. Physical agent modalities (PAMs), such as the use of biofeedback and neuromuscular electrical stimulation, may also be used in conjunction with these approaches to facilitate improved physical posturing.

Motor learning approaches also emphasize remediation of motor impairment in the stroke patient. These approaches theorize that skilled, smooth movements are the result of several complex interactions from the CNS, musculoskeletal system, and biomechanics. The main premise of a motor learning approach is that the control of movement is centered on goal-driven, functional activities. The importance of involving the participation of the patient in the treatment goals and tasks is crucial because without active patient involvement, improved motor control will not be attained. This is a relatively new model of treatment that still has not demonstrated validity in stroke patients, but it is suggested as an adjunct to traditional facilitation approaches (Sabari, 1991).

Compensatory approaches to self-feeding are the same as in dysphagia treatment. The goal is to enhance function in order to make the patient as independent as possible, but they do not focus on remediating the motor deficits. Adaptive techniques and equipment, in addition to environmental modifications, are commonly used in compensatory treatments.

SUMMARY

Three points are made in summary of this chapter on compensation:

1. Application of compensatory techniques must be based on the swallowing physiology demonstrated by the individual patient. Because of the widely varying nature of dysphagic symptoms, no assumptions can be made about management until individual patient physiology is understood.
2. Patients with cognitive impairment offer great challenges for the clinician in developing a management plan that is feasible and efficacious. Creativity in environmental manipulation will be required to maximize the patients potential for recall and execution of compensatory strategies.
3. Management of the patient with dysphagia is an interdisciplinary issue. A narrow focus on swallowing physiology without attention to postural and nutritional aspects will likely be ineffective.

Whether compensatory approaches are used for short-term or long-term management, the goal is to maximize potential for safe oral intake and improved quality of life.

7

Malnutrition and Dehydration in Dysphagia

This chapter discusses the nutrient and hydration requirements in the elderly and define the terms nutrition, malnutrition, and dehydration. The causes, indicators, risk factors, and effects of aging on malnutrition and dehydration are given. The presence of dysphagia can impact the nutrient and hydration needs of a patient. The role of speech-language pathologists is discussed with respect to the nutritional management of dysphagia. Specific coaching tips are provided to clinicians.

There are many reasons a patient may become malnourished or dehydrated. Dysphagia may or may not play a role in precipitating these significant health problems. It is a complex task to diagnose and manage a patient's nutritional status. Consequently, it is often difficult to discern the role of dysphagia in the management of nutritional status. Nutrition intervention often involves many components, with dysphagia intervention usually one of many initiatives offered to manage nutritional status. Many other factors may contribute to the success or failure of managing nutritional status. Therefore, successful dysphagia intervention may or may not result in improved nutritional status, and it is difficult to ascertain how important dysphagia intervention is in producing the observed effect. Given the complex nature of managing nutritional status, outcome measurements that attempt to demonstrate a clear association between improved nutritional status and successful dysphagia intervention are difficult to establish. It is hoped that as clinicians begin to appreciate the complexities involved in diagnosing and managing malnutrition and dehydration, especially in the elderly population, they can better understand their role in improving nutritional status as they provide dysphagia intervention.

MALNUTRITION

Nutrient Intake in the Elderly

The published recommended daily allowances (RDAs) most commonly referenced by the public were developed from studies of healthy young adults, not healthy elderly (Granieri, 1990; Kerstetter, Holthausen, & Fitz, 1993). Estimating calorie intake for the elderly is not easy, since many physiologic changes occur with aging that affect nutritional needs.

The recommended caloric needs for the elderly need to be individually calculated by the dietitian. Dietitians commonly use a cut-off point of two-thirds or three-quarters of the RDA to identify inadequate intake levels, since the original RDAs are based on two standard deviations above the average requirement for an individual, with the exception for energy requirements (Kerstetter et al., 1993). This formula was used to encompass individual variability and meet the needs of 98% of the population.

However, meeting the RDAs does not necessarily mean elderly patients have met their nutritional requirements, just as low intake does not indicate a deficiency. Intake below the RDA indicates only greater risk for a deficiency. The variability of medical problems, medications taken, metabolic rate, and overall functional problems of the elderly make estimation of caloric needs a complicated task.

Definition of Nutrition and Malnutrition

Poorly defined terminology in the fields of dysphagia and nutrition is frequently the cause of confusion among disciplines. Since communication is crucial between team members, it is important to examine the definitions of common terminology to avoid misunderstandings and enhance implementation of the treatment plan. Just as "dysphagia" has many definitions in the literature, "nutrition" and "malnutrition" also have numerous definitions. These definitions refer to the processes or stages of taking in nutrients (nutrition) and any disorder that may alter these processes (malnutrition), resulting in impaired absorption, assimilation, or use of the nutrients (Table 7–1).

Extent of Malnutrition in the Elderly

Malnutrition is reported to be quite common in hospitals and chronic care facilities. Hospitalized patients and long-term care residents have the greatest incidence of malnutrition compared to other populations, with as many as 40% of the patients and residents in these settings documented to have malnutrition (Table 7–2). It is difficult to estimate accurately the extent of malnutrition in the elderly who live in the community, since this diagnosis alone does not usually lead a patient to seek medical attention. However, even this population is reported to have a 25% incidence of malnutrition.

National efforts to increase public awareness of nutritional health have been developed by a national advisory committee, under the leadership of the American Dietetic Association, American Academy of Family Physicians, and the National Council on the Aging, Inc. This committee developed a manual for professionals who work with older Americans, depicting

Table 7–1. Definitions of nutrition and malnutrition.

Term	Definition
Nutrition	The sum of the processes involved in the taking in of nutrients and in their assimilation and use for proper body functioning and maintenance of health. The successive stages include ingestion, digestion, absorption, assimilation, and excretion.[1]
	The study of food and liquid requirements of human beings or animals for normal physiologic function, including energy, need, maintenance, growth, activity, reproduction, and lactation.[2]
Malnutrition	Any disorder of nutrition. It may result from an unbalanced, insufficient, or excess diet or from the impaired absorption, assimilation, or use of foods.[1]
	Faulty nutrition resulting from malabsorption, poor diet, or overeating.[2]

Sources: [1]From *Mosby's medical dictionary*, 4th ed., 1994, St. Louis: Mosby-Yearbook, Inc. [2]From *Stedman's medical dictionary*, 26th ed., 1995, Baltimore: Williams & Wilkins.

Table 7–2. Incidence of malnutrition in different populations.

Population	Percent Incidence	Source
All hospitalized patients	40	Roubenoff, Preto, and Balke, 1987
Elderly hospitalized patients	35–55	Barrocas et al., 1995; Bennet, 1992; Bistrian, Blackburn, Vitale, Cochroan, and Naylor, 1976; Nutrition Screening Initiative 1992, 1994; Kamath, Lawler, Smith, Kalat, and Olsen, 1986; Mowe and Behmer, 1991; Reilly, Hull, Albert, Waller and Bringardener, 1988
Long-term-care residents	40	Bernstein and Jordan, 1995; Hart and Associates, 1993; Keller, 1993
Elderly in the community	25	Coats, Morgan, Bartolucci, and Weinsier, 1993; Codispoti and Bartlett, 1994; North Carolina Department of Human Resources, 1993; Roubenoff, Preto, and Balke, 1987; U.S. Department of Health and Human Services, 1994

a variety of nutrition screening tools and interventions (Nutrition Screening Initiative, 1992).

It is interesting to note that one nutrition screening tool to provide early warning signs of poor nutritional health includes several factors associated with the presence of dysphagia, such as the presence of an illness or condition that changes the kind and/or amount of food eaten, tooth or mouth problems that make it hard to eat, or unintentional weight loss (Table 7–3). This tool is designed to help determine a person's nutritional risk only, and cannot determine the actual presence of malnutrition. Likewise, dysphagia cannot be determined from this screening tool, but it may help a person seek more timely diagnosis and treatment.

Causes of Malnutrition

Malnutrition is caused when any deficiency, imbalance, or excess of nutrient(s) occurs within the body, in a variety of combinations and degrees

Table 7–3. National screening test for malnutrition in the elderly.

	Yes
I have an illness or condition that made me change the kind and/or amount of food I eat.	2
I eat fewer than 2 meals per day.	3
I eat few fruits or vegetables, or milk products.	2
I have 3 or more drinks of beer, liquor, or wine almost every day.	2
I have tooth or mouth problems that make it hard for me to eat.	2
I don't always have enough money to buy the food I need.	4
I eat alone most of the time.	1
I take 3 or more different prescribed or over-the-counter drugs a day.	2
Without wanting to, I have lost or gained 10 pounds in the last 6 months.	2
I am not always physically able to shop, cook, and/or feed myself.	2
TOTAL	

Total Your Nutritional Score. If it's

0–2	Good! Re-check your nutritional score in 6 months.
3–5	You are at moderate nutritional risk. See what can be done to improve your eating habits and lifestyle. Your office on aging, senior nutrition program, senior citizens center or health department can help. Recheck your nutritional score in 3 months.
6 or more	You are at high nutritional risk. Bring this checklist the next time you see your doctor, dietitian or other qualified health or social service professional. Talk with them about any problems you may have. Ask for help to improve your nutritional health.

Source: From *Nutrition intervention manual for professionals caring for older americans* by Nutrition Screening Initiative, 1992, Washington, DC: Author.

(Cope, 1996). There are many etiologies of malnutrition, with dysphagia playing a major or minor role at times. The consequences of malnutrition can be severe, with overall decreased mental and physical function and even death. Therefore it is important to understand all the reasons why malnutrition may occur so that the role dysphagia may play can be more accurately determined and managed.

Indicators of Malnutrition

Indicators are defined as signs or symptoms of a problem. The presence of one indicator does not necessarily indicate the presence of malnutrition, but it does increase the possibility of malnutrition. Dysphagia is one of many possible indicators of malnutrition, which can include weight loss, poor oral/dental status, and cognitive loss, among others. (Table 7–4).

According to a national assessment tool used in nursing homes called the Resident Assessment Instrument (RAI) (see Chapter 12), the following indicators of nutritional status would be flagged for further investigation and possible intervention (Cameron, 1997, p. 45):

1. Significant weight loss
2. Presence of taste alterations
3. Presence of parenteral or intravenous (IV) feeding
4. Diet order for mechanically altered diet, syringe feeding, or therapeutic diet

Table 7–4. Major and minor indicators of malnutrition.

Major Indicators	Minor Indicators
Weight loss of 10 lbs.+	Alcoholism
Under-/overweight	Cognitive Impairment
Serum albumin below 3.5 g/dl	Chronic renal insufficiency
Change in functional status	Multiple concurrent medications
Inappropriate food intake	Malabsorption syndromes
Mid-arm muscle circumference < 10th percentile	Anorexia, nausea, dysphagia
Triceps skinfold < 10th percentile or > 95th percentile	Change in bowel habit
Obesity	Fatigue, apathy, memory loss

Nutrition-related disorders
  Osteoporosis
  Osteomalacia
  Folate deficiency
  B_{12} deficiency
	Poor oral/dental status
	Dehydration
	Poorly healing wounds
	Loss of subcutaneous fat or muscle mass
	Fluid retention
	Reduced iron, ascorbic acid, zinc

Source: From *Malnutrition in the elderly: A national crisis* by K. Cope, 1996, p. 8, Washington, DC: U.S. Government Printing Office.

5. Twenty-five percent of food left uneaten at most meals
6. Presence of pressure ulcers

Obviously, the presence of any of these indicators would "trigger" or flag the need for further investigation in any setting. In the nursing home setting, specific guidelines are given to assess any of these indicators further. These guidelines are called Resident Assessment Protocols (RAPs). The RAPs provide guidelines regarding various parameters that may require further assessment of nutritional assessment. The following indicators would require further evaluation (Cameron, 1997, p. 46):

1. Weight change (unintentional loss or gain) of 1 to 2% or more in 1 week, 5% or more in 1 month, 7.5% or more in 3 months, or 10% or more in 6 months
2. Possible fluid imbalance
3. Signs and symptoms of malnutrition, including muscle or fat wastage; bilateral edema; reduced urine output; pale skin, mucosa, or nail beds; poor skin turgor; dull eyes; swollen lips or gums; swollen and/or dry tongue with scarlet or magenta hue
4. Abnormal laboratory test results, including serum albumin, prealbumin, hemoglobin, hematocrit, transferrin, total lymphocyte count, blood urea nitrogen (BUN), glucose, sodium, potassium, magnesium, thyroid status, calculated serum osmolality, and calculated creatinine clearance
5. Possible drug-nutrient interactions
6. Hydration status
7. Pressure ulcers

In addition, it is important to assess other types of problems that may affect nutritional status. These may include dementia, paranoia (fear that food is poisoned), pacing, feeding dependency, communication problems that affect ability to make needs known, and ill-fitting dentures (Cameron, 1997). Similar to the diagnosis of dysphagia, the diagnosis of malnutrition involves the clinical interpretation of a variety of indicators. In particular, the elderly have special nutrition needs that are complex to diagnose and manage, requiring a medical team approach.

Risk Factors of Malnutrition

The risk factors for malnutrition are complex and diverse, ranging from physiologic, psychological, and socioeconomic factors to the simple lack of information regarding nutrition, due to poor access (Table 7–5). Anything that interferes with the body's intake of adequate nutrient(s) at the

Table 7–5. Risk factors for malnutrition.

Physiologic Factors	Psychological Factors
Presence and severity of dysphagia	Depression
Acute/chronic diseases or conditions	Mental/cognitive problems
Medication use	
Oral/dental problems	
Sensory changes	
Physical disabilities	
Advanced age (80+)	
Socioeconomic Factors	**Lack of Nutritional Knowledge**
Poverty	Poor access to information
Social Isolation	
Dependency/disability	

Source: From *Malnutrition in the elderly: A national crisis* by K. Cope, 1996, pp. 8, 11, Washington, DC: U.S. Government Printing Office.

cellular level may cause malnutrition, and is considered to be a potential risk factor.

Processes Involved with Nutritional Status

The processes involved in providing adequate nutrition are ingestion, digestion, absorption, metabolism, assimilation (getting the nutrients to the tissues), and excretion (Cope, 1996). The progressive effects of malnutrition lead to physical and psychological decline, and eventually cause death.

Presence of Acute or Chronic Medical Problem(s)

Increased risk of malnutrition is present whenever an elderly patient has an acute medical problem, such as a urinary tract infection, or a chronic medical problem, such as chronic obstructive pulmonary obstructive disease (COPD) (Granieri, 1990). Any medical condition can cause decreased food intake in the elderly, as a result of increased fatigue. In patients with COPD, poor intake can result from the increased effort necessary to eat

(Granieri, 1990). Whenever a patient does not feel well, he or she may not eat well.

Feeding Dependency

Physical or cognitive impairments may result in the need for a patient to be fed. However, poor nutritional intake is common in these patients, possibly in relation to caregiver feeding practices and philosophy (Sanders et al., 1992). The many issues and challenges surrounding the management of feeding dependent patients with dysphagia are discussed at length in Chapter 10.

Social Isolation and Poverty

The death of a spouse or physical disability can lead to depression, immobility, and poor eating habits (Granieri, 1990). The social isolation and decreased finances due to these losses can directly impact the nutritional status of a person. While these factors will not directly cause dysphagia, they may be present in a patient with dysphagia.

It is a great challenge to manage patients with dysphagia who are emotionally and/or physically isolated from a social support system, and who may lack sufficient funds to purchase nutritious foods. Clinicians need to remember that the basic needs for survival must be met before dysphagia intervention can be implemented with any chance of success. These factors would certainly be evaluated during the informal assessment of the patient and weigh heavily in the management plan.

Use of Medications

It is well known that certain medications result in unpleasant side effects, such as decreased appetite (anorexia), dry mouth, nausea, and diarrhea (Feinberg, 1996). All of these factors may decrease oral intake, causing decreased nutritional status.

A medication designed to improve one medical condition can create or exacerbate dysphagia. Drug-induced confusion is common due to medication as well. All of these factors can interfere with a patient's overall rehabilitation (Feinberg, 1996). Careful consultation with the physician and pharmacist is strongly recommended, to help determine the possible effect of the patients' medications on their oral intake and plan appropriate intervention, including the best manner of administration.

Effect of Aging on Malnutrition

Metabolic, Biochemical, and Physiologic Changes with Aging

It is generally agreed that many metabolic, biochemical, and physiologic processes change with increasing age (Nelson, Moxness, Jensen, & Gastineau, 1994). These changes may adversely affect the nutritional status of the elderly. The ability to digest and absorb nutrients decreases in the gastrointestinal tract. There are body composition changes that occur with aging, such as decreased lean body mass, total body water and decreased bone mass. These body composition changes occur simultaneously while adipose tissue and plasma volume increase. A decline in the ability to tolerate carbohydrates, in combination with a lower metabolic rate, make the elderly more vulnerable to obesity and diabetes. All of these physiologic changes with aging, and others as listed in Table 7–6, may introduce the elderly patient to greater nutritional risk.

Nutrient needs also change with aging and challenge the notion of what dietary recommendations are appropriate for the elderly. The need for Vitamin A decreases with age and makes the elderly susceptible to toxicity with supplements. Yet other nutrient needs increase with age, such as protein (American Dietetic Association, 1996). Maintaining adequate nutrition in the elderly is a challenge for all health care providers.

Decreased Perception of Hunger with Aging

Decreased perceptions of hunger and thirst have been observed with aging, which may predispose even a healthy older person to anorexia and dehydration (Rolls, 1989; Rolls & Phillips, 1990). Decreased hunger in the elderly may also be influenced by multiple medical conditions and the use of medications. Clinicians need to be aware that these factors may contribute to low nutrient intake, in addition to dysphagia.

Dental and Vision Changes with Aging

Fifty percent of those over 65 years of age are edentulous (Granieri, 1990). This fact, coupled with poorly fitted dentures, can contribute to a patient's inability to manage a variety of food textures. In addition, the elderly frequently suffer from decreased vision, because of cataracts, diabetic retinopathy, or macular degeneration (Granieri, 1990). Visual loss can impact a patient's ability to prepare food or self-feed, leading to poor nutritional status.

Table 7–6. Physiologic changes with aging.

Physiologic Changes	Potential Impact on Nutritional Status
Decreased volume and viscosity of saliva; atrophy of taste buds	Dry mouth, difficulty chewing and initiating swallow, decreased taste sensation, anorexia, pain and irritation from foodstuffs → avoidance of many food items → decreased food intake
Atrophy of olfactory receptors	Decreased sense of smell and taste sensation, foods lose appeal → decreased food intake
Missing teeth, periodontitis	Poorly fitting dentures cause difficulty chewing → restricted variety of food or decreased food intake. Dentures interfere with sense of taste → food loses appeal → decreased food intake
Impaired vision and hearing	Interferes with socialization at mealtimes, difficulty in food preparation → diminished enjoyment of food → decreased intake
Decreased secretion of acid in stomach, enzymes in small intestine, and decreased peristalsis	Diminished digestion and absorption of some nutrients
Decreased capacity of kidney to concentrate urine	Dehydration and need for increased water to prevent azotemia
Decreased intestinal motility, weakened abdominal and pelvic muscles, and decreased sensory perception	Chronic constipation → decreased or altered food intake
Decreased lean body mass, increased increased adipose tissue, lower metabolic rate	Vulnerable to obesity
Decreased breathing capacity	Limited activity → decreased caloric expenditure → obesity or decreased food intake → wasting
Decline in glucose tolerance	Vulnerable to development of diabetes → restricted dietary selections decreased food intake

Source: From *Mayo clinic diet manual: A handbook of nutrition practices,* 7th ed., p. 59, by J. K. Nelson, K. E. Moxness, J. D. Jensen, & C. F. Gastineau, 1994, St. Louis: Mosby-Year Book, Inc. Reprinted by permission.

Taste and Olfactory Changes with Aging

Decreased taste and olfactory acuity occur with aging (Granieri, 1990). In the elderly, the ability to taste flavors may be decreased because of the decreased number of papillae or taste buds per papillae, or as a result of taste bud atrophy (Cooper, Bikash, & Zubek, 1959; Liss & Gomez, 1958). Decreased volume and viscosity of saliva may also contribute to decreased taste sensation and difficulty chewing and swallowing foods (Nelson et al., 1994). In addition, decreased texture can diminish taste (Jaime, Mela, & Bratchell, 1993; Overbosch, Afterof, & Haring, 1991; Schiffman, 1973), and thereby result in poor intake. The inability to chew certain textures, because of oral, dental, or swallowing problems, may affect food choices and thus decrease intake (see Chapter 9).

Role of Protein-Calorie Malnutrition Causing Dysphagia

An interesting question regarding the role protein-calorie malnutrition (PCM) may play in causing dysphagia has been discussed by Veldee and Peth (1992). They suggest that the presence of PCM in an individual with dysphagia may negatively affect patient morbidity and mortality.

Although it is known that muscle mass decreases with age (Kerstetter et al., 1993), PCM can also lead to decreased muscle mass, inadequate immune response, and marked functional decline noted within muscle cells (Young, 1990; Young, Munro, & Fukagawa, 1989; Veldee & Peth, 1992). No research has yet specifically addressed how the muscles and neural pathways for deglutition may be affected by malnutrition.

However, Veldee and Peth (1992) suggest that while the underlying disease or condition causing dysphagia may mask the contributions of PCM, the presence of PCM in patients with dysphagia may have clinical relevance. They argue that PCM in a patient with dysphagia can increase the incidence of aspiration episodes and subsequent risk for pneumonia, exacerbate the severity of the dysphagia, or interfere with a patient's ability to recover from aspiration pneumonia.

Nonoral Nutrition for Patients with PCM

Based on this hypothesis, they recommend that patients with dysphagia and subsequent malnutrition initially receive nonoral nutrient intake. Repletion of nutrient store to the muscle cells may quickly improve swallowing ability, although this has not been demonstrated empirically. In addition, they caution that attempts to feed malnourished patients with dysphagia orally, even when the diet is modified, may actually increase the risk of aspiration because of the effects of PCM on the dysphagia.

DEHYDRATION

Hydration in the Elderly

Pure water is an essential body nutrient. In general, dietitians calculate the recommended fluid requirements for the elderly using the standard of 30 ml/kg of desired weight (Kerstetter et al., 1993). However, a recent study compared this standard with two other established standards to determine adequacy of fluid intake in the institutionalized elderly. Chidester and Spangler (1997) found that this standard resulted in unrealistically low fluid recommendations for underweight residents and too high of a recommendation for overweight residents.

A New Standard for Determining Fluid Requirements in the Elderly

Chidester and Spangler (1997) suggest a standard of 100 ml/kg for the first 10 kg, 50 ml/kg for the next 10 kg, and 15 ml/kg for the remaining kg body weight. This standard adjusts for extremes in body weight and is more reasonable for all patients, regardless of whether they are underweight, of normal weight, or overweight.

Definition of Dehydration

Dehydration is defined as a deficit of pure water, an essential body nutrient (Levinsky, 1987). The loss of body water affects several important physiological functions, such as increasing the risk of infection, renal failure, increased falls, and related injury and confusion (Table 7–7). These consequences of dehydration are serious and can dramatically affect the health and mental well-being of a patient.

Extent of Dehydration in the Elderly

The extent of dehydration in elderly individuals who reside in the community has not been established (Rolls, 1989). However, dehydration has long been recognized as a problem in the elderly, especially for those individuals who reside in institutions (Hoffman, 1991; Lavizzo-Mourey, 1987; Lavizzo-Mourey, Johnson, & Stolley, 1988; Leaf, 1984; Warren et al., 1994).

Dehydration is present in 25% of nonambulatory geriatric patients, according to one study (Spangler, Risley, & Bilyew, 1984). These patients were found to be dehydrated initially in this study, as measured by specific gravity of the urine. An intervention consisting of regular verbal prompts

Table 7–7. Effect of dehydration on body function.

Increased risk of infection

Renal failure

Decreased skin turgor, with skin breakdown

Increased falls and related injury

Confusion

Lethargy

Constipation with impaction

Xerostomia

Decreased body regulation

Toxicity of water-soluble medications

Increased thirst

Sources: Adapted from "Nutrition and the older adult" by E. Granieri, 1990, *Dysphagia, 4,* 199; "Dehydration in the elderly: Insidious and manageable" by N. B. Hoffman, 1991, *Geriatrics, 46*(6), 35; "Nutrition and nutritional requirements for the older adult" by J. E. Kerstetter, B. A. Holthausen, and P. A. Fitz, 1993, *Dysphagia, 8,* 54.

and assistance with fluids completely eliminated dehydration in these subjects. This simple, but apparently powerful, treatment deserves careful consideration by all health care providers.

Causes of Dehydration

Dehydration may be caused by a variety of problems. Abrams, Beers, and Berkow (1995) list the following etiologies for dehydration:

1. Decreased food or fluid intake
2. Febrile illness
3. Diabetes Mellitus
4. Vomiting
5. Diarrhea
6. Chronic renal disease
7. Use of diuretics
8. Nasogastric suction

The causes of dehydration may also result in a phenomenon called volume depletion. This occurs after the body loses water and sodium, and, subsequently, extracellular fluid (ECF) is decreased (Abrams et al., 1995). As Abrams and colleagues (1995) describe, there is a complex hormonal system that regulates body fluid. Body sodium content is regulated by a balance between dietary intake and renal excretion, since fluid loss due to sweat and stool are normally small. The body self-regulates the amount of ECF through thirst perception and secretion of antidiuretic hormone (ADH, or vasopressin), the major hormone to regulate water balance. In addition, other hormones contribute to maintaining ECF, such as hormones that regulate sodium excretion, blood pressure, renal blood flow, glomerular filtration rate, and kidney sympathetic nerve activity and response system.

Indicators of Dehydration

There are many indicators that physicians, nurses, and dietitians use to diagnose dehydration. A patient may present with increased body thirst, dry mouth, decreased skin turgor, constipation, lethargy, confusion, and decreased body temperature regulation. The lack of adequate body fluid can cause an excessive response to heat and cold, inducing hyperthermia or hypothermia (Kerstetter et al., 1993). Frequently, physicians and dietitians rely on certain serum (blood) lab values to indicate dehydration. These are electrolyte and blood urea nitrogen (BUN)/creatinine blood tests, which measure the amount of sodium and protein in the blood, respectively (Henderson, 1991).

When dietitians assess a patient for possible dehydration, they collect a variety of important data before contacting the physician. They evaluate the amount of fluid intake ingested daily, body weight and any changes, medications being administered, medical diagnoses, and the results of various lab values. The normal and acceptable range for various tests that indicate possible dehydration will vary, according to every lab performing the tests. Therefore, dietitians usually use the cut-off points provided by their facility's lab to determine when a value is abnormal and should be brought to the physician's attention.

Recognizing that every lab may provide a slightly different range, Nelson and colleagues (1994) place the normal range value for sodium between 135 and 145 mEq/L. Serum creatinine can overestimate renal functioning in the elderly, and therefore a ratio of serum BUN/creatinine is recommended to assess renal function more accurately. The serum BUN/creatinine ratio generally needs to be 25 or higher to indicate dehydration (Hoffman, 1991).

Depending on the cause of dehydration, the lab values for the amount of sodium in the blood will differ. If patients have poor intake of body fluids, their serum sodium level will be too high. This is called *hypernatremia.*

If patients lose a vital amount of body fluid quickly, such as with diarrhea or nausea, their blood sodium may rapidly decrease as the sodium is washed out of the body. This condition is called *hyponatremia*. Because diarrhea can occur with tube feedings, this cause for dehydration must be monitored carefully. Therefore, the presence of hypernatremia or hyponatremia may indicate dehydration but is due to different causes, either too little or too much body fluid in relation to sodium content.

In addition, another common form of hyponatremina in the elderly may occur when sodium content is normal but water is retained, because of increased ADH secretion (Abrams et al., 1995). This may occur when underlying disorders that lead to low fluid intake increase ADH secretion. In this case, fluid intake is too low to produce dilutional hyponatremia. However, when fluid intake increases, such as when fluids are encouraged due to fever or low intake, the increase in body water may lead to the rapid development of hyponatremia. If serum sodium values are too low (< 115 mEq/L) and drop quickly, sudden death may occur (Abrams et al., 1995). Another common cause for hyponatremia in the elderly is the use of nutritional supplements, such as Isocal, Ensure, or Osmolite since these formulas are extremely low in sodium (Abrams et al., 1995). Therefore, the presence of hyponatremia (low sodium in the blood) may be due to dehydration or "overhydration." Given the complexities of these nutritional issues, clinicians need to rely on their medical team for appropriate interpretation of any abnormal lab values or dehydration indicators.

Risk Factors of Dehydration

The risk factors associated with dehydration are numerous, with dysphagia, feeding dependency, impaired communication, and cognition skills listed, among others, in Table 7–8. Clinicians should be aware of these risk factors in their patients, especially since elderly patients are at risk of dehydration even when dysphagia is not present.

Living in an Institution

Many studies have suggested that individuals who are institutionalized may receive inadequate fluid (Hoffman, 1991; Lavizzo-Mourey, 1987; Lavizzo-Mourey et al., 1988; Leaf, 1984; Warren et al., 1994). Residents in an institution may not receive proper hydration for a variety of reasons related to their overall health status, poor access to fluids, and caregiver dependence. For more information regarding the impact of feeding dependency on dysphagia, see Chapter 10.

Table 7–8. Risk factors of dehydration.

Decreased water access due to immobility, poor visual ability, and/or altered mental status

Presence and severity of dysphagia, leading to fear of oral intake

Fear of urinary incontinence, leading to diminished fluid intake

Administration of diuretics

Previous dehydration episodes

Anorexia, as the poor eater is usually the poor drinker of fluids

Acute illness superimposed on chronic disability

Feeding dependency

Impaired communication skills

Impaired cognitive skills

Low frequency of medications

Low percentage of meal consumption

Poor fluid intake, taken from *both* beverages and solid foods

Administration of either IV radiographic contrast agents or high protein enteral feeding, causing an osmotic diuresis

Sources: Adapted from "Fluid intake in the institutionalized elderly" by A. C. Chidester and A. A. Spangler, 1997, *Journal of the American Dietetic Association, 97*(1), 27; and "Dehydration in the elderly: Insidious and manageable" by N. B. Hoffman, 1991, *Geriatrics, 46*(6), 35.

Use of Medications

Interestingly, one study found that increased fluid intake between meals was noted in institutionalized elderly, in direct correlation to the number and frequency of medications administered to them (Chidester & Spangler, 1997). In other words, the more medications they received, the less likely they were to have poor fluid intake. Their findings suggest that adequate fluid intake in long-term care elderly residents may be dependent on receiving fluid with their medications. On the other hand, the use of some medications such as diuretics, can actually increase dehydration (Hoffman, 1991). Therefore, it appears that the presence or even the absence of medications administered to patients may increase the risk of dehydration.

Physical/Cognitive Limitations

Many elderly, especially those who reside in long-term care settings, lack the physical and/or cognitive ability to hold a glass of water independently, or reach the water faucet to get something to drink (Russell, 1997). In these cases, staff must be encouraged to offer fluids throughout the day, perhaps with each visit to the bathroom or through facility programs that encourage increased hydration, such as a Happy Hour where bulk refreshments are delivered daily to nursing home residents on their unit in a social atmosphere (Musson et al., 1990; Russell, 1997). Cup holders attached to wheelchairs may also increase access and motivation to drink adequate fluids for those patients who are wheelchair bound.

Self-Imposed Fluid Restriction

Clinicians need to remember that some elderly may self-restrict fluid intake in an effort to avoid "accidents" of incontinence and maintain dignity. These patients are usually acutely aware of their health problems. They may increase their risk of dehydration, rather than risk social embarrassment. Solutions to decrease the frequency of incontinence can be developed by the medical team, such as the use of a daily toileting schedule. For example, a patient may be offered an opportunity to be toileted every 2 hours initially, and upon success of remaining continent, the time between opportunities is gradually increased. A referral to a urologist and review of medications being administered may also be indicated.

Effect of Aging on Dehydration

Fluid Loss in Aging

There are changes that occur in total body fluid over time. Total body water has been found to decrease with age, in relation to decreased lean body mass (Cope, 1996; Schoeller, 1989; Watson, Watson, & Batt, 1980), making the elderly more susceptible to dehydration. A newborn infant is 80% water, but a mature adult is approximately 70%, decreasing to less than 60% in senescence (Reiff, 1989). It is unclear whether this decline is due to extracellular or intracellular decline (Kerstetter et al., 1993). This change may contribute to the difficulty the elderly have in maintaining adequate hydration.

Increased ADH Secretion

ADH (vasopressin) is the major hormone that regulates water balance in the body. With aging, the ability of the body to secrete ADH increases, which in turn leads to the loss of body fluid. It is hypothesized that the cause of increased ADH secretion may be impaired baroreceptor function, which normally inhibits ADH release. This increases the risk of hyponatremia in the elderly when fluid intake is increased, leading to a syndrome called syndrome of inappropriate secretion of ADH (Abrams et al., 1995).

Decreased Perception of Thirst in Aging

Decreased perceptions of thirst have been found in healthy elderly persons, increasing their risk for dehydration (Rolls, 1989; Rolls & Phillips, 1990). The reason why the elderly have diminished thirst is not fully understood. However, this impaired perception may result in a greater risk of decreased nutritional status, and increased risk for morbidity and mortality (Siebens et al., 1986). This is a complex problem that is not easily corrected. The key to maintaining adequate hydration in the elderly appears to be moderation and careful monitoring.

Decreased Ability to Conserve Free Water and Sodium

Healthy, elderly individuals exhibit a decreased ability to conserve free water and sodium (Abrams et al., 1995). In other words, aging predisposes otherwise healthy individuals to lose water and sodium when fluid intake is limited, thereby increasing the risk of dehydration. Since decreased thirst perception is present in aging, which leads to low fluid intake, healthy elderly individuals are easily prone to hyponatremia. The effects on body function of hyponatremia can include anorexia and weight change, among other factors (Table 7–9). Hyponatremia has been reported to be present in 22.5% of the patients admitted to a chronic disease unit, of whom most were elderly (Kleinfeld, Casimir, & Borra, 1979), and up to 11% of geriatric medicine department admissions (Sunderam & Mankikar, 1983). In one longitudinal study over 12 months, hyponatremia among elderly long-term care residents was about 50% (Abrams et al., 1995).

NUTRITIONAL MANAGEMENT AND DYSPHAGIA

The Medical Team: Roles and Importance

Given all the complexities of diagnosing and managing malnutrition and dehydration, speech-language pathologists must work within a medical team. The members of the team minimally are the physician, dietitian,

Table 7–9. Effect of hyponatremia on body function.

Postural hypotension

Weakness

Anorexia

Dry mucus membranes

Weight change

Mental confusion

Source: Adapted from "Nutrition and the older adult" by E. Granieri, 1990, *Dysphagia, 4*, 199.

speech-language pathologist, and patient. Depending on the setting and problems of every patient, additional team members may be involved, including nurse, dentist, otolaryngologist, pulmonologist, neurologist, gastroenterologist, radiologist, case manager, and social worker, to name just a few.

The registered dietitian and physician on the team provide the expertise regarding the diagnosis and management of malnutrition and dehydration. While speech-language pathologists are not trained to determine the nutritional status of a patient or the necessary nutrient content of their diet, clinicians should have a basic understanding of the terminology and management issues regarding various nutrient intake options to be an integral team member.

Every member brings a certain expertise to the team, and strengthens the ability of the team to identify the cause(s) and appropriate intervention(s) quickly and correctly, to manage malnutrition and dehydration. In keeping with a coaching analogy, the professional members of the medical team are similar to an entire coaching staff assembled for an athletic team. All coaches must share information and insights regarding the patient—the player—and decide together with the patient which intervention is best to manage their dysphagia, malnutrition, and/or dehydration.

Role of Speech-Language Pathologist in Nutrition Management

Speech-language pathologists provide information regarding the diagnosis and management of oropharyngeal dysphagia. Speech-language pathologists are trained to provide information about whether a patient with dysphagia can eat orally, and if so, *how* food and liquids can be swallowed safely. This does not automatically mean foods and liquids must be modified in some manner. Recommendations may include any of the various intervention options discussed in this text.

Clinicians can also provide information to the medical team regarding the endurance and ability of patients to meet their nutritional needs orally. Fatigue or a slow rate of ingestion can dramatically affect adequate, safe oral intake. The integration of this information by the team is crucial to develop an appropriate care plan to meet the nutritional needs of a patient with dysphagia.

The decision of whether a patient should be fed orally, nonorally, or by a combination of both is discussed fully in Chapter 8. The role of the speech-language pathologist is crucial in evaluating these options with the patient and other medical team members. The prevention and management of malnutrition and dehydration in patients with dysphagia are complicated.

Prevalence of Malnutrition, Dehydration and Dysphagia

Patients with dysphagia are obviously at risk for malnutrition and dehydration (Finestone, Greene-Finestone, Wilson, & Teasell, 1995; Ganger & Craig, 1990; Sitzmann, 1990; Sitzmann & Mueller, 1988). Dysphagia has been reported in 12 to13% of hospitalized patients, and 40% in long-term care facilities (Groher & Bukatman, 1986). As many as 90% of hospitalized patients with dysphagia can exhibit clear nutritional compromise (Moqhissi & Teasdale, 1980). Speech-language pathologists play an important role in diagnosing and managing dysphagia, and thus, they can have an impact on a patient's nutritional status. Therefore, they need to be informed and concerned about nutritional intake and the many issues surrounding malnutrition and dehydration. Aspiration pneumonia is not the only negative consequence of oropharyngeal dysphagia.

Coaching Tips

Be careful only to make recommendations regarding HOW to improve oropharyngeal dysphagia. Do not suggest the nutrient content of a diet. A dietitian once expressed great anger with a speech-language pathologist who recommended the use of a total nutrition liquid supplement in a patient with dysphagia and liver failure. Patients in severe liver failure cannot digest the high-density nutrients in this type of supplement. Speech-language pathologists must be careful to make dietary recommendations with regard to diet consistency only, and the effect of fatigue or endurance on maintaining adequate oral intake. Refer to the team dietitian for nutrient recommendations and the possible need for nutritional supplements.

Always know the type and frequency of medications administered to your patient. Evaluate the role medication may play in causing dysphagia, malnutrition, and/or dehydration in a patient. Review the medical chart for current and previous medications administered. Explore what medications may be useful as an intervention for dysphagia.

All medication questions need to be discussed with the physician and/or pharmacist. Be careful not to recommend specific drugs in evaluation reports, since the prescription of medication is not within the scope of practice of speech-language pathology. However, clinicians must discuss the possible side effects of a patient's medication(s) with the physician. Physicians need to consider how certain medications may cause a dysphagia, exacerbate its severity, affect oral intake or medication administration, or even improve dysphagia. It is the legal and ethical duty of clinicians to explore all possible causes and effects of medication on dysphagia, and bring them to the attention of the health professionals caring for the patient.

Don't forget to refer to the dentist, oral surgeon, optometrist, or ophthalmologist when necessary. A sore mouth, decayed teeth, or ill-fitting dentures can make bolus formation and transport nearly impossible for patients. These patients may exhibit a severe oral dysphagia, but the intervention is not dysphagia therapy. Refer to the dentist or oral surgeon. Likewise, poor self-feeding skills or a lack of interest in eating may be due to decreased vision and embarrassment about eating without spilling, requiring the attention of an optometrist or ophthalmologist. Refer to the appropriate professional when necessary.

Remember that the decision for nonoral nutrition involves many factors. Consult your team dietitian and physician. Be careful when interpreting malnutrition and dehydration information regarding your patient. Do not overstep the scope of practice within speech-language pathology in diagnosing malnutrition/dehydration or unilaterally determining the best intervention(s). The decision for nonoral nutrition involves many factors (see Chapter 8). Develop the best intervention option(s) only after consulting with patients, their caregivers/family, and the medical team.

Be careful not to "force fluids" in a patient with dysphagia. Rapid development of hyponatremia, with sudden death, may occur if fluids are increased too quickly. This is particularly important for patients who receive IV fluids or have congestive heart failure or other edematous medical conditions. Be sure to develop an appropriate intervention with the entire medical team to manage dehydration.

CONCLUSION

Patients with dysphagia are at great risk for malnutrition and dehydration. Timely identification and management of malnutrition and dehydration are crucial for all patients. The complications and consequences of malnutrition and dehydration are severe, and need to be taken into consideration when dysphagia is present.

The decision of what constitutes adequate nutrient and fluid intake for an elderly patient with dysphagia must be made individually and carefully by the registered dietitian and physician. Many physiologic and social changes occur with aging that need to be taken into consideration if the intervention plan is to succeed. Nutritional management of dysphagia can be accomplished through nonoral or oral options, or a combination of these two approaches.

Speech-language pathologists are important members of the nutritional management team, to provide information regarding *how* patients may continue to eat orally, estimate the risk of aspiration/obstruction, and determine whether the patient appears to possess adequate skills to maintain his nutritional needs by oral means. Physicians and dietitians determine *what* patients may eat, with regard to nutrient content. The nutritional management of patients with malnutrition, dehydration, and dysphagia is complicated and best performed within a medical team approach.

CHAPTER

8

Nonoral Nutrition

This chapter describes the various types of nonoral nutrition approaches available to patients with dysphagia. Enteral and parenteral feeding options are defined, and the indications, contraindications and complications of each option are given. The rationale and ethics of enteral feeding, especially with the chronically ill elderly, are discussed. In addition, the role of the speech-language pathologist in the management of dysphagia and nonoral nutrition is addressed.

The risk of aspiration due to oropharyngeal dysphagia can be high. In studies of patients who have suffered strokes, the incidence of patients who aspirated because of pharyngeal dysphagia has been reported to vary from 33 to 51% (Horner et al., 1988; Veis & Logemann, 1985). The mortality rate of pneumonia caused by aspiration is over 60% (Cameron & Zuidema, 1972). Given the great risks involved of aspiration due to dysphagia, nonoral methods of nutrient intake are sometimes recommended in an effort to reduce aspiration risk . There are many different ways to administer adequate nutrition and hydration nonorally. A description of various nutritional support options, including enteral and parenteral feeding, are listed in Table 8–1.

ENTERAL FEEDING

Definition

Enteral feeding is the term used to describe delivery of hydration and nutrients into the gastrointestinal (GI) tract. By strict definition, the gastrointestinal tract encompasses the digestive anatomy from the mouth to the anus.

Table 8–1. Description of various nutritional support options.

Nutritional Support Option	Definition
Enteral feeding	Delivery of hydration and nutrients anywhere along the gastrointestinal tract
Nasogastric feeding (NG)	Placement of a tube for nutrient ingestion via the nose
Operative gastrostomy (OG)	Surgical placement of a tube through the abdominal wall directly into the stomach for nutrient ingestion or suctioning out gastric contents
Percutaneous endoscopic gastrostomy (PEG)	Endoscopic placement of a tube through abdominal wall directly into the stomach for nutrient ingestion or suctioning out gastric contents
Jejunostomy (J-tube)	Surgical placement of a tube for nutrient ingestion through the abdominal wall directly into the jejunum
Percutaneous endoscopic jejunostomy (PEJ)	Endoscopic placement of a tube for nutrient ingestion through the abdominal wall directly into the jejunum
Cervical esophagoscopy/ pharyngoscopy	Surgical placement of a tube through lateral pharyngeal wall directly into upper esophagus for nutrient ingestion
Total parenteral feeding (TPN)	Administration of nutrients via a central vein
Peripheral parenteral feeding (PPN)	Administration of nutrients via a peripheral vein
Intravenous hydration (IV)	Administration of fluids for hydration only

However, enteral feeding usually refers to tube feedings that are placed directly into the gastrointestinal tract (American Gastroenterological Association, 1995). Tube placement can occur through the nose, esophagus, stomach, jejunum, or duodenum. While the duodenum can be used for tube placement, it does not usually occur because the position of the duodenum in the body gives it a tendency to swing backward. This makes tube placement in the jejunum difficult (Whitney & Cataldo, 1983).

Indications

Enteral feeding is indicated within 1 to 2 weeks of no nutrient intake, when a patient is not able to orally ingest nutrients adequately and/or safely, and if access can safely be attained (American Gastroenterological Association, 1995). Many factors are taken into consideration before enteral feeding is administered as an option for nutritional support. The overall medical status of a patient must be assessed and his or her wishes for artificial nutrition must be known. Enteral feeding may be a temporary or permanent source of nutritional support. All risks and benefits need to be discussed with a patient, in consultation with the physician.

Placement of tube feedings directly into the stomach (via the nose, esophagus, or stomach) allows the stomach to begin the process of digestion at a controlled rate. This subsequently gives the intestine adequate time to absorb the nutrients (Whitney & Cataldo, 1983). Allowing the stomach to begin digestion is always preferred if enteral feeding is used for nutrition.

Placement of tube feedings farther down the GI tract, such as into the jejunum, bypass the stomach. Since the stomach controls the rate of emptying gastric contents into the intestine and begins the digestive process, it is a more difficult task to regulate enteral feedings that bypass the stomach. Greater adjustments must be made regarding formula selection, rate of delivery, and feeding schedules to achieve adequate nutrition and absorption. Diarrhea is a common complication when feedings bypass the stomach (Nelson et al., 1994).

Contraindications

Mechanical obstructions that prohibit the placement of a tube are the only absolute contraindications of enteral feeding, according to the American Gastroenterological Association (1995). However, enteral feeding may also be contraindicated if a patient has severe vomiting or upper gastrointestinal bleeding (Heymsfield, Horowitz, & Lawson, 1980). In addition, enteral feeding requires a functional gastrointestinal tract. If a patient is not able to digest nutrients via the GI tract, enteral feeding is not an option.

Nasogastric Feeding (NG tube)

Definition

Nasogastric feeding is a type of enteral feeding that involves placement of a feeding tube through the nose into the stomach.

Indications

Nasogastric tube placement is indicated when enteral feeding is required for only a short period of time. This situation may occur when a patient has suffered an acute medical condition but rapid recovery is expected or possible. Nasogastric tube placement is typically chosen when the estimated length of time for its use is less than 30 days (American Gastroenterological Association, 1995). If enteral feeding is determined to be required for a longer period of time, other methods of enteral feeding are usually discussed with the patient.

Contraindications

NG tube placement is contraindicated if there is facial trauma or nasal obstruction that prohibits transnasal placement. Prior to insertion, a careful assessment of the patient's individual attributes to tolerate the placement of an NG tube must also be taken into consideration. Confused or agitated patients may not cooperate with the procedure to allow correct placement of the tube. Many patients will not be able to manage the discomfort and/or embarrassment of having a tube remain in their nose all the time. These factors may preclude NG feeding as a nonoral feeding option.

Placement of NG Tube

The placement of a nasogastric tube does not require surgery. Patients are asked to "swallow" the tube as it is pushed through the nose into the stomach (NG placement), duodenum (ND placement), or jejunum (NJ placement). The literature reports that most patients tolerate this procedure very well, with the exception of the disoriented or agitated patient (Whitney & Cataldo, 1983). However, nurses who have performed this procedure anecdotally report that NG tube placement can be quite challenging and traumatic at times, even with willing, alert patients.

Pliable tubes that are resistant to gastric acids, and sometimes weighted at one end to help passage from the stomach to the intestine during peristalsis, are used. It is important to verify placement of the tube into the stomach to avoid the serious complication of endotracheal feeding tube placement. Feeding tube sizes are identified by using the term *French* plus a number to indicate diameter size. The smaller the number, the smaller the diameter tube size. For example, a French 7 tube is a smaller diameter tube than a French 12. The term French is not a brand name or a unit of measure, but it is the common term applied to tube diameter. The smallest diameter tube possible to adequately administer the tube formula is used.

Complications of NG Tube Placement

Gastrointestinal and mechanical complications can occur with nasogastric enteral feeding, such as vomiting, cramping, diarrhea, and kinking of the tube in the GI tract (Table 8–2). While many of the gastrointestinal complications can be prevented or resolved by altering formula selection and the rate of delivery, there is still the risk of self-extubation (patient removes the NG tube) or increased aspiration risk if the tube is inappropriately placed into the trachea rather than the esophagus (Sitzmann & Mueller, 1988).

Gastrostomy Feeding (G-Tube)

Definition

The term *ostomy* is used to describe a surgical opening through which a tube can be placed. *Gastrostomy* is the term for a surgical opening into the stomach to allow the placement of a feeding tube. It is the most prevalent type of long-term enteral feeding. It can remain permanently or be removed at any time, if a patient's condition improves.

Indications

Gastrostomy feeding is indicated in patients who cannot or will not orally eat, and if the resumption of oral eating is not expected within a relatively short period of time (< 30 days). In addition, these patients must have a functional gastrointestinal tract and a safe method of access for tube placement (American Gastroenterological Association, 1995).

In general, a G-tube is used when it can benefit a patient by providing time to treat an underlying medical condition, clarify prognosis or when prolongation of life is feasible and desirable (Lo & Dornbrand, 1992). Since dysphagia can directly affect a patient's ability to safely manage oral eating, gastrostomy feeding may be indicated when dysphagia is present.

Table 8–2. Nasogastric enteral feeding complications.

Types of Complication(s)
Mechanical Complications
Obstruction of tube lumen
Kinking of tube in GI tract
Patient discomfort leading to self-extubation
Esophageal erosions
Aspiration of GI contents
Gastrointestinal Complications
Vomiting
Cramping
Diarrhea
Metabolic (Fluid and Electrolyte) Complications
Inability to assimilate (utilize at the cellular level) nutrient load

Source: From "Enteral and parenteral feeding in the dysphagic patient" by J. V. Sitzmann and M. Mueller, 1988, *Dysphagia, 3,* 39.

Contraindications

As with the contraindications for nasogastric feeding, gastrostomy feeding is contraindicated if patients do not have a functioning gastrointestinal tract or if they possess mechanical obstructions prohibiting tube placement (American Gastroenterological Association, 1995). The question of whether feeding tubes are contraindicated in patients with severe irreversible illness, especially in the elderly, is controversial (see "Ethics of Tube Feedings" in this chapter on page 189). A patient should discuss the contraindications of feeding tube placement with his physician.

Placement of a Gastrostomy Feeding Tube

A gastrostomy feeding tube can be inserted using a surgical or endoscopic procedure. The surgical procedure is called an operative gastrostomy (OG) or surgical gastrostomy (SG), while the endoscopic procedure is called a percutaneous endoscopic gastrostomy (PEG).

Both procedures insert a feeding tube into the stomach. The difference between the two procedures is the method of insertion. One involves surgery (OG), while the other visualizes the abdominal wall, using a fiberoptic endoscope passed into the stomach, as a feeding tube is either pushed or pulled in place (PEG). A prospective randomized trial comparing the pull and push methods of PEG were found to have similar outcomes in terms of complications, morbidity, and mortality (Hogan, deMarco, Hamilton, Walker, & Polter, 1986).

The decision of whether a patient with dysphagia receives an OG or PEG is decided by a patient and his physician. The use of PEG, rather than OG, as the preferred route of enteral feeding has increased the overall incidence of feeding tube placement, according to one community-based study by Bergstrom, Larson, Zinsmeitster, Sarr, and Silverstein (1995). It was also found to be cheaper than OG.

Complications of PEG and OG Tube Placement

Since the introduction of PEG in 1981, a great deal of attention has been given in the literature regarding the relative benefits and risks of PEG and OG, especially when used with the elderly (Ciocon, Silverstone, Graver, & Foley, 1988; Kaw & Sekas, 1994; Mitchell, Kiely, & Lipstiz, 1997). When compared to OG, PEG is generally less expensive, takes less time to perform and does not require surgical removal. These benefits, and others, often make PEG placement preferred for patients rather than OG (Table 8–3). However, while many perceive PEG outcomes to be better than OG, several studies have confirmed that similar outcomes can be expected given OG or jejunostomy (Bergstrom et al., 1995; Jones, Santanello, & Falcone, 1990; Rogers & Bowden, 1992; Samii & Suguitan, 1990). It was found that patients who require enteral feeding have multiple comorbid conditions that influence outcome, regardless of whether a PEG or OG was placed (Bergstrom et al., 1995).

Therefore, attention may need to focus on the overall medical condition of the patients in whom a feeding tube is placed. If a feeding tube is placed at all, Bergstrom et al. (1995) recommend the decision for a PEG, rather than OG, be based primarily on cost and the local expertise available in tube placement techniques. In patients in whom PEG is not indicated or local expertise is not available, similar outcomes can be expected with OG placement.

Jejunostomy Feeding (J-tube)

Definition

A *jejunostomy* is the placement of a feeding tube through the abdominal wall into the jejunum.

Indications

The main indication for J-tube placement is in patients who have a previous history of tube-feeding aspiration pneumonia or reflux esophagitis (American Gastroenterological Association, 1995). Jejunostomy is also

Table 8–3. Comparison of operative and percutaneous endoscopic gastrostomy procedures.

Operative Gastrostomy (OG)	Percutaneous Endoscopic Gastrostomy (PEG)
Requires 52–55 min to perform[e,k,r,s]	Requires 11–27.5 min to perform[e,k,r,s]
22–66% use of general anesthesia[c,e,u]	87 % use of local anesthesia[t]
Higher cost than PEG	One-third to one-half less expensive than OG[k,u,v]
Complications: internal leakage, failure to decompress, migration, nausea, diarrhea wound dehiscence, gastric hemorrhage, intraperitoneal leakage, fistula; prolonged ileus	Complications: gastric wall hematoma, gastrocolic fistula, periostomal leakage, tube migration, wound infection[h,k,r,t,w–z,1a]
Overall complication rate: 0.3–17%[a–e,f,i–o]	Overall complication rate: 0–18%
Mortality rate: 0.3–16%[a–c,e,h,n–q]	Mortality rate: 1%[1b]
Surgical removal	Nonsurgical removal

Source: Adapted from "Enteral and parenteral feeding in the dysphagic patient," by J. V. Sitzmann and M. Mueller, 1988, *Dysphagia, 3,* 39. Copyright by Springer-Verlag New York.

Note: Data from [a]Haws, Sieber, and Kiesewetter, 1966; [b]Campbell and Sasaki, 1974; [c]Wasiljew, Ujiki and Beal, 1982; [d]Shellito and Malt, 1985; [e]Ruge and Vazquez, 1986; [f]Hinsdale, Lipkowitz, Pollock, Hoover, and Jaffe, 1985; [g]Wilkinson and Rickleman, 1982; [h]Stern, 1986; [i]Parrish and Cohen, 1972; [j]Senac and Lee, 1983; [k]Miller, Kummer, Kotler, and Tiszenkel, 1986; [l]Webster, Carey, and Ravitch, 1975; [m]Smith and Farris, 1961; [n]Holder and Gross, 1960; [o]Holder, Leape, and Ashcraft, 1972; [p]Gallagher, Tyson, and Ashcraft, 1973; [q]Burtch and Shatney, 1985; [r]Strodel, Lemmer, Eckhauser, Botham, and Dent, 1983; [s]Russell, Brotman, and Norris, 1984; [t]Ponsky, Gauderer, Stellato, and Aszodi, 1985; [u]Kummer, Tiszenkel, Kotler, and Miller, 1985; [v]Randall, 1984; [w]Kozarek, Ball, and Ryan, 1986; [x]Stellato, Danziger, Nearman, and Creger, 1984; [y]Larson, Fleming, Ott, and Schroeder, 1983; [z]Thatcher, Ferguson, and Paradis, 1984; [1a]Moore, Curreri, and Rodning, 1986; [1b]Larson, Burton, Schroeder, and DiMagno, 1987.

performed when there is some reason that the stomach cannot be used, such as fistula, previous resection, obstruction, gastric atony, or severe reflux (Sitzmann & Mueller, 1988).

Jejunostomy is the preferred type of nutritional support when severe reflux and emesis are present, since aspiration of these GI contents is virtually eliminated, because of the negative pressure present below the pyloric sphincter. This makes it very difficult for any contents to flow upward in the GI tract. However, patients with dysphagia may still aspirate their own oral secretions. Clinicians must be careful to remember that tube placement, even a J-tube, does not eliminate aspiration of oral secretions. Aspiration of gastric contents, but not oral secretions, is eliminated with J-tube placement.

Contraindications

Contraindications for jejunostomy are similar to those for any surgical procedure, when feeding tube placement is chosen as the nutritional mode of treatment. The overall medical condition of the patient, and need for J-tube placement, needs to be carefully assessed by the physician, in coordination with the speech-language pathologist, dietitian, and nurse.

Placement of a Jejunostomy Feeding Tube

Surgery is required for placement of a jejunostomy feeding tube. There are a number of procedures used to perform J-tube placement, and an optimal procedure has not yet been identified (American Gastroenterological Association, 1995). It is expected that refinements to the procedure will continue to occur over time.

Complications of J-tube Placement

Complications of jejunostomy feeding may involve diarrhea, peritoneal leakage, obstruction of the tube, wound drainage and infection, and volvulus (American Gastroenterological Association, 1995). Volvulus is a twisting of the intestine causing obstruction. Diarrhea may occur because of a patient's difficulty in regulating absorption via the intestine, and can be controlled with careful monitoring of formula administration and composition.

PARENTAL (INTRAVENOUS) NUTRITION

Definition

Parenteral and *intravenous nutrition* are synonymous terms that describe the administration of nutrient requirements via a vein. The central and peripheral veins can be used to deliver parenteral nutrition. The central veins, such as the superior vena cava, are the large diameter veins located close to the heart. The peripheral veins, such as those found in the arms and legs, are the smaller diameter veins which bring blood to the extremities.

Total parenteral nutrition (TPN) and peripheral parenteral nutrition (PPN) describe the administration of nutrients via a central or peripheral vein, respectively. The technique of administering nutrients by vein is complicated, since the smaller veins can become quite irritated and collapse when exposed to the nutrient solutions. The use of a central vein is less irritating and decreases the risk of collapse, since its larger diameter and volume of blood can rapidly dilute the nutrient solution. Its irritating effect is substantially reduced by the time it reaches the peripheral veins.

The use of peripheral intravenous solutions, also called intravenous hydration fluid (IVF), involves the delivery of simple parenteral solutions via a peripheral vein. These IV solutions contain water and combinations of dextrose, electrolytes and sometimes other nutrients (Whitney & Cataldo, 1983). IVF is commonly used in hospitals to maintain fluid and electrolyte balance in well-nourished patients who are expected to eat orally within a few days, such as postsurgical patients. It also can provide a short-term solution to meet nutrient requirement in patients with dysphagia, as the need for enteral feeding is evaluated

Indications

Parenteral nutrition is indicated when patients have a nonfunctional gastrointestinal tract or when the GI tract needs to rest. Some common medical conditions that may indicate a need for parenteral nutrition are severe malnutrition or burns, bowel obstruction, ileus, or cancer treatment that requires surgery, or radiation treatment that results in a nonfunctional GI tract (Ganger & Craig, 1990; Whitney & Cataldo, 1983). Since nutrient solutions are administered directly into the vascular system, TPN and PPN eliminate the possibility of aspiration of formula, but not oral secretions.

Contraindications

PPN or TPN is contraindicated in patients who have a functional gastrointestinal tract, since enteral feeding is always desired over parenteral feeding.

Placement of Parenteral Nutrition in a Peripheral or Central Vein

Any health care professional trained to insert an IV may initiate placement of parenteral nutrition in a peripheral vein. Many facilities have a policy regarding who may initiate PPN in a patient. Therefore, the professional required to initiate PPN may differ from one facility to another.

In contrast, TPN requires surgery by a physician to insert the tube into a central vein. In some facilities, only specially trained physicians insert and manage TPN in patients. Local anesthesia is usually given, and sterile conditions are maintained in and around the catheter for the duration of TPN. No blood is drawn nor medications given via the catheter to prevent bacterial contamination (Whitney & Cataldo, 1983).

Complications of Parenteral Nutrition

The major complication of PPN is related to catheter-related sepsis (Nelson et al., 1994). Sepsis is the presence of disease-causing bacteria in the blood. Other complications may be due to technical or metabolic problems, as with the difficulties experienced with TPN.

The complications related to TPN insertion and use are numerous and dangerous, such as fluid, air, or gas in the chest or a variety of metabolic complications related to inappropriate blood levels of glucose, magnesium, calcium, phosphorus, ammonia, and potassium (Table 8–4). Sepsis is a major complication of TPN. Other documented complications are congestive heart failure, liver compromise, acid-base or electrolyte abnormalities, vitamin deficiencies, and pneumothorax (Fischer, 1983; Sitzmann, Townsend, Siler, & Bartlett, 1985).

Although severe malnutrition can be reversed rapidly using this method without surgery or a major procedure, it obviously does carry serious possible complications as well. It is a complex and costly therapy, usually administered to the patient with dysphagia with advanced malnutrition in the hospital on a short-term basis (Sitzmann & Mueller, 1988). Given the number of serious complications observed with parenteral nutrition, this form of nutritional support is generally not preferred over the gastrointestinal system as an alternate mode of nutrition.

COMPLICATIONS OF ENTERAL FEEDING

Aspiration

Aspiration is one of the most controversial and significant complications associated with enteral feeding (American Gastroenterological Association, 1995). The incidence of aspiration pneumonia associated with tube feeding has been reported to vary from 2 to 95%. This wide range of prevalence may possibly be due to poorly defined criteria for aspiration in the literature. It is important for clinicians to realize that a recommendation for nonoral nutrition will not necessarily eliminate aspiration in the patient.

Table 8–4. Complications associated with TPN.

Complications Related to Catheter Insertion or Care

Fluid in the chest (hydrothorax)

Air or gas in the chest (pneumothorax)

Blood in the chest (hemothorax)

Catheter tip breaks off, obstructing the blood flow (catheter embolism)

Air leaks into catheter, obstructing blood flow (air embolism)

Hole or tear made in heart by catheter tip (myocardial perforation)

Catheter inadvertently placed in subclavian artery (arterial puncture)

Improper position of catheter tip

Sepsis

Blood clots (thrombosis)

Metabolic Complications

Elevated blood glucose (hyperglycemia) or low blood glucose (hypoglycemia)

Dehydration

Coma from excessive glucose load (hyperosmolar, hyperglycemic, nonketotic coma)

Low blood magnesium (hypomagnesemia) or low blood calcium (hypocalcemia)

High blood phosphorus (hyperphosphatemia) or low blood phosphorus (hypophosphatemia)

Low blood potassium

Essential fatty acid deficiency or trace element deficiencies

High blood ammonia levels (hyperammonemia)

Acid-base imbalances or elevated liver enzymes

Source: From *Understanding normal and clinical nutrition,* by E. N. Whitney and C. B. Cataldo, 1983, p.779. New York: West Publishing Company. Copyright 1983 by West Publishing Company. Reprinted by permission.

There are many different reasons purported why enteral feeding has such a high association of aspiration.

Aspiration of Oral Secretions

In the case of severe oropharyngeal dysphagia, the main source of pulmonary aspiration is from the aspiration of oral contents. Oral contents may consist of food, liquids, *and* oral secretions. Tube feeding can eliminate aspiration of oral nutrition, but not oral secretions. Therefore, tube feeding may not eliminate the primary source of pulmonary aspiration in some patients with severe neurogenic oropharyngeal dysphagia (Lazarus, Murphy, & Culpepper, 1990). Clinicians need to carefully evaluate the benefit of enteral feeding in the management of oropharyngeal dysphagia, prior to tube placement.

Aspiration Caused by Tube Position and Reflux

There are limited data regarding the relationship between tube position and reflux (American Gastroenterological Association, 1995). However, Mittal, Stewart, and Schirmer (1992) have suggested that increased gastroesophageal reflux may occur if a tube is passed through the pharynx (as occurs in nasogastric feeding), since this may lead to transient relaxation of the lower esophageal sphincter. This is an important question that requires further study.

Aspiration Caused by Body Position

Studies have shown an increased incidence of aspiration or episodes of tracheal aspiration in the supine position using nasogastric tubes; however a semirecumbent position reduced the incidence of reflux and aspiration by 34% but did not prevent it (Ibanez et al., 1992; Torres et al., 1992). All clinicians are intuitively aware of the effect of body position on aspiration when eating. The importance of body position during enteral feeding is just as significant. It is important to monitor the maintenance of upright positioning, as high as tolerated, every time a clinician sees a patient who receives tube feeding.

Effect of Gastric Emptying Dysfunction Caused by Disease or Injury

Some diseases or injuries may contribute to a dysfunction in gastric emptying, leading to gastric distention and aspiration due to increased risk of reflux. Therefore, it is important to consider the underlying disease pathophysiology of a patient with dysphagia, including the presence of gastric emptying dysfunction, prior to choosing a method of nutrient intake (American Gastroenterological Association, 1995).

Enteral Feeding Regimens

There are several different ways enteral feeding can be administered to a patient, and numerous feeding schedules can be used. The administration rate and schedule of enteral feeding can increase gastroesophageal reflux of the feeding, which can subsequently increase the risk of aspiration.

Bolus Enteral Feeding

Bolus enteral feeding refers to the administration of formula intermittently throughout a day, using a syringe, pump, or gravity. Syringe bolus feeding is termed "rapid bolus feeding" since the rate of administration is controlled solely by the professional who pushes the syringe, and this tends to be much quicker than the other options. Rapid bolus feedings have been shown to decrease lower esophageal sphincter pressure to such low levels that it is associated with free gastroesophageal reflux to the sternal notch and vomiting (Coben, Weintraub, DiMarino, Jr., & Cohen, 1994; Nelson et al., 1994). Despite this risk, rapid bolus feedings are generally preferred by ambulatory, independent patients and those who are outpatients, since these feedings do not take long to administer independently and, therefore, patients can control when and where to feed themselves.

Continuous Enteral Feeding

Enteral feedings can also occur continuously. The speed of continuous enteral feeding can be best controlled using an electric pump, although gravity is also a reliable rate of administration. Continuous enteral feeding is standard practice if tube placement is through the jejunum, since this slow, controlled rate of administration improves nutrient absorption (American Gastroenterological Association, 1995). Interestingly, Mullan, Roubenoff, and Roubenoff (1992) recommend slow continuous drip feeding to reduce aspiration risk, regardless of tube placement. Ultimately, the decision of continuous or bolus enteral feeding is made by a patient's physician, in consultation with the nurse and dietitian.

Advantages and Disadvantages of Feeding Regimens

A gradual progression from continuous to bolus feeding is advantageous, since it normalizes the body's consumption of nutrients and allows a patient more convenience and independence. In addition, it may prepare the patient emotionally and physiologically for resumption of a more normal feeding schedule as well. However, care should be taken not to progress too quickly. Increased risk of reflux aspiration or gastrointestinal complications can occur with bolus feedings as compared to continuous feedings, especially if progression is made too quickly (Table 8–5).

Determining the Rate and Schedule of Formula Delivery

The registered dietitian and physician are responsible for determining the rate and schedule of formula delivery. They will need to work closely with the speech-language pathologist, especially if the patient with dysphagia is beginning to tolerate small oral feedings. Overload on the gastrointestinal tract could occur, causing discomfort and a lack of appetite if the rate and schedule of formula delivery are not altered as oral feedings begin. This can be prevented using a coordinated team approach.

Medication Absorption

Drug absorption and metabolism may be altered or interrupted during tube feedings (American Gastroenterological Association, 1995). Some drugs may show decreased potency when mixed in a formula while others are unchanged (Plezia, Thornley, Kramer, & Armstrong, 1990; Strom &

Table 8–5. Comparison of continuous and bolus enteral feeding.

Continuous Tube Feeding	Bolus Tube Feeding
Enhanced nutrient absorption	Increased rate of gastrointestinal complications: diarrhea, abdominal distention, delayed gastric emptying
Decreased aspiration risk	Increased risk of recurrent pulmonary aspiration of formula
Preferred feeding schedule for jejunostomy	"Normalizes" digestive system; preferred method when possible
Increased convenience for staff in long-term care settings	Increased mobility for patient between feedings Easier for patients to manage independently

Sources: From "Safe and effective tube feeding of bedridden elderly," by C. T. Henderson, 1991, *Geriatrics, 46*(8), 58; D. Acox, *Personal communication,* June, 1997; M. L. Huckabee, *Personal communication,* August, 1997.

Miller, 1990). In addition, some medications do not mix well with formula, and result in a gel or viscous mass that cannot be administered via a tube. Clinicians need to be mindful of this fact as they consider nonoral nutrition for a patient. They need to compare the risk of orally presenting medications (increasing aspiration risk) to the possibility that a patient may not be able to consume the medication at all, if nothing is allowed by mouth.

Diarrhea

Diarrhea is a common complication of enteral feeding, with its reported incidence varying from 2.3 to 68% (Cataldi-Betcher, Seltzer, Slocum, & Jones, 1983; Ganger & Craig, 1990; Kelly, Patrick & Hillman, 1983). Numerous causes for diarrhea with tube feeding have been postulated (American Gastroenterological Association, 1995).

Severity of Illness

The presence of severe illness may predispose patients to diarrhea. It has been suggested that critically ill patients may suffer from diarrhea because of overall, reduced physiologic function, and not directly as a result of the use of tube feeding formulas (Kandil, Opper, Switzer, & Heiser, 1993). This is an important finding that clinicians need to remember.

Medications

Many patients who are receiving enteral feeding may also be receiving multiple medications. Diarrhea may be induced by the use of certain medications, and be totally unrelated to the use of formula.

Altered Bacterial Flora

Reduced gastric and small bowel motility theoretically may lead to small intestine bacterial overgrowth and an alteration in intestinal microflora (American Gastroenterological Association, 1995). Unfortunately, it is difficult to study bacterial overgrowth conclusively in critically ill patients, since multiple medical problems occur simultaneously in these patients, which hinder investigation of the cause of diarrhea.

Hypoalbuminemia

Low serum albumin levels may predispose patients to diarrhea, although it has not been conclusively determined that hypoalbuminemia causes diarrhea since the sickest patients may be susceptible to diarrhea for many reasons (American Gastroenterological Association, 1995).

Formula Composition

The typical formula composition used in tube feedings does not produce significant diarrhea in normal volunteers, even when administered at the extremely fast rate of 340 mL/h (Kandil et al., 1993). Most continuous tube feedings are 60 to100 cc/hr. Therefore, it is postulated that diarrhea induced by tube feeding in the critically ill may be due to altered physiologic function, rather than the formula.

A controversy regarding the benefit of adding fiber to formula is noted in the literature. Some studies investigating the use of fiber-containing formulas failed to show improvement in controlling diarrhea (Fischer et al., 1985; Frankenfield & Beyer, 1989; Guenter et al., 1991). Another study demonstrated positive results of adding fiber to tube feeding formulas (Frank & Green, 1979). This controversy has caused the American Gastroenterological Association (1995) to conclude in their technical review paper that the benefit of fiber to control diarrhea is "unsettled" (p. 1292). The decision of whether fiber will be beneficial to enteral feeding formula clearly is not within the realm of speech-language pathology, and clinicians must defer to the dietitian and physician to make the best decision for patients.

Formula Contamination

If a formula becomes contaminated with microorganisms and enters the gastrointestinal tract, it could possibly cause diarrhea (American Gastroenterological Association, 1995). However, contaminated formula resulting in diarrhea is questionable, because of the protective mechanism of gastric acid and if normal sanitation procedures are used when handling the formula.

DYSPHAGIA AND NONORAL NUTRITION: MAKING THE DECISION

Who Makes the Decision?

The decision to provide nutrient intake and hydration using a nonoral method is not as clear-cut and easy as some would think, especially in patients with severe neurogenic dysphagia. In some cases, the decision may be made quickly by a physician, to meet an acute need. At other times, the decision is gradually made over time with the medical team and patient, as nutritional status and oral intake slowly decline. In either case, the primary decision should be left to the patient, if possible. If a patient is deemed incompetent to make the decision, or unable to do so at the time when a decision must be made, his or her family or surrogate should make the decision based on what they believe the patient would want.

Criteria for Making the Decision for Nonoral Nutrition

Speech-language pathologists need to be extremely careful when discussing nonoral nutrition options with a patient or their caregivers. There are many factors that must be evaluated and weighed before nonoral nutrition is recommended to manage dysphagia.

Comprehensive Formal and Informal Assessment

Prior to discussing the option of nonoral nutrition, a careful and comprehensive dysphagia assessment should occur. In addition to collecting formal data regarding swallowing physiology and overall medical condition, it is critical to evaluate a patient's personal attributes, and those of the caregivers that may care for the patient. This information is necessary to help determine a prognosis for recovery, and the variety of intervention options possible. It provides a complete evaluation of a patient's strengths, weaknesses, and what the best intervention strategies are for the patient. In some instances, nonoral nutrition may not be the best management decision, even when severe aspiration or obstruction risk is present. For example, terminal illness may lead a patient to decide to continue oral eating for quality of life, despite probable risk of aspiration pneumonia or airway obstruction. The severity of the dysphagia does not automatically determine the mode of nutrient intake. Clinicians must gather all pertinent information regarding a patient, including his or her wishes regarding dysphagia intervention.

Patient Competency

Since the decision of whether to manage dysphagia through nonoral nutrition is ultimately up to the patient, it is important to determine whether the patient can fully understand the risks and benefits of each option available. Determining the competency of a patient is not within the realm of speech-language pathology. Physicians and psychologists are legally able to determine competency, and clinicians need to refer to these professionals for guidance in this area. Preferably, documentation will be provided in the medical chart identifying whether a patient is competent to make his or her own medical intervention decisions. If a patient is deemed incompetent, the chart should clearly identify who is legally able to make health care decisions. Clinicians need to know this information so they can educate the appropriate person(s) regarding the results and recommendations of their comprehensive dysphagia evaluation.

Prognosis for Recovery

Whenever nonoral nutrition is recommended as an option to manage dysphagia and nutritional status, patients and physicians want to know a reasonable prediction for recovery. This is a very difficult task, since recovery from dysphagia is often directly related to the prognosis for recovery from the medical condition(s) that caused it. Clinicians can develop a reasonable prediction for dysphagia recovery by carefully synthesizing all the data from the comprehensive assessment of dysphagia, taking into account the medical condition(s) that caused the dysphagia. In this manner, a prognosis for recovery from dysphagia can be determined.

In addition, the prognosis of recovery from dysphagia without resorting to nonoral nutrition should be discussed. It is clear that many factors other than the presence of dysphagia contribute to the serious health complications of aspiration pneumonia (Langmore et al., 1998), malnutrition and dehydration (Cope, 1996). In some cases, continued oral eating in the presence of dysphagia certainly may be possible with no serious health consequences. Clinicians must synthesize all data carefully and present an objective picture of the risks and benefits of every option to a patient.

The Ethics of Tube Feedings in Chronically Ill Elderly

Interestingly, there has been some controversy in the literature surrounding the use of feeding tubes in chronically ill elderly patients (Ackerman, 1996; Ciocon et al., 1988; Sheiman, 1996). The question has been raised whether the use of a nasogastric (NG) tube, or any feeding tube, may be contraindicated in patients with severe irreversible illness who are unable to orally eat.

Physician Practice Patterns and Attitudes

Quill (1992) conducted a physician questionnaire and retrospective twelve month medical chart review study of physician practice patterns and attitudes regarding the use of NG tubes with hospitalized, chronically ill elderly patients. These patients were admitted to the hospital with a primary diagnosis of cerebrovascular accident, organic brain syndrome, or metatastic cancer, were over 70 years old, and received a nasogastric feeding tube.

Although most physicians believed a patient's wishes should guide the decision for tube feeding, a review of the hospital medical records revealed that oral or written consent by the patient was documented in only 2 of 51 NG tube insertions. Seven charts documented consent given by a surrogate, but only one surrogate stated approval was given in consideration of the patient's actual wishes.

Rationale for Tube Placement

Quill (1992) reported that physicians stated biomedical concerns were the primary clinical reason leading to NG tube placement, rather than concerns regarding a patient's quality of life (8:1 ratio). Biomedical concerns are those that address the patient's medical condition, such as dehydration or malnutrition. Although 38% of the physicians reported that NG tube placement was conducted for patient comfort, the chart review showed that 53% of the patients required restraints to keep the NG tube in place. Of those patients in whom NG tube placement was performed to provide patient comfort, 90% (19/21) of these patients died in the hospital. Overall, 64% of these patients died in the hospital.

Legal and Ethical Implications

The legal and ethical implications drawn from this important study are many. Lo and Dornbrand (1992) believe that Quill's findings should be required reading for judges, physicians, patients, and families. They do not believe tube feedings should be viewed as "basic, humane care that must always be provided" (p. 72) since Quill's study indicates no demonstrable benefit can be observed with their use. In fact, it is recommended by all of these authors that if a patient pulls out a feeding tube, it is a nonverbal indicator the patient does not give consent for the tube. If a patient does give consent for a feeding tube, a gastrostomy or jejunostomy tube is less likely than a nasogastric tube to be pulled out (Lo & Dornbrand, 1992).

Recommendations for Feeding Tube Use with Chronically Ill Elderly

Quill (1992) offered several recommendations to professionals when considering the use of NG and other feeding tubes. The following suggestions from Quill (1992) may be good guidelines for clinicians and the entire dysphagia team, as they struggle with the difficult decision of whether to insert a feeding tube for nutrition:

1. *Develop formal policies regarding the use of feeding tubes.* Hospitals need to develop policies for the use of all feeding tubes that include formal, written informed consent for the procedure by the patient. A patient must be educated regarding his or her condition, prognosis, and personal benefits/burdens of this intervention.
2. *Make decisions based on a patient's wishes.* If a patient is deemed incompetent to give informed consent, a family member or other surrogate must make a decision regarding treatment based on what the patient's wishes would be, if he or she were able to understand the pros/cons of feeding tube placement in his or her current condition.
3. *Try tube placement for a short period of time when recovery is uncertain.* NG tube placement can be used for a short period of time and later discontinued, if the burdens appear to outweigh the benefits. This may be useful in cases where no clear-cut decision can be reached regarding the potential for medical improvement. (However, NG tubes do have a high discomfort level and, therefore, this option may not be accepted by the patient.)
4. *Do not use restraints when a patient removes a feeding tube.* Physical or chemical restraints should not be used if a feeding tube is removed by the patient. Rather, careful reevaluation of the benefits and burdens of continued tube feedings should occur.

How to Progress from Nonoral to Oral Nutrition

Clinicians obviously want to progress a patient to oral nutrition as quickly and safely as possible. Many different philosophies are held regarding how best to proceed from tube feeding to oral eating. For example, Groher and McKaig (1995) suggest that bolus feedings continue for 3 to 5 days before oral trials are attempted, to allow the stomach time to "stretch" and reinitiate the hunger cycle. They recommend that one meal be introduced orally for 1 week, with more meals added as the patient is able to tolerate oral eating. Tube feedings are adjusted when necessary to supplement a patient's nutritional needs, as he or she is able to eat more each day. Finally, once a patient is able to meet nutritional needs orally, they suggest that appropriate maintenance of the tube should occur for up to 90 days before the tube is removed.

Although Groher and McKaig (1995) provide one philosophy of how to progress from tube feeding to oral nutrition, clinicians may determine that patients may advance more rapidly or slowly than recommended in their guidelines. The introduction of oral food requires frequent consultation with the medical team to monitor health, nutritional status, and any significant changes. Criteria necessary for increased oral nutrition will include assessment of various indicators of nutritional status, such as fluid and caloric intake, and overall health status, such as strength, endurance, and respiratory condition. It is imperative that clinicians work in concert with all of the medical team to advance oral nutrition in a safe and responsible manner, as rapidly as possible.

Coaching Tips

Intravenous hydration fluid may be indicated as a short-term intervention for some patients, when rapid recovery from dysphagia is expected. The use of IVF may be an appropriate and useful intervention in patients with dysphagia who require an alternate mode of nutrition for only a short period of time, such as postsurgical patients or those with acute, reversible illness. Clinicians must remember to evaluate the cause(s) of dysphagia and potential for recovery when considering nonoral nutrition options. This option allows a clinician and patient time to determine whether oral nutrition may resume or a more permanent solution to nonoral nutrition should be explored.

Recognize that a recommendation for nonoral nutrition will affect many aspects of a patient's care and overall health. Clinicians must know that nonoral nutrition may not achieve all the benefits desired for a patient. In fact, this form of nutrition can increase the health problems of a patient. Aspiration of oral secretions is not remedied with tube feeding. Difficulties in tolerating and receiving tube feedings can result, causing aspiration, diarrhea, and problems in medication administration and absorption. Careful consultation must occur with the patient, his or her physician, nurse, and dietitian before nonoral nutrition is recommended. Continuous communication among all health care professionals must occur if nonoral nutrition is implemented.

Before discussing the option of nonoral nutrition with a patient, be sure to consult with his or her physician first. The ultimate decision regarding nonoral nutrition must be decided by a patient, in consultation with his or her physician. Since many dysphagia management options involve a clear understanding of the patient's overall medical condition and prognosis, it is imperative that clinicians consult with the physician regarding their dysphagia evaluation results, prior to discussing nonoral nutrition as a management option with a patient. If a physician disagrees with a dysphagia intervention recommendation, clinicians must try to educate the physician to the rationale behind their recommendation, and clearly document their differing opinions. The legal and ethical obligations of clinicians regarding what to do when physicians, patients or families disagree with their management recommendations are discussed in Chapter 12.

Work closely with your patient, the physician, nurse, and dietitian to progress a patient from tube feeding to oral nutrition. While it is tempting and comforting to follow a predetermined schedule for progressing a patient from tube feeding to oral eating, meeting the nutritional needs of a patient requires a multidisciplinary, coordinated approach. General guidelines can be followed, but patients don't always follow the guidelines. Changes in formula schedules and rates are not within the realm of speech-language pathology. Always work directly with the health professionals involved with the patient, to progress a patient from enteral to oral nutrition.

CONCLUSION

Enteral and parenteral nutrition are two interventions available to patients with severe dysphagia who cannot safely ingest food or liquids orally. Enteral nutrition involves the administration of nutrients directly into the gastrointestinal tract via a tube; parenteral nutrition administers nutrients through a peripheral or central vein. Both methods of nutrient administration have benefits, but they also carry the risk of serious complications that require careful monitoring by the physician, nurse, and dietitian.

Clinicians need to carefully evaluate the necessity of nonoral nutrition in their patients with severe dysphagia, in consultation with their patients and their health care providers. While nonoral nutrition options provide alternatives to oral eating, they do not eliminate all aspiration risk. Aspiration of oral secretions is not eliminated with tube feedings, and many medical complications can occur with tube feedings.

The ethics of using tube feedings with chronically ill elderly patients has been raised. Patients need to make the decision of whether they choose nonoral nutrition as a treatment. They need to be informed about their current medical condition and severity of dysphagia, and the risks/benefits of all available treatments. The decision of treatment is ultimately theirs and must be respected. Clinicians must provide timely, comprehensive assessments and information to patients so they can make an informed decision regarding the choice of nonoral nutrition intervention to manage their dysphagia.

9

Oral Nutrition Interventions for Dysphagia

This chapter discusses the terminology and management issues involved with diet modification as an intervention option for oropharyngeal dysphagia. Suggestions are given to standardize terms used in liquid and food modification, and improve communication among all team members. The use of dairy products and free water in dysphagia diets is discussed.

Oral nutrition intervention options for the patient with dysphagia can involve food texture and/or liquid viscosity modifications. Modifications can be extreme, with all foods pureed and liquids thickened to a pudding-like consistency, or minor, involving only an avoidance of certain foods or very thin liquids. Diet modifications may be temporary and introduced as an adjunct to rehabilitative treatments. Conversely, they may be permanent, especially for individuals with degenerative diseases or intractable dysphagia. Diet modification may be the primary compensatory option for some patients and the only way they can continue to eat orally and avoid aspiration.

Diet modification has been suggested to be the last treatment option, owing to poor patient acceptance (Logemann, 1993). However, for some patients, diet modification may be accepted early in the rehabilitation process since it allows safe, continued oral eating. Some patients may initially modify their diets to eliminate just difficult foods, as they work to improve their swallowing skills. Others may choose diet modification to eat safely, rather than rely on certain postures or strategies with every swallow. Clearly, these decisions are ultimately up to every individual patient. The choice of diet modification, and the management issues involved in implementing it as an intervention option, are complex.

DIET MODIFICATION

There are many benefits of diet modification as a dysphagia intervention. Eating is a highly social and cultural event that provides great pleasure. Diet modification can allow patients the continued pleasure of sharing a meal with friends and family. It can mark time in a day for confused patients, as three daily meals are served. The value of continued oral eating cannot be underestimated since so many pleasurable events in our lives are centered around food, such as celebrations or meetings for a cup of coffee or lunch with a friend. Food even has many cultural and religious meanings, with the withholding of food considered unacceptable in some religions (Shoemaker, 1997). The quality-of-life issues surrounding diet modification are complex, since most patients wish to avoid tube placement and continue to enjoy the pleasure of eating. Extreme fatigue, physical weakness or paralysis, or severe illness may lead some patients to welcome diet modification as an option to continue oral eating. When patients are aware of their chewing difficulty or experience problems trying to swallow certain foods or liquids, they often will eliminate these items from their diet. While all patients wish they didn't have to modify anything in their diet, they will accept this option since they derive no pleasure trying to eat these foods. These patients are often highly motivated to rehabilitate their swallowing skills, if possible, and they willingly maintain diet modifications during the intervention process.

However, modifying the diet is not accepted by all patients. Poor compliance of diet modification is also common, and may increase their risk for malnutrition. If a patient refuses to drink thickened liquids, the likelihood of dehydration can also increase (Layne, 1990). There are many reasons why a patient may reject diet modification. These include factors such as poor texture, taste, and appearance, as well as the cost and inconvenience of obtaining or preparing modified food.

Texture, Taste, and Appearance

If the food does not look or taste appealing, it will not be consumed. The visual appearance of food can significantly contribute to the acceptance or rejection of diet modification by patients. In addition, the importance of texture to food consumption was highlighted by a study of healthy, young adult subjects who could only identify 40.7% of 29 foods presented, when they were pureed and strained to eliminate textural cues (Schiffman, 1973). When patients complain to clinicians that food does not taste"right"when pureed, perhaps they have a point.

The act of mastication may contribute to the acceptance of diet modification. Chewing releases flavor and is a highly enjoyable sensation, which even appears to have a noticeable soothing effect (Bourne, 1982). Many behaviors associated with anxiety, such as finger tapping and leg swinging, have been observed to decrease greatly during mastication. Mastication is a process that begins digestion. It breaks food down into smaller pieces, mixes with saliva, brings the food to near body temperature, and "imparts pleasurable sensations that fill a basic need" (Bourne, 1982, p. 24). Therefore, the lack of texture or the need to chew may greatly influence the compliance of patients to eat a modified diet.

It has been noted that of the four properties inherent in food (appearance, flavor, texture, nutrition), only nutrition is not considered a"sensory acceptability factor," since it is not perceived by the senses (Bourne, 1982). Since nutrition is not perceived by the senses, many patients may choose the increased risk of malnutrition, aspiration, or even obstruction rather than accept the decreased appearance, taste, and pleasure of diet modification.

Convenience and Cost on Food Consumption

Last, it is important to remember that individuals purchase and consume foods based not only on taste and individual/cultural preference, but on convenience and cost as well (Wilke, 1993). Most people consume foods that are easy to purchase or prepare, and are low in cost. Similar factors may impact whether an individual with dysphagia, or a facility charged with the responsibility of caring for that individual, will actually"pay the price"of implementing diet modifications. It takes time and money to prepare pleasing, flavorful texture modifications. In some instances, diet modifications may be rejected for these reasons, even though the patient and a facility understand and accept their need.

TERMINOLOGY ISSUES IN DIET MODIFICATION

The lack of standardization of diet modification terminology within the field of speech-language pathology creates tremendous problems with this intervention option, and often causes confusion and miscommunication with other disciplines, as well as within the profession itself. One of the greatest challenges in the field is to standardize the terminology and methodology for thickening liquids. The names given to each degree of thickness and what it represents are numerous, undefined, and highly subjective. A survey conducted among nine dysphagia programs revealed no consistency between the label used (thin versus thick) and the actual viscosity tested during videofluoroscopy across facilities (Mills et al., 1992). Furthermore, there was no correlation between the test materials and actual dietary foods and liquids. Until a standard is established for labeling viscosity, it will be difficult to test what is safe for a patient to consume reliably, or to communicate the desired recommendations to the patient and caregivers.

In addition, diet "stages" that recommend only certain foods, with specific preparation instructions, need to be critically evaluated during assessment and carefully generalized to dietary foods available. For instance, it is not known how to generalize a patient's skill in managing a Lorna Doone cookie to other dietary foods, such as bread, nuts, fresh apple, or chili. Clinicians try to generalize entire diet recommendations of what foods and liquids can be safely consumed, usually after only a small number of trials during the evaluation process. The addition of barium to foods and liquids alters the actual taste, texture and viscosity of the foods and liquids tested. Fiberoptic endoscopic evaluation of swallowing allows testing of dietary foods and liquids in their natural state, but even this test cannot examine all desired foods and liquids for a dysphagic diet. The variety of food textures and fluid viscosities available in a "normal" diet is beyond the ability of clinicians to test during an instrumental evaluation.

Furthermore, some terms used in diet modification are jointly used by other disciplines, but have vastly different meanings to each professional. For example, speech-language pathologists and dietitians use terms such as *regular* or *soft diet,* with very different definitions (Table 9–1). The use of these terms without clarification among all staff members can be confusing and even dangerous, if a diet order is misunderstood. Dietitians describe a patient's diet primarily in terms of what nutrients are allowed and can be digested. For example, a dietitian would use the term "regular

Table 9–1. Common terminology and definitions used in dietetics and speech-language pathology.

Term	Dietetic Definition	Speech-Language Pathology Definition
Regular diet	No nutrient restrictions	No texture/viscosity restrictions
Mechanical soft/soft	Elimination of foods difficult to digest in GI tract	Foods easily chewed into cohesive bolus
Therapeutic diet	Nutrient modifications	Specific texture/viscosity modifications and feeding techniques
Diet progression	Increasing ability to digest nutrients	Increasing ability to manage food texture and thin liquids; increasing oral intake

Source: Developed in conjunction with Donna Acox, MA, RD.

diet" to mean no nutrient modification is necessary. Nutrient modification refers to the amount of fat, sodium, sugar, calories, and so on allowed in the diet per day. In contrast, speech-language pathologists describe a "regular diet" to mean that no texture modifications are necessary. Speech-language pathologists describe a dysphagia diet in terms of what food texture, viscosity, or feeding techniques should be used to eat safely.

Last, use of a standard to estimate meal consumption is also needed, with specific criteria established to estimate the percentage of food and amount of liquid consumed. This would result in more reliable nutrient intake information and nutritional planning. Staff members within a facility often are required to document the percentage of a meal consumed for every resident, and the exact amount of liquid consumed in metric measures. However, the most common error observed in determining meal consumption is an overestimation of total consumption (Rouse, 1994). This occurs when a total entrèe is consumed but no other food is touched, when food is pushed around the plate, or if the judgment is based on how much is usually consumed by the patient, rather than actual consumption. Visual aids that depict various pictures of meals, according to the percentage eaten, may be helpful to train and help caregivers accurately determine the amount of food and liquid actually ingested (Figure 9–1).

Definitions of Texture and Viscosity

Speech-language pathologists define a food's texture according to a patient's amount of difficulty in forming and propelling it as a cohesive

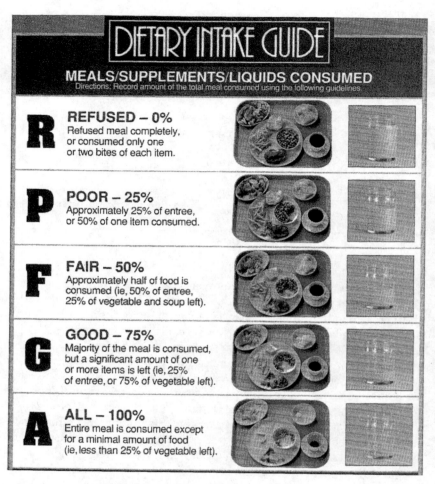

Figure 9–1. Dietary intake guide.
(From "Dietary intake guide," by Jennifer Rouse, 1994, Columbus, OH: Ross Products Division, Abbott Laboratories. Reprinted by permission.)

bolus, in a safe and timely fashion. Viscosity is defined according to actual dietary foods that vary in consistency, using terms such as syrup, nectar, honey, and pudding. The use of these descriptions is widespread within the field, yet they lack any objective measurement or standardization as to their meanings. To help clinicians find the structure and standardization they are searching for in diet modification, the definitions and methodology used in the field of food science may be beneficial.

The field of food science has extensively studied food texture and fluid viscosity for many decades. Food scientists have long recognized the importance of textural properties of food and liquids for consumer acceptance in their research, as they develop or evaluate new food products for food companies. People will not buy or eat anything they do not like. Similarly, patients with dysphagia will not prepare or eat anything they do not like, even if it provides them with all their nutrition needs, in a safe manner.

Food science has developed specific definitions and classifications to describe food texture and fluid viscosity parameters. For example, food scientists have calculated the viscosity of catsup to make sure it always pours out of the bottle but is not runny. They use objective and subjective methodology to help them analyze and study these parameters, to learn how to replicate a desired food for mass production. In addition to learning how to replicate textures and viscosities reliably, food scientists are concerned with the "sensory acceptability" of a food or liquid. A food or liquid must be pleasurable to eat. The ability to replicate desired viscosities and textures for dysphagia evaluations, and increase acceptability of diet recommendations, is sorely needed. The field of food science may provide the structure, definition, and methodology sought by clinicians who provide dysphagia management.

Food Science Definitions

Food scientists define *texture* as consisting of many different physical sensations, rather than a single parameter as speech-language pathologists tend to do (Szczesniak, 1987). The relation between textural parameters, as described by food scientists, and popular nomenclature is listed in Table 9–2. Texture is a group of properties that are sensed by touch, usually by the mouth and occasionally by the hands. It is not related to the chemical senses of taste or odor and can be measured in terms of its physical properties (called *rheology*) and perceived properties (*haptaestheis*).

Viscosity is defined as "the internal friction of a fluid or its tendency to resist flow" (Bourne, 1982, p. 13). Food scientists use mathematical equations and the laws of physics to define and measure viscosity and texture. The conventional unit of viscosity is called a poise, but since this is a rather large unit of measure, viscosity is typically described in terms of centipoise (cP). Water is 1.0 cP at 20°C. This level of specificity is certainly different from the definitions clinicians now use to describe viscosity in dysphagia management. While clinicians are not expected to become food scientists as they evaluate and manage dysphagia, a basic understanding of this terminology and methodology may help clinicians develop better definitions to the terms commonly used in dysphagia management.

Table 9–2. Relations between textural parameters and popular nomenclature.

Mechanical Characteristics		
Primary Parameters	**Secondary Parameters**	**Popular Terms**
Hardness		Soft → firm → hard
Cohesiveness	Brittleness	Crumbly → crunchy → brittle
	Chewiness	Tender → chewy → tough
	Gumminess	Short → mealy → pasty → gummy
Viscosity		Thin → viscous
Elasticity		Plastic → elastic
Adhesiveness		Sticky → tacky → gooey
General Characteristics		
Class		**Examples**
Particle size and shape		Gritty, grainy, coarse, etc.
Particle shape and orientation		Fibrous, cellular, crystalline, etc.
Other Characteristics		
Primary Parameters	**Secondary Parameters**	**Popular Terms**
Moisture content		Dry → moist → wet → watery
Fat content	Oiliness	Oily
	Greasiness	Greasy

Source: From "Classification of textural characteristics," by A. S. Szczesniak, 1963, *Journal of Food Science, 28,* 385–389. Copyright 1963, by Institute of Food Technologists. Reprinted by permission.

Although it appears initially that texture refers to solid foods, and viscosity to liquids, this distinction is not clear and separate. Many solids will act like a liquid if enough "stress" is placed on them, and it is important to realize the nature of solids and liquids frequently overlap (Bourne, 1982). The definition of *stress* in food science is a measurement of the amount of force applied to a material. Therefore, the act of mastication makes all solid foods become more "liquid" in the mouth, prior to swallowing the bolus. Clinicians are also well aware of the liquid nature of certain "solid" foods, such as applesauce and yogurt. Thus, the distinction between solid foods and liquids is often obscure and should be evaluated carefully in all diet modification recommendations.

MODIFYING LIQUID VISCOSITY

As clinicians modify liquids to aid compensation or assess a patient's ability to safely swallow liquids, it is important to understand what factors can influence liquid viscosity. The factors affecting viscosity of fluids are temperature, the concentration and molecular weight of a solute, and the amount of suspended matter in the fluid. In addition, flavor has been shown to decrease with increased viscosity or mechanical strength of foods and beverages (Baines & Morris, 1987; R. C. Clark, 1990; Godshall & Solms, 1992; Guinard & Marty, 1995; Jaime et al., 1993; Mann & Wong, 1996; Overbosch et al., 1991).

It is well known that as temperature increases, viscosity decreases (Bourne, 1982). Therefore, more thickener is necessary to achieve the same desired consistency in a hot liquid than a cold liquid. Liquids increase in thickness because of the slowing of the molecules as they cool. For this reason, refrigerated liquids will appear thicker initially after being taken out of the refrigerator. Stirring the liquid will usually return the liquid to its previous consistency. Clinicians need to be aware of the serving temperatures of foods and liquids, and even the temperature of swallowing samples during instrumental evaluation. The change in viscosity observed over time, due to changes in temperature, is a major problem in facilities. In many facilities, there is a lapse of time between kitchen preparation and delivery to the patient. This will result in warming the cold drinks and cooling the hot drinks, thus changing the viscosity of the thickened liquids.

A direct, nonlinear relationship between the concentration and molecular weight of a solute and the viscosity of the liquid is usually observed (Bourne, 1982). The concentration and molecular weight of material in a liquid can be likened to pieces of fruit within gelatin. The size and number of fruit pieces in the gelatin relate to the concentration and molecular weight of the substances within a liquid. In addition, the suspension of matter will affect viscosity. This term refers to the distribution of matter in a liquid. For example, is the fruit all at the bottom of the gelatin or evenly distributed throughout? Obviously, all of these factors may affect the viscosity of a liquid and how it will respond to commercial thickening. Clinicians commonly see the effect of these factors as they try to mix barium with various liquids. The inherent properties of barium often are heavier than the liquids they are mixing it with, and it is difficult to maintain even distribution throughout the liquid. Barium often falls to the bottom of the liquid mixture.

Furthermore, viscosity can be affected by a time dependency factor called *thixotropic*. A thixotropic factor is when the apparent viscosity of a fluid decreases at the time of mixing, but reverts to its original state after standing (Bourne, 1982). This is commonly observed when using commercial thickening agents, whereby a fluid appears thin while mixing but thickens after standing. A thixotropic factor usually encourages the use of too much thickening agent, since it requires standing time to reach the desired viscosity. Thickened liquids are reported to continue to absorb liquid and swell for up to 30 minutes (Casper, Tobochnik, Brown, & Mills, 1996). The starch in the liquid is being hydrated during this process, but the liquid eventually stabilizes its thickness and remains constant over a 24-hour period. It has also been reported that higher acidity will make a liquid thicken faster and thicker than water, although the thickness will lessen slightly over time (Casper et al., 1996). Most fruit juices have a low pH value, which indicates high acidity. Water is neutral (7.0 pH).

Given all of these factors, it is not surprising that commercial thickeners have been found to be unreliable in producing certain desired viscosities with different liquids and to have poor acceptability in terms of taste, given current clinical practices (Pelletier, 1997). Clinicians must learn to control and understand a liquid's inherent chemical properties, temperature, mixing technique, standing time, and flavor to lend more reliability to the various liquid viscosities used in dysphagia intervention. These factors are critical regardless of the thickening agent used.

Thickening Agents

When compared to various foods used to thicken liquids, the modified cornstarch thickeners were found superior in one study since they did not increase volume, stayed suspended over time, and were moderate in cost (Stanek, Hensley & VanRiper, 1992). However, natural food thickeners are sometimes preferred from a nutritional point of view, since patients will not "fill up" on modified cornstarch and, thus, they have some opportunity for additional nutrients through their liquids. Natural food thickeners may also be preferred for their lower cost, easy availability, and adequate performance in thickening. Some possible natural thickeners are applesauce, instant potatoes, miso, or any softened fruit (Shoemaker, 1997). Regardless of which thickening agent is used, clinicians need to evaluate critically which viscosity is imperative for safe swallowing and which dietary foods or liquids provide this viscosity in their natural state. In addition, they should be mindful of the sensory acceptability of a thickened liquid.

Line-Spread Test for Measuring Viscosity

Recently, an objective measurement test of viscosity developed many years ago by food scientists has been tested for use by clinicians who are assessing and recommending thickened liquids to patients with dysphagia. The line-spread test, also called the U.S. Department of Agriculture Consistometer, was originally developed as an alternative to trained sensory panels to assess viscosity of foods and beverages by food scientists (Bourne, 1982). A trained sensory panel is a group of individuals who have been extensively trained in standard rating scales and have demonstrated the ability to reproduce a texture "profile" of a simple food product successfully. This type of evaluation has actually proven to be quite reliable, but it does require a great amount of time and concentration by the individuals on the panel (Bourne, 1982). The line-spread test is based on measuring the amount of fluid flow due to gravity, over a flat surface. In a study by Mann and Wong (1996), the line-spread test was evaluated for use in formulated foods and beverages in dysphagia diets and found to be a reliable, objective tool to measure viscosity.

A premeasured amount of various foods and thickened beverages was allowed to travel for 1 minute over a diagram of premeasured concentric circles, underneath a sheet of clear plexiglass that was leveled to assure it was lying flat on the surface (Figure 9–2). The results of the line-spread

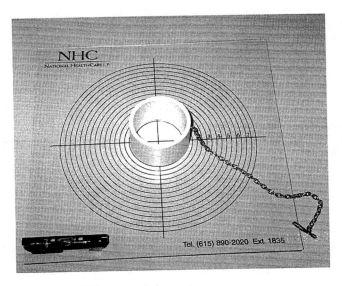

Figure 9–2. Commercial line-spread viscometer.
(Courtesy of National HealthCare, 1997, Murfreesboro, TN.)

test were compared to a trained sensory panel. Both the sensory panel and line-spread test values indicated significant differences among the samples and a strong positive correlation between the two types of results. This would indicate strong predictive validity for this method of viscosity measurement.

It has previously been recommended that viscosity measurements be standardized for use during modified barium swallow studies, so that a reliable "test kit" could be consistently used during dysphagia evaluations (Li, Brasseur, Kern, & Dodds, 1992). Pelletier and Huckabee (1997) tested the ability of the line-spread test to provide viscosity measurements with dietary foods, liquids (thickened and unthickened), and various barium dilutions, using the protocol described by Mann and Wong (1996). While this test does not appear appropriate for thin liquids, it did provide an objective measurement for other viscosities. Terms such as nectar and honey were defined according to the distance traveled over 1 minute on a flat surface. These terms provided an objective measurement that could be easily replicated by patients and caregivers in all settings.

Therefore, the line-spread test may prove beneficial to clinicians who are seeking a stable, objective, low-cost tool to assess viscosity. Viscometers that provide measurement in terms of centipoise are an alternate tool and significantly more precise, but they are expensive and therefore are not likely to be readily used in clinical settings. The inexpensive materials required for the line-spread test are available at most hardware and department stores (Table 9–3), although some of the materials are even now available commercially. The concept and methodology are easy to understand and perform (Table 9–4). While the data are still crude compared to expensive viscometers, the measurement terms are less subjective than the dietary terms typically used. However, this test does

Table 9–3. Materials required for line-spread test.

Concentric circles (0.5 cm apart), with 5 cm inner circle, and 2 lines bisecting circle like a cross to form 4 equal quadrants

Paper cups (9 oz), with bottom cut out of them

Bubble level (carpenter's level)

Clear glass or plexiglass to cover circle diagram

Metric measuring cup (50 ml)

Temperature probe

Clock/stopwatch/timer

Table 9–4. Collecting viscosity measurements using the line-spread test.

1. Record core *serving* temperature of liquid using thermometer probe.

2. Measure 50 ml of liquid.

3. Level concentric circle diagram, placed under sheet of glass/plexiglass, using bubble level.

4. Place hollow 9-oz paper cup in center circle of diagram (5 cm diameter).

5. Hold cup firmly against glass/plexiglass as liquid is poured into cup.

6. Slowly and carefully raise cup upward approximately 3 inches to allow liquid to flow. For thicker viscosities, scrape liquid into cup. Allow cup to remain over center until all drips stop.

7. After 60 seconds, record distance traveled at each of 4 quadrants. *The liquid must completely fill the circle to be rated at that distance. If only a portion of the circle is covered, the previous numbered circle is recorded.*

8. Determine the distance traveled by averaging all 4 data points from each quadrant.

9. Repeat two more times and take average of all three trials. This is the line-spread measurement for that liquid viscosity, when measured at the recorded temperature.

have limitations since it does not provide reliable data with thin liquids. Further study is needed into the application of this tool to help define viscosity terminology.

MODIFYING FOOD TEXTURE

The management issues of modifying food texture in dysphagia diets are a major source of frustration and concern by all professionals concerned with the nutritional status of patients. The development and preparation of dysphagia diets, based on a gradual progression of food properties designed to increase eating safety, is not well defined nor agreed on by clinicians. The decision of how and what foods must be modified to reduce aspiration risk is a clinical one, usually based on the evaluation of physiologic need. However, not all food textures can be evaluated during an instrumental examination, and patient variability from meal to meal may affect swallowing skills. Patient acceptance is also a major concern and problem. Since the nutritional status of the patient can obviously be affected by the presence of a modified diet, patients, caregivers, and the medical dysphagia team often look to the speech-language pathologist for guidance regarding what foods are allowed or not allowed. Therefore, clinicians need to weigh carefully all the data they collect, including a patient's wishes and desires, before they recommend a dysphagia diet.

At one end of the continuum in dysphagia diets is the recommendation for pureed food. Food that is pureed is very smooth and pudding-like. The use of pureed food textures is often recommended for patients with difficulty forming and propelling a cohesive bolus safely. However, pureed textures may also have inadequate taste, temperature, texture, and pressure to elicit an adequate pharyngeal swallow (Miller & Groher, 1982). Some authors have even advocated for the substitution of pureed foods with high-moisture semisolid foods to decrease the aspiration risk associated with the use of pureed diets (Curran & Groher, 1990).

The long-term use of pureed diets has also been criticized with regard to its effectiveness in maintaining adequate nutritional needs, resulting in protein-calorie malnutrition (Cluskey, 1989). Groher and McKaig (1995) demonstrated that many nursing home patients may be inappropriately placed or maintained on modified diets. In a review of two nursing homes with 212 residents suspected of having feeding or swallowing problems, 31% of the residents were found via chart review to have been placed on a mechanically altered diet. Ninety-one percent of those residents were receiving a diet more mechanically altered than was indicated by their swallowing physiology, as assessed by a speech-language pathologist. Four percent were at a dietary level higher than they could manage safely, and 5% were found to be at the appropriate level. The two nursing homes used in the study did not have a speech-language pathologist on staff or as a consultant. It appears that the need for specialized evaluation and reevaluation of long-term residents on diet modifications is essential not only to prevent medical complications and decreased intake, but to normalize the diet whenever possible. In fact, increased intake with better nutritional status and decreased complications may occur when the appropriate diet is recommended and normalized in a timely fashion.

The opposite end of the continuum in dysphagia diets is what is termed a regular diet, where no food restrictions are imposed with regard to textural properties. Clinicians do need to be aware that cultural and individual preferences may play a role in determining textural preferences for certain foods. While chewing is a highly enjoyable activity for healthy individuals, little is known about how long a food can be chewed before it is no longer considered pleasurable. Food scientists have researched what properties of food increase acceptance or rejection of a certain food. They have coined the term "swallowing threshold" to describe what size the food pieces must be in the mouth before a person will swallow it. In other words, what size and consistency must a bolus of food be before it is swallowed, and how does that affect acceptability of that food?

One comparison of unpublished data examined the number of chews a Filipino and an American panel took to swallow the same foods (Szczesniak & Bourne, 1982). The Filipino panel required more chews than the American panel to eat the same foods. It was hypothesized that the Filipino panel required more chews because they were culturally used to a softer textured diet. The question of what food texture is necessary for sensory pleasure needs to be individually considered for patients as dysphagia is assessed. It has been reported that individuals will reject a food texture if they require more than 10 seconds to complete the oropharyngeal phases of the swallow (O'Gara, 1990). Yet, it appears clinicians may need to reconsider this time frame and assumption,, since cultural and individual preferences may influence bolus formation, transport, and pleasure. Clinicians need to investigate individual, cultural, and religious preferences prior to recommending any diet modification, and include as many traditional, favorite foods as possible.

FOOD FOR THOUGHT:

How does dysphagia influence "swallowing thresholds"? Since cultural and individual preferences may alter how long a patient will chew before swallowing, what constitutes an appropriate length of time to form and propel a bolus? What time frame would constitute "excessive chewing"?

Dysphagia Diets

A plethora of dysphagia diets, usually described in terms of levels or stages, exist for use by patients. Unfortunately, no standardization or agreement of terms, levels or stages exists today. Therefore, it is impossible to provide specific levels in this text that all clinicians should follow. However, a major initiative to provide this information is currently being studied and developed by a group of dietitians, speech-language pathologists, food scientists, and the food industry. This initiative is called the National Dysphagia Diet Project. The objective of this diet is "to rapidly progress the patient to as normal a food texture as possible while maintaining safety" (National Dysphagia Diet Task Force, 1997).

According to their Internet newsletter (www.dysphagia-diet.com), food properties have been placed on a continua, with anchors set at each end, of actual food choices and measurable values. Four levels have been proposed for both solids and liquids. The solid diet levels are dysphagia pureed, dysphagia mechanically altered, dysphagia advanced, and regular. The liquid levels are termed thin, nectar-like, honey-like, and spoon-thick. There are seven textural properties that appear to influence the quality of a swallow and the overall health status of patient, according to research conducted by Med-Diet Laboratories, Inc. The seven textures are (republished with permission of Don Tymchuck, Med-Diet Laboratories, Inc.):

1. *Adhesiveness*—the work required to overcome the attractive forces between the surface of the food and another contacted surface, such as the palate
2. *Biteability (fracturability)*—the force with which a solid sample breaks, such as between the incisors
3. *Chewability (hardness)*—the force required to compress a solid food to attain a certain deformation, as in biting and chewing
4. *Cohesiveness*—the degree to which the product deforms rather than shears when compressed, such as between the tongue and palate
5. *Firmness*—the force required to compress a semisolid, such as between the tongue and palate
6. *Springness*—the degree/rate that a sample returns to its original shape when compressed
7. *Viscosity*—the rate of flow per unit force, such as required to draw the food between the lips and spoon

The goal of this project is to provide ultimately a comprehensive program that can be used by all professionals concerned with meeting the nutritional needs of the patient with dysphagia. This would include evaluation and documentation tools and recommendations for patient education and staff training (National Dysphagia Diet Task Force, 1997). The participation of all the critical players in dysphagia management to develop this much needed tool make this project laudable. Clinicians can only hope that their efforts will prove fruitful and beneficial in the near future.

Although the textural properties of solids are important, food appearance and taste are also vital for patient acceptance. Many food companies now manufacture food molds, puree food thickeners to enhance texture and appearance, and prepared pureed meals that are frozen and reconstituted prior to serving. There are various cookbooks available with ideas of how to prepare dysphagia diets with modified texture, adequate nutrient content, and, most important, pleasing appearance. It is hoped that many reluctant patients may accept a textural modification if it is presented in an appetizing manner on the plate, with the right temperature and recognizable items. However, the cost and inconvenience of preparing pureed meals with high visual appeal may deter even a highly motivated individual or facility to implement these suggestions.

SPECIAL ISSUES: USE OF MILK AND WATER IN DYSPHAGIA DIETS

Occasionally, recommendations for diet modification as a treatment option for patients with dysphagia will also give rise to questions regarding the use of milk and dairy products and free water in the modified diet. It has been hypothesized that milk and other dairy products may produce increased mucus, thereby exacerbating an oropharyngeal dysphagia and making it difficult to swallow safely. Consequently, patients with this apparent mucus reaction are sometimes not allowed any dairy products for consumption. In addition, patients with documented aspiration of thin liquids frequently are recommended to eliminate all free water from their diet, because of the increased risk of pneumonia. Yet the hypothesis of whether the aspiration of small amounts of free water will actually increase the risk of pneumonia is often questioned. Given the importance of maintaining nutrient and hydration status in patients with dysphagia, the elimination of all dairy products and/or free water may have a significant effect on the health status of a patient if the substitutions are not accepted. Therefore, clinicians should understand what is known about these issues, and educate patients regarding the risks involved as patients choose their dysphagia diet.

Milk and Mucus

It has been believed for decades that drinking cow's milk increases the production of mucus (Tufts University, 1993). Studies in Australia found that 30% of the population hold this belief, with an associated 38% reduction in liquid milk intake observed (Arney & Pinnock, 1993). Unfortunately, there are no clinically controlled studies that have specifically addressed the effect of milk and dairy products in increasing mucus and difficulty swallowing in patients with dysphagia. However, the "milk makes mucus" theory has been studied in other groups. Athletes commonly report a cottonmouth feeling drinking milk, creating dryness, discomfort, and thick white saliva in the mouth. In studies with athletes, it was concluded that the cottonmouth feeling was associated with fluid loss and emotional stress during competition and practice, and not due to drinking milk (N. Clark, 1990; National Dairy Council, 1991). It is known that as body water is lost, the flow and composition of saliva change. Therefore, it was hypothesized that the athletes' complaint of increased mucus due to milk may actually be due to the amount of water lost during strenuous exercise.

Other studies have investigated the effect of milk on respiratory symptoms. Pinnock, Graham, Mylvaganam, and Douglas (1990) reported that no association was observed among milk intake, respiratory symptoms, and nasal secretion weights in adults injected with a cold virus. Asthmatic children who were given high milk instead of a milk-free diet showed a small increase in nasal congestion, but no other symptoms of congestion, wheeze, or peak flow measurements were found related to the milk diet, compared to the milk-free diet (Pinnock, Martin, & Mylvaganam, 1989).

Healthy individuals who believe that milk makes mucus were found to report more respiratory symptoms and consume less milk and dairy products than those who were nonbelievers of this theory (Arney & Pinnock, 1993). Interestingly, both believers and nonbelievers reported identical increased mucus symptoms when drinking cow's milk and an identically flavored placebo of a soy-based product (Pinnock & Arney, 1991). This placebo was indistinguishable from milk in pretesting. Since these reported increased symptoms occurred in the milk and placebo groups, the authors concluded that the effect of increased mucus, if real, is not specific to milk. It can be duplicated with a similarly formulated milk substitute.

These studies raise interesting questions, as clinicians think about dysphagia and the possible effect of milk on mucus production. It is known that elderly individuals, healthy and sick, have difficulty maintaining adequate hydration. It is not known what effect the presence of dehydration and the emotional stress of illness may play in a patient with dysphagia in producing mucus. Could these factors influence saliva production and composition and cause increased mucus? What is the risk of increased mucus in patients with dysphagia? While the answers to these questions are not yet known, it does appear that many factors other than milk alone may be involved in producing milk-mucus symptoms.

Free Water

For some patients restricted in their liquid intake to thickened liquids or tube feedings, the craving for water is overwhelming. For patients who refuse thickened liquids, they may become dehydrated and crave water to quench their thirst. Although adequate hydration may actually occur via a feeding tube or even thickened liquids, some patients continue to request ice chips or free water for oral satisfaction. They demand water, even when it is understood that aspiration occurs with thin liquids. Their compliance and satisfaction with their dysphagia intervention plan can be quite low. Unfortunately, there are no controlled studies that have investigated the efficacy of patients with drinking water when aspiration of thin liquids is documented.

A recent review of the literature regarding the use of water to maintain hydration in nursing home patients who aspirate thin liquids concluded that patients should be assessed individually and managed carefully, incorporating all relevant information gained from their medical history, current status, cognition, and swallowing deficits (Batchelor, Neilsen, & Sexton, 1996). It is reported that small amounts of saliva or water aspirated in healthy individuals may pose no health problem, but it is strongly believed by some authors that this is not true for individuals who are ill or bed-ridden (Batchelor et al., 1996; Langley, 1989; Logemann, 1983).

Water is neutral in acidity. Minute amounts of water aspirated into the lungs can be rapidly absorbed by the body (Batchelor et al., 1996). According to Batchelor and colleagues (1996), the problem for patients with dysphagia may reside in the change in water composition as it enters the oral cavity and is aspirated into the lungs. The oral cavity has anaerobic bacteria living in its crevasses, around dentures and natural teeth (Terry & Fuller, 1989; Batchelor et al., 1996). Poor oral hygiene and dental caries also contribute to bacteria growth in the mouth. These bacteria can be easily washed into the lungs as a patient aspirates free water. Severe respiratory distress can occur if liquid enters the lungs (DePaso, 1991). Many nursing home patients may suffer severe consequences if anaerobic bacteria enters their lungs, since their immune systems and pulmonary functions may already be compromised (Batchelor et al., 1996).

Many questions are raised by the use of water in dysphagia management. While aspiration of oral saliva in patients with dental decay or poor oral care appears associated with increased risk of pneumonia (Langmore et al., 1998), it is not known whether patients would be able to manage the aspiration of small amounts of free water safely if their oral care was aggressively addressed. Increased patient satisfaction and even perhaps better compliance with the use of other thickened liquids may occur. Some clinicians have anecdotally reported no increased pneumonia in their patients who were allowed free water between meals, but this observation has not been tested in large controlled clinical trials (Hartlage & Panther, 1992). There has been one randomly controlled study that has evaluated the effect of uncontrolled oral water intake in two groups of 10 patients, all with identified aspiration (Garon, Engle, & Ormiston, 1997). While one group was allowed oral water and one was not, neither group developed pneumonia. However, the sample size of this study is too small to determine definitively the effect of uncontrolled water intake in patients who aspirate. It should be viewed by clinicians as interesting pilot data only.

Clearly, the benefits perceived by patients and families given the ability to consume free water would be great. However, these benefits need to be weighed against the potential risk of pneumonia, given the current state of knowledge regarding this issue. Again, it is ultimately the patient, not clinician, who must decide whether the risks outweigh the benefits of drinking free water when pharyngeal dysphagia is present.

CONCLUSION

The use of diet modification in the treatment of oropharyngeal dysphagia presents many challenges. The lack of standardization in the terminology used in diet modification creates confusion among the field of speech-language pathology, patients, and other disciplines involved in managing the nutritional status of the patient. The discipline of food science has established definitions and methodologies regarding food texture and liquid viscosities that may prove beneficial to speech-language pathology. It is clear that clinicians must now focus on improving their terminology and communication with others as they recommend diet modification as a nutritional option for dysphagia. In addition, attention must be paid to the factors that influence patient acceptance of diet modification, such as taste, texture, appearance, cost, and convenience. The efficacy of using dairy products or free water in dysphagia diets is still not known. These important clinical issues still need to be evaluated, using controlled clinical trials, before their risk can be fully understood.

10

Special Issues of Feeding Dependency

Being dependent for feeding appears to be a major risk factor for developing aspiration pneumonia. It has implications for the prevention of malnutrition and dehydration as well. The many management issues surrounding caregivers who feed patients and what role clinicians can play in implementing proper feeding techniques with patients are the subject of this chapter.

The risk of developing aspiration pneumonia is almost 20 times greater for a patient who is dependent on others to be fed, than for people who can feed themselves (Langmore et al., 1998). While dysphagia is an important risk factor for aspiration pneumonia, Langmore and colleagues found that its presence is generally not sufficient to cause pneumonia unless other risk factors are present as well. Interestingly, the best predictors of aspiration pneumonia in elderly subjects were dependency for feeding, dependency for oral care, tube feeding, number of decayed teeth, number of medications, more than one medical diagnosis, and smoking. Feeding dependency was the best single predictor of pneumonia.

The implications for dysphagia management are significant. It appears that clinicians must direct their attention to the issues surrounding feeding dependency, in addition to providing traditional rehabilitative and compensatory interventions. Minimizing the amount of material aspirated, whether it be food, liquid, or saliva, appears to be crucial in preventing pneumonia (Langmore et al., 1998). Thus, it appears that *how* caregivers are feeding patients and providing their oral care, among other factors, may be vital in preventing pneumonia. In addition, caregiver training and implementation of the care plan may be important to prevent malnutrition and dehydration. Clinicians need to focus equal attention to caregivers and patients dependent on feeding to maximize success of the dysphagia management plan.

PATIENTS AND THEIR CAREGIVERS

While caregivers are a critical component of the management plan for feeding dependent patients, patients themselves are critical to the success of the care plan. Through verbal or nonverbal communication, or quality-of-life directives, they can indicate their wishes regarding their desire to be fed. They can physically resist feeding presentations, spit food out, and verbally or physically strike out. The legal and ethical issues surrounding the eating-dependent patient are great. The staff caring for patients who are dependent for feeding must be trained to respect their wishes at all times. Careful documentation and discussions with staff and the patient should occur (see Chapter 12).

Caregivers are responsible for maintaining and implementing the appropriate dysphagia management recommendations for patients who are dependent on others for feeding. They may be family members, close friends, employed staff at facilities where a patient is living, or even a volunteer at a local nursing home or hospital. They may be involved in the care temporarily or permanently, depending on the setting and relationship. They are involved only when patients are not able independently to implement the care plan themselves. They may serve a minor role to the patient or be solely responsible for the dysphagia intervention.

The importance of caregiver attitudes, training, and motivation when feeding patients who are dependent for feeding appears critical to safe, adequate oral intake. Caregivers can be instrumental in enhancing or reducing enjoyment in eating. They can encourage or discourage acceptance of the feeding strategies. They can diligently introduce appropriate feeding techniques for every meal, or they can ignore them. They can be knowledgeable about a patient's likes or dislikes, or ignorant about them. They can choose to cooperate with the care plan or not. They are essential to the success or failure of the care plan.

Feeding a Patient: Incidence and Importance

Although feeding dependency can occur in any setting, it is well known that long-term care facilities increasingly rely on staff to assist patients in feeding, with 50 to 66% of the residents requiring some form of assistance (Dwyer et al., 1987; Siebens et al., 1986; Silver, Morley, Strome, Jones, & Vickers, 1988). Because of limited physical movement, poor physical endurance, or low cognition/responsiveness, some patients must have someone else feed them. It is not unusual for one staff member to be responsible for 8 to 10 patients per meal, with tremendous pressure placed on staff members to maximize oral intake and speed of eating (Musson et al., 1990).

It appears that feeding dependency may play an important role in the incidence of malnutrition, dehydration, and aspiration pneumonia in the nursing home setting. Malnutrition and dehydration are common problems in this setting, with a reported incidence of 12 to 70% (Cooper & Cobb, 1988; Kolasa, Schmidt, & Bartlett, 1989; Sandman, Adolfsson, Nygren, Hallmans, & Winbald, 1987). Feeding dependency has been suggested as one explanation for these problems (Cooper & Cobb, 1988; Sandman et al., 1987). The incidence of aspiration pneumonia in nursing homes is also high, accounting for 13 to 48% of all infections in this setting (Crossley & Thurn, 1989; Zimmer, Bentley, Valenti, & Watson, 1986). The social embarrassment of being fed may also contribute to poor nutritional intake (Levy, 1993).

CAREGIVER FEEDING PRACTICES
AND PHILOSOPHIES

Since caregiver feeding practices may directly relate to the incidence of aspiration pneumonia, malnutrition, and dehydration in patients, a careful observation into common feeding practices may yield important information for clinicians. An interesting study by Sanders, Hoffman, and Lund (1992) regarding feeding practices of caregivers may help provide clinicians with greater insight into the complexities surrounding this management issue and give them insight into what can be done to improve it.

Sanders et al. (1992) conducted a comparison of feeding practices between five dependent eaters and five independent eaters in a nursing home setting. Dependent eaters were defined as those residents who were physically or cognitively unable to feed themselves, as assessed by nursing personnel. Independent eaters were able to feed themselves and sit in a dining room to eat, requiring assistance only to set up the meal (opening milk carton, buttering bread, and so on). Caregivers were individuals who actually helped set up the meal or feed the dependent eaters. They were registered and licensed nurses, nursing aides, and family members. There were 15 caregivers involved in setting up the meal or feeding the residents.

Observations of the feeding practices of caregivers and the intake of residents were conducted for 3 meals daily and the evening snack, over 3 consecutive days, for a total of 45 meals for each group. The residents and caregivers were aware of being observed for some of the meals, but not all of the meals. An interview was conducted with all caregivers, which included direct questions regarding their feeding practices and philosophy. The results of this study provide some interesting data regarding a variety of factors compared between dependent and independent eaters, such as time factors to receive and eat a meal, size of the utensil used to feed, food texture and temperature, and caregiver knowledge and use of appropriate feeding techniques (Table 10–1).

Time Factors

Time factors, in terms of waiting to eat and the speed of being fed, differed between the groups. Dependent eaters waited approximately 14 minutes longer than independent eaters for their meals, making their meals lukewarm approximately half of the time. Independent eaters were served acceptable food temperatures all the time. Dependent eaters were fed more bites/min than the independent eaters fed themselves. A tablespoon, rather than teaspoon, was used to feed dependent eaters for a majority of the meals while independent eaters used a tablespoon less than half of the time. The speed of eating observed for each group was not significantly differently in this study and averaged approximately 17 minutes. However, when caregivers were questioned regarding the average length of time it took them to feed a patient, a third of the caregivers reported the duration of a meal could take as long as 5 to 10 minutes.

A wide variation in the duration of time necessary to feed someone has been reported in the literature, ranging from 5 to 99 minutes to complete a meal. Hotaling (1990) suggests 30 to 50 minutes are necessary to

Table 10–1. Comparison of feeding practices between dependent eaters and independent eaters in 45 meals for each group.

Factor	Dependent Eaters	Independent Eaters
Waiting for meal (min)*	22.7 ± 2.3[a]	9.2 ± 0.7
Duration of meal (min)	17.3 ± 2.2	17.7 ± 1.0
No. of bites/min*	5.5 ± 0.1	4.4 ± 0.2
Size of utensils used*		
Tablespoon	30[b]	19[b]
Teaspoon	15	26
Swallowing difficulty*	22	2
Acceptable food temperature*	23	45
Patient's posture during meal < 45° angle*	28	None
Caregiver's distance from patient during feeding		
Full arm's length	37	NA[c]
Forearm's length	8	NA
Position of meal tray from patient*		
Front of patient	6	45
Side of patient	39	None
Caregiver knows of patient's food preference	18	17
Texture of diet served*		
Puree	37	None
Solid	8	45

[a]Mean ± standard error.

[b]Number of meals of total of 45.

[c]NA = not applicable.

*Significant at the .05 level or better.

Source: From "Feeding strategy for dependent eaters" by H. N. Sanders, S. B. Hoffman, and C. A. Lund, 1992, *Journal of the American Dietetic Association*, 92 (11), 1389. Copyright 1992, by American Dietetic Association. Reprinted by permission.

feed a patient without rushing. A study of 214 dependent eaters in a nursing home in Sweden (Backstrom, Norberg, & Norberg, 1987) showed that the average duration of a meal fed by a caregiver was approximately 20 minutes. Hu, Huang, and Cartwright (1986) reported that caregivers in a nursing home spent 18 minutes per day feeding patients who were severely demented, while similar patients fed at home were fed for 99 minutes. Even within the nursing home, Hu et al. (1986) reported differences were found regarding the duration of feeding by staff and family caregivers. Staff members took an average of 14 minutes per day to assist a patient who was mild to moderately demented, while family members took 28 minutes. It is obvious that the emotional bond between caregiver and patient may affect the amount of time taken to feed a meal. What constitutes an appropriate length of time to safely feed a patient is still not known, since every patient and situation differs.

Position Factors

Improper positioning for feeding may lead to increased dysphagia symptoms, despite being fed a pureed diet (Athlin, Norberg, Axelsson, Moller, & Nordstrom, 1989). Sanders et al. (1992) reported that dependent eaters were fed at $< 45°$ angle 28 out of 45 meals while independent eaters fed themselves always in an upright position. During the caregiver interview, all caregivers indicated they knew the appropriate position to feed a patient ($> 45°$ angle), yet this was observed in less than half of the meals served dependent eaters. It appears that while caregivers know that feeding position may influence aspiration risk, they frequently do not safely position the patient to feed them.

Food Texture Factors

It has been suggested that the use of pureed diets may not prevent the incidence of aspiration pneumonia in selected patients (Groher, 1987) and it may contribute to poor nutrient intake (Cluskey, 1989). Sanders et al. (1992) reported the majority of dependent eaters were fed a pureed meal while all independent eaters ate solid food. It has also been reported that 15 to 20% of residents in long-term care settings receive a pureed diet (Hotaling, 1992).

It is not known whether the lack of texture and, therefore, a decrease of sensory input, contributes to the increase the risk of aspiration. It is also not known whether feeding practices or the medical conditions that contribute to the necessity of being fed lead to increased risk of aspiration. However, it does appear that the use of food texture modification is prevalent in dependent eaters and it warrants careful scrutiny in the management of these patients. Pureed consistency may not prevent aspiration in some patients, and it may even contribute to malnutrition and dehydration if the patient does not accept the diet modification.

Caregiver Philosophies

Perhaps most intriguing in the Sanders et al. study (1992) are the responses by caregivers to questions regarding their own feeding practices and philosophy. They recognized that a patient may choke by being fed an inappropriate bolus food size or being fed too quickly. They also knew that a medical condition such as a stroke or presence of dysphagia may increase a patient's chance of choking. However, no caregiver listed his or her own feeding practices as a reason for a patient choking.

The majority of caregivers used patients' diagnosis or ability as the basis for determining their need for feeding. Nine of 15 caregivers listed the main priority in feeding was to maintain energy and fluid intake, while the rest reported the need to prevent choking or aspiration as top priority. Only 4 out of 15 of the caregivers felt that noise during a meal would bother a patient; all others believed noise would have no effect on food intake. Three caregivers received formal training on feeding practices during school, while seven received no training. The rest received an orientation only.

This study raises some important points. Why don't caregivers practice the safe feeding skills they know? How much do caregivers really know about the rationale and importance of safe feeding practices? According to the Sanders et al. study (1992), caregivers do not really understand these issues. The vast majority of caregivers (13 out of 15) stated some patients do not feed themselves because they crave attention, while the remaining caregivers stated they did not know the reason why patients are feeding dependent. These caregivers listed a variety of methods to correct these attention-seeking behaviors. Some caregivers refused to feed these patients, some gave in and fed them, and some encouraged the patients to feed themselves independently.

Sanders et al. (1992) concluded that proper training of caregivers was important to implement correct feeding techniques and maximize nutritional intake. However, it appears that basic knowledge of "how to feed" may not be enough. More emphasis must be given to caregivers regarding the reasons for feeding a patient and the importance of getting to know the patient. Most caregivers relied on a patient's facial expression or body language to determine a patient's feeding preferences, while only one caregiver asked a family member (Sanders et al., 1992). Caregivers often are unclear how to increase oral intake or modify their feeding technique to help patients eat difficult foods. They may try to soak difficult foods in liquid or coach or reward the patient. They may decide not to feed patients difficult foods, or refuse to feed them at all. Of great concern is the response by some caregivers that they would "try not to force the patient to eat." Forcing patients to eat in an effort to increase oral intake must never occur. Patients have the right to refuse food and liquid and the act of forcing food or liquid into their mouth violates that right. It also may increase their risk of aspiration or obstruction, as patients fight the placement rather than coordinate a safe swallow. Finally, this act certainly contributes to a negative eating experience rather than a pleasurable event. For all of these reasons, no patient should ever be forced to eat or drink. It is imperative to listen to what the patient is saying, even if it is by nonverbal communication.

The appropriate interventions to manage these problems must be based on a comprehensive evaluation of the patient, his or her particular needs, personality, and the nature of the disordered swallowing physiology. It is hoped that once caregivers understand the rationale for feeding dependency, appropriate feeding practices can be individually developed and implemented with reliability.

ENHANCING PATIENT ACCEPTANCE

When patients refuse to be fed, clinicians need to evaluate the reason(s) for patient rejection. Rejection may revolve around many problems such as the appearance, temperature, and texture of food and liquids (see Chapter 9). Clinicians may improve patient acceptance to diet modifications and feeding dependency if attention is given to these factors. In addition, clinicians must evaluate the patient's readiness to eat, which includes alertness, oral care and status, a pleasant eating environment, and appropriate body position. Also, the use of backward chaining as a feeding technique may increase patient acceptance and provide self-feeding training. This is a common technique employed in occupational therapy that involves using the "end product" as the beginning task, by guiding the patient's hand directly to his or her mouth initially and then gradually declining assistance to the mouth. Since clinicians must rely on caregivers to implement the care plan judiciously, attention must also be given to caregiver training and feeding techniques. Clinicians need to evaluate the ability for the patient to manage finger foods safely, and how placement of food into the mouth can enhance bolus control. All of these factors may improve acceptance of being fed (Table 10–2).

Alertness

Patients must be awake and alert to their environment to be fed. They do not have to be responsive verbally, but they must be able to indicate readi-

Table 10–2. Techniques to enhance acceptance of feeding.

Position properly first.

Check alertness: Is patient awake and ready to eat?

Approach patient calmly and appropriately to his or her mood.

Investigate whether patient can use any finger foods safely.

Enhance food and liquid appearance, taste, and temperature.

Place small amount of food on lips and encourage licking it off.

Place bolus of food correctly in mouth, according to physiologic need, to enhance control.

Create a pleasant atmosphere that increases appetite.

Try backward chaining feeding technique.

Decrease all distractions.

ness to receive food into their mouth. The decision of whether a patient is awake enough to accept oral food is a clinical judgment. Food or liquid should not be offered to a patient who is not alert enough to ingest the material safely. Eyes may be closed, but clinicians must judge carefully the readiness of the patient to accept oral food or liquid. Patients may indicate readiness by licking off a taste of food to the lips or by accepting an empty spoon to the lips or mouth. If a patient does not respond to these attempts with some appropriate oral movements (closure around the utensil, sucking movements, and so forth), oral feeding should not occur.

Oral Care

All patients need to practice good oral hygiene to eliminate bacteria in their mouths, prevent infection and dental decay, and maximize their ability to eat comfortably and safely. Patients who are dependent for feeding may also be dependent for their oral care, leaving this essential daily task to the responsibility of a caregiver. Since patients who are dependent for oral care have been found to be almost three times more likely to get pneumonia than those who can independently perform this task, the importance of practicing adequate oral hygiene appears crucial (Langmore et al., 1998). The reasons for not providing adequate oral care in the nursing home have been investigated and are numerous. Some reasons reported include poor physical health, poor manual dexterity, poor access to dental services, negative attitude of dentists caring for the elderly, and a lack of knowledge and skill regarding how to provide adequate oral care by the nursing home staff (Empey, Kiyak, & Milgrom, 1983; Napierski & Danner, 1982).

Adequate oral care must involve several components. Teeth should be brushed at least twice a day and flossed at least once every 24 hours. Power toothbrushes may be helpful to patients with impaired motor function (Wilkins, 1989), and suction toothbrushes are beneficial to patients who cannot voluntarily spit after brushing. It is recommended that only a pea-sized amount of toothpaste be used on a toothbrush, without water, to decrease foaming and increase the abrasive cleaning action. An oral suction machine can be used to remove excess foaming, which eliminates the need for a water rinse. Removal of any food residue after eating is important, even with a patient who is edentulous. A fluoride rinse or anti-bacterial mouthwash may be used when soaked in a sponge toothette and wiped in the mouth. Antibacterial toothpaste, mouthwash, and even gum are now available in nonprescription form (*Biotene,*™ Laclede Research Laboratories) to destroy oral cavity bacteria and provide lubrication.

Xerostomia

Xerostomia, the clinical manifestation of salivary gland dysfunction, is a common problem reported in healthy elderly that results in a feeling of dryness, alternations in taste, and difficulty with mastication and swallowing (Kaplan & Baum, 1993). This is a common problem in patients who have severe dysphagia and may need to be fed. Xerostomia may be due to a variety of medical conditions, such as medications, radiation therapy, diabetes, stress, depression, and autoimmune disorders. It does not appear to be due to increased age, as previously believed (Atkinson & Fox, 1992; Kaplan & Baum, 1993). Saliva serves many important functions. It regulates the composition of the oral flora, begins the breakdown of food for digestion, acts as a solvent and vehicle for taste to the taste buds, and protects the teeth and oral mucosa, by neutralizing the high acid environment produced by oral bacteria (Kaplan & Baum, 1993). When patients do not produce enough saliva, it can be painful and difficult to eat and swallow. A variety of products are available that may provide relief to xerostomia, such as lubricating gels and artificial saliva sprays. Interestingly, milk has even been suggested as a treatment for xerostomia (Herod, 1994). Because milk is nutritious and anticariogenic, it may provide the extra moisture necessary to aid mastication, taste, and swallowing when eating food.

Eating Environment

Hotaling (1990) outlines specific recommendations for assessing the eating environment in a nursing home, and enhancing appetite and intake. She suggests that poor nutritional intake, for independent and dependent feeders, may be improved by creating a positive mealtime experience. The use of nutritional supplements may be avoided if appetite is enhanced during mealtimes. The use of aromas (coffee brewing in the room, cookies baking, and so on) may increase patients' interest. According to Hotaling (1990), a pleasant atmosphere can be attained in any setting with a little effort. Low music may be pleasant, but this should be carefully assessed. For some cognitively impaired individuals, music may be beneficial to rouse them for a meal. On the other hand, it may be overstimulating and result in behavior problems. Patients need to be carefully assessed to determine the environment they need to increase their interest and ability to eat orally. Although clinicians may suggest ideas to improve the eating environment, the decision for implementing these suggestions usually is not under their direct control.

Body Position

The importance of appropriate positioning for eating, whether the patient eats in the dining room or in bed, is critical and should be the first step prior to feeding a patient. Appropriate positioning will improve a patient's ability to self-feed if it is possible, aid in airway protection, and provide maximal comfort (Hotaling, 1990).

Patients should be positioned for feeding with the pelvis and shoulder girdle straight and upright. When this body position is obtained, correct placement of the extremities and head and neck for eating can occur. Whenever possible, a patient should be sitting upright with the pelvis as far back as possible in a solid chair, with solid arms. This will add stability and allow upper extremity movement for self-feeding. The hips should be at a 90° angle, with both feet placed flat on the floor and shoulders slightly forward. The arms of a patient should be supported on the table or arms of the chair, with the height of the table and chair appropriate for the patient. The head should be upright and aligned with the trunk (Koltin & Rosen, 1996).

Backward Chaining

The use of "backward chaining," a specific training technique used in occupational therapy, has anecdotally been quite successful in combating resistance to being fed. The goal of backward chaining is to increase patient control and awareness of oral intake, as the clinician gradually decreases the amount of guidance necessary for the patient to reach his or her mouth. This idea and technique are common in occupational therapy for retraining a variety of activities of daily living, such as dressing or tying a shoe (Pedretti, 1996). Rather than feeding a patient by placing a spoonful of food to the mouth, clinicians place the spoonful of food in the patients' hand and help them guide it to their own mouth. In this manner, patients receive the same hand-to-mouth movement required when feeding oneself. Eliciting hand-to-mouth movements in the patient may help individuals who are cognitively impaired realize that oral intake is about to begin (Logemann, 1997). For those with hearing or visual losses, they may not become as startled when the spoon touches their mouth. Assistance is gradually withdrawn from guiding their hand to their mouth, as patients learn to regain the ability to feed themselves again.

A referral to the occupational therapist is indicated for suggestions regarding how to retrain feeding skills and maximize feeding independence. Adaptive utensils and materials, such as dycem to hold a plate in place, sipper cups, and swinging spoons, can be useful in aiding independent feeding skill. The use of finger foods also may be beneficial to many patients who are relearning how to feed themselves. If a patient can safely manage the texture of finger foods, their use may greatly increase nutritional intake in a patient who resists being fed.

Caregiver Training

Caregivers who are family members or employees of an institution present different training issues. Since caregivers within a patient's home are solely responsible for implementing diet modifications, Pardoe (1993) suggests that educational material be carefully developed for each diet stage and liquid modification. The instructions must be designed with great clarity as well, since many patients and family members are advanced in age and the risks involved for noncompliance may be severe. Likewise, continuous education and monitoring must occur in health care settings for staff members who are responsible for producing and serving modified diets (Pardoe, 1993). Once staff is made aware of the importance of their actions in maintaining appropriate diet recommendations, it is not uncommon for them to return unsatisfactory food to the production area, report difficulties, or offer suggestions for improvements. This is a positive and welcome sign that the caregivers are knowledgeable and diligent in their understanding of dysphagia interventions.

Given the enormous responsibility of nursing home staff to provide feeding assistance to many residents, the introduction of volunteer programs and multidisciplinary treatment teams has developed. Musson et al. (1990) developed three interdisciplinary programs within a nursing home to address the prevention of malnutrition and dehydration in residents who required feeding assistance. A volunteer program called "Silver Spoons" was developed that recruited, trained, and supervised community volunteers to feed nursing home patients. A "Happy Hour" time each afternoon was instituted that involved the delivery of bulk refreshments and snacks to a nursing unit to increase hydration and socialization. Group activities were conducted during happy hour to promote the social aspects of eating and drinking, and increase appetite and thirst. The final program developed was "Second Seating," in which lunch in the dining room was provided at an alternative time, for selected patients who required special modifications of eating style, food texture, or timing. These patients had previously been fed in their rooms because of their feeding requirements, but during "Second Seating," they were fed lunch in the dining room when the greatest staff or volunteer assistance was available and when time was not an issue.

The training of volunteers for "Silver Spoons" was similar to another training program described by Lipner, Bosler, and Giles (1990). Both programs involved the following components:

1. All volunteers must complete a training program before feeding a patient.
2. The training program consisted of a 90-minute lecture and practical experience.
3. Specific training objectives were outlined and volunteers were evaluated to meet the established criteria prior to feeding a patient.
4. Some form of recognition was given to the volunteer to wear when feeding a patient (button, pin, or apron), to allow staff to identify volunteers who have completed the training and to provide a sense of team recognition.
5. Quarterly or annual recognition program of volunteer service was conducted, usually at a dinner or special meeting.

Evaluating Caregiver Training Programs

Do these training programs work? Do they prevent malnutrition, dehydration, or pneumonia in patients who require feeding? Unfortunately, there are few data regarding the effectiveness of volunteer training programs in preventing these significant complications. Musson et al. (1990) did report that weight gain was noted in those patients who participated in her programs, with greater weight gain documented as the number of programs they attended increased. Lipner et al. (1990) reported an increased prominence for the role of the speech-language pathologist in evaluating and treating dysphagia within long-term care facilities, but no improvement was documented for the patients. More medical requests for swallowing evaluation consultations were made and it was believed that nursing staff was able to provide improved patient care to feeding "high-risk" patients, given the use of trained volunteers to help feed other residents.

Martens, Cameron, and Simonsen (1990) reported on a prospective study conducted in a neurology/neurosurgery unit to determine if a dysphagia program would improve caloric intake and body weight, improve self-feeding ability, or decrease the frequency of aspiration pneumonia. A time series design was implemented in which the control group was treated by staff who had not received dysphagia treatment training. In addition, the control group was not assessed by a dysphagia team. The treated group received bedside and videofluoroscopic examinations to determine the specific swallowing disorder. Nursing staff were trained in general dysphagia management and how to implement an individualized treatment plan.

Significant weight gain and increased caloric intake occurred in the treated group, but no incidence of aspiration pneumonia was reported in either group. It was speculated that the absence of aspiration pneumonia in either group may have been due to the excellent care delivered in the acute hospital setting and the greater attention given to both groups regarding prevention.

SPEECH-LANGUAGE PATHOLOGISTS AND FEEDING DEPENDENCY

The responsibilities of the speech-language pathologist in managing patients who are dependent for feeding are great. As Langmore et al. (1998) suggests, intervention cannot be solely focused on managing patients' physiologic impairments of swallowing. Attention needs to be given to the caregivers who feed and provide oral care for their patients. In keeping with a coach analogy, clinicians need to assess the other "team" players surrounding the patient and determine what is needed to implement the plan. Who will be responsible for feeding the patient? What is the relationship of the patient to the caregiver? How many caregivers will be responsible for feeding the patient? What is the prognosis for self-feeding in the future? What are the current feeding and oral care practices?

Caregivers often anticipate or experience a variety of problems as they try to implement a care plan. They may decide the intervention is not appropriate or feasible for a variety of reasons, and quietly implement what they think is right. Training on the mechanisms of the intervention plan may not be enough to guarantee appropriate feeding practices. In addition, one reason for poor follow-through of the management plan may be the low level of authority clinicians have over important components of the care plan. It is rare for clinicians to have supervisory authority over staff who feed patients. In addition, clinicians typically do not make purchasing decisions regarding foods, liquids, or thickeners. They do not decide the time or manner of preparation. Clinicians must rely on others to follow the feeding techniques recommended, and present the appropriate diet in an acceptable manner.

There is often a high level of frustration and "burn-out" experienced by clinicians working with feeding-dependent patients and their caregivers. Many clinicians become discouraged as they realize the amount of training and *retraining* necessary with caregivers. Clinicians often feel powerless to ensure that feeding recommendations are implemented for every meal and that appropriate oral hygiene practices are followed afterward.

Development of Negotiation Skills

Given the difficulties observed in caregiver feeding practices, clinicians may need to learn how to "sell" the management plan to caregivers, in addition to providing basic information regarding feeding practices. Speech-language pathologists may find that they will benefit from learning basic negotiation skills. These skills will help prepare clinicians on ways to anticipate problems, engage others in problem-solving exercises, and learn the art of successful negotiation. These skills are typically not trained in dysphagia workshops or courses, yet they may be crucial for successful implementation of a management plan to feed a patient.

Clinicians can maximize successful training of caregivers and implementation of the care plan, especially those in long-term care settings, when they

1. Anticipate and acknowledge problems in all aspects of feeding dependent patients
2. Develop a structured program for training caregivers
3. Discuss ways to solve problems with caregivers and those people with the authority to approve solutions
4. Attend workshops to improve personal communication skills in group dynamics, art of negotiation, and problem-solving skills
5. Encourage continuous feedback and suggestions for improvement

Coaching Tips

Assess the entire "team" environment, which includes all caregivers who prepare the meal and/or feed the patient, prior to developing a dysphagia management plan. A comprehensive management plan can only be developed when the patient and his caregivers are involved and agree to implement the plan. In medical facilities, caregivers may include not just those who feed a patient, but those people who prepare and serve the food as well. Clinicians cannot develop care plans for a patient in isolation of his environment. This is imperative for the safety of the patient who is dependent on caregivers for eating and oral care.

Respect the patient's wishes regarding being fed at all times. Patients can make their wishes known regarding feeding preferences verbally and nonverbally. Clinicians and caregivers must not ignore their communication, even when they do not agree with or like what is being communicated. Be sure to evaluate carefully all possible reasons for rejection with the patient and caregivers, but stop all efforts if patients refuse. This is a patient's legal and ethical right.

Focus training efforts with caregivers on the rationale for feeding techniques, not just "how to feed." It appears that if caregivers understand the rationale behind certain feeding techniques, and the consequences of their feeding practices, better compliance might occur.

Learn negotiation techniques. The best management plan, developed from astute clinical diagnostic skills and expertise, will not work if it is not implemented. Clinicians must "sell" their plan to caregivers, and sometimes even to facility administration to gain professional respect and legitimacy. These skills are typically not learned by clinicians in academic settings or dysphagia workshops. However, further study into these valuable social skills may provide an avenue for clinicians to gain authority and respect within their facilities. Consequently, they may be able to implement appropriate dysphagia management programs more easily within their facilities.

CONCLUSION

It appears that dependency for feeding and oral care can increase a patient's risk for pneumonia. Furthermore, dependency for feeding may also influence a patient's risk for malnutrition and dehydration. Careful training of caregivers, whether they be family members, staff, or volunteers who feed patients, appears crucial to maximize safety, intake, and pleasure in eating. The use of a structured training protocol in long-term care settings, with ongoing supervision and recognition of staff and volunteers who participate in feeding patients, may improve caloric intake and weight gain. If patients reject being fed, the possible reasons for refusal should be explored, such as positioning, food appearance and temperature, and oral/dental status. Clinicians may want to learn negotiation techniques to enhance their legitimacy and respect within facilities so that dysphagia management programs are appropriately implemented.

Successful management of the feeding dependent patient is complicated. It requires careful consideration of patient rights and wishes, caregiver cooperation and diligence, and clinician leadership. There is not a formula for success that can be applied to every patient, caregiver, or clinician. It is achieved only through ongoing communication and hard work.

CHAPTER

11

Surgical Management of Dysphagia of Neurogenic Origin

Guest Author: Mark A. Varvares, MD

Often management of the person with a neurogenic dysphagia requires a variety of medical, behavioral, and surgical managements. In this chapter, selected surgical managements are described. Knowing what is possible from surgery gives the management team the maximum possible number of options, especially for persons whose dysphagia does not improve with other treatment or time.

INTRODUCTION

The management of the patient with dysphagia of neurogenic origin is a difficult problem in which sometimes only incremental improvements in patient function can be met. Since very often the pharyngeal lesion is just one component of a constellation of degenerative processes, the management team must communicate realistic expectations to the patient and family prior to initiating surgical management. In general, the more progressive the disease process, the more limited are the possibilities of restoring normal deglutition with normal respiration. Because these patients represent a management challenge, a multidisciplinary approach is a necessity. Coordination between the speech-language pathologist, neurologist, internist, and head and neck surgeon is paramount to seeing that the appropriate therapeutic modalities are implemented to result in an improved patient outcome.

Full Evaluation Precedes Management

It is essential that all patients who are being evaluated for dysphagia of neurogenic origin as surgical candidates have the etiology of their dysphagia clearly outlined. It is absolutely imperative that these patients be ruled out for the presence of an upper aerodigestive tract malignancy. It is an all-too-frequent occasion that patients are referred to the head and neck surgeon for management of dysphagia that is felt to be of neurogenic origin, only to be diagnosed with a slowly progressive upper aerodigestive tract carcinoma. It is for this reason that any patient with dysphagia, be it of neurogenic or other etiology, be subjected to a complete head and neck evaluation.

Structural and functional evaluation needs to include very careful inspection of the nose, nasopharynx, oral cavity, oropharynx, hypopharynx, larynx, and neck. The examiner must assess the patient for the presence of anatomic lesions, the presence or absence of normal sensation to the mucosa of the upper aerodigestive tract, and abnormalities of motor function. Hypopharyngeal and laryngeal examination should involve a direct fiberoptic nasopharyngoscopy that allows an extended evaluation of the laryngopharynx to assess mobility on both swallowing and phonation, and for evidence of neurogenic or anatomic obstruction presenting as pooled secretions in the hypopharynx and esophageal inlet. Nasopharyngoscopy also allows the evaluation of soft palate mobility and any evidence of velopharyngeal insufficiency. Examination of the neck should include an assessment of laryngeal elevation on swallowing. The examiner should also note changes in the soft tissue of the neck, such as the fibrosis seen following radiation therapy. Careful palpation of the visceral compartment for evidence of either intrinsic or extrinsic masses of the upper digestive system should be performed.

Once the office exam has assured that there is no evidence of a neoplastic cause for dysphagia, an appropriate radiologic workup can be done.

In most cases, a modified barium swallow will be performed objectively to assess deficits in the patient's swallow. In addition, a functional endoscopic evaluation of swallowing done at the bedside with the speech-language pathologist may be helpful. A chest X ray should be performed to evaluate the patient for evidence of pulmonary complications, such as pneumonia or other infiltrative processes.

All patients that are to undergo surgical management of dysphagia require a direct examination of the upper aerodigestive system under anesthesia. This should include direct laryngoscopy and rigid esophagoscopy. This will definitively rule out a neoplastic lesion of the laryngopharynx and esophagus that could mimic a neurogenic cause of dysphagia. These evaluations may be done immediately preceding the planned surgical intervention.

SURGICAL MANAGEMENT OF SPECIFIC LESIONS

Management of Isolated Upper Esophageal Sphincter Hyperfunction

The surgical management of isolated upper esophageal sphincter (UES) hyperfunction has a high likelihood to restore normal deglutition in properly selected patients (Berg, Persky, Jacobs, & Cohen, 1985). In general, patients with isolated upper esophageal sphincter hyperfunction will respond well to cricopharyngeal and inferior constrictor myotomy. However, patients who have neurogenic lesions involving the pharynx and cervical esophagus will have a lesser degree of success following this procedure. An example of this can be seen in the success of patients who undergo cricopharyngeal and inferior constrictor myotomy for oculopharyngeal muscular dystrophy (Montgomery & Lynch, 1971). For patients who present early in the disease process where the major lesion is cricopharyngeal dysfunction, cricopharyngeal and inferior constrictor myotomy has a high rate of restoring normal deglutition. However, as the disease process progresses, and increasing areas within the pharynx become dysfunctional, the best performed myotomy will still be unsuccessful.

Patients with Zenker's diverticulum will respond well to cricopharyngeal and inferior constrictor myotomy. Such patients have an isolated lesion of the cricopharyngeus which leads to formation of a pharyngeal pouch. By either suspending or resecting the pouch and performing a complete cricopharyngeal and inferior constrictor myotomy, these patients are able to enjoy a significant improvement in their deglutition (Montgomery, 1989).

Patients who may not benefit to as dramatic a degree are those who have lesions of the brain and cranial base that have led to multiple cranial neuropathies. Patients who have undergone surgery for skull base tumors that involve the jugular foramen and cranial nerves IX, X, XI, and possibly XII, for instance, may have some improvement in their deglutition following cricopharyngeal myotomy combined with vocal cord medialization (Montgomery, Hillman, & Varvares, 1994). These patients will still require significant intervention by the speech and language pathologist to implement compensatory mechanisms to allow them to swallow safely. This is due to the nature of lesions in this area which leave the patient with not only motor deficits, but sensory deficits as well.

The Myotomy Procedure

The surgical technique for cricopharyngeal and inferior constrictor myotomy is straightforward (Blakeley, Garety, & Smith, 1968; Montgomery, 1989; Montgomery et al., 1994; Stevens & Newell, 1971; Wilkins, 1964). Montgomery emphasizes the importance of not only dividing the cricopharyngeus muscle, but dividing the entire inferior constrictor muscle fibers extending into the upper cervical esophagus. This surgical philosophy blends well with the concept of the UES functioning primarily as a unit made up of a region within the hypopharynx and cervical esophagus, rather than a specific muscle (Shapiro & Martin, 1995). This procedure is done with the patient under general anesthesia. Following the induction of general anesthesia, the patient undergoes rigid esophagoscopy. The surgeon advances the rigid esophagoscope to the gastroesophageal junction and then slowly withdraws it, looking for evidence of mucosal or extrinsic lesions of the upper digestive system. A large (#9) endotracheal tube is placed into the esophagus to help locate the esophagus during the myotomy. The patient is placed on a shoulder roll and the head is turned to the right. The left neck is chosen in most cases for this procedure, as the esophagus is more readily accessed in the left neck.

Two incisions are possible. One option for incision is one that parallels the anterior border of the sternocleidomastoid muscle. Another is a horizontal incision at the junction between the lower and middle one-third of the neck. Regardless of which of these two incisions is made, the incision is extended down through the platysma muscle until the investing layer of deep cervical fascia is encountered. This is then incised. The sternocleidomastoid muscle is then identified and mobilized laterally along with the internal jugular vein, carotid artery, and vagus nerve. The omohyoid muscle is divided along its central tendon. The posterior border of the thyroid cartilage is then identified. Using a double skin hook, this posterior border is grasped and mobilized away from the surgeon. Blunt dissection in the plane between the constrictor muscles and the prevertebral fascia allows further mobilization of the laryngopharynx away from the surgeon so that the posterior aspect of the laryngopharynx can be visualized directly. The endotracheal tube is now easily palpated in the hypopharynx and cervical esophagus.

The inferior constrictor muscle is then identified at its superior edge where it is superficial to the middle constrictor muscle. The inferior constrictor muscle takes origin off the oblique line of the thyroid cartilage, which can be a useful landmark for locating the upper edge of the muscle. Using a hemostat, the plane between the constrictor muscle and the submucosa of the hypopharynx and cervical esophagus is established in the posterior midline. The key to avoiding injury to the recurrent laryngeal nerve is to create the myotomy in the posterior midline of the hypopharynx and cervical esophagus. Once this plane is located, the muscle is divided. This is continued from inferior to superior until complete division of the inferior constrictor, cricopharyngeus and upper esophageal muscle fibers have been achieved. At the conclusion of the myotomy, the endotracheal tube should be clearly visible through the mucosa of the hypopharynx and cervical esophagus. The wound is then drained with closed suction drains and closed in multilayers.

Postoperatively, the patient should be able eat the evening following surgery. Initially, there still may be some residual dysphagia because of perioperative edema and pain in the neck and pharynx. Oral intake is instituted based on the patient's overall swallowing function. Patients with isolated UES lesions should be returned to a near-normal diet in a short period of time. Patients with multiple deficits in the pharynx, however, will still require extensive rehabilitation.

The possible complications following cricopharyngeal and inferior constrictor myotomy are injury to the recurrent laryngeal nerve, hypopharyngeal or esophageal perforations with cervical abscess and mediastinitis, or hemorrhage. When this technique is done carefully and in experienced hands, the complication rate is extremely low.

An alternative to open treatment of UES dysfunction with Zenker's diverticulum is the endoscopic Dohlman procedure (Dohlman & Mattsson, 1960). This technique is used infrequently and is reserved for patients who are unable to withstand the longer open procedure.

Management of Aspiration

There exists a wide spectrum of severity of the neurologic lesion in the patient with dysphagia and aspiration. In some patients, the glottis is incompetent from the loss of the innervation to the intrinsic laryngeal musculature through the recurrent laryngeal nerve. These patients will have relatively mild aspiration that can be compensated for, either with reha-bilitation or with surgical intervention. Patients who have undergone ma-jor neurologic insults, however, will have an incompetent glottis related to complete loss of sensory input, motor response, and laryngopharyngeal coordination. In these patients, the degree of aspiration is much more se-vere, and the surgical approaches to prevent this disorder are much more involved. In this section, a graded surgical intervention is described, based on the components involved in the neurologic deficit.

Vocal Cord Medialization for Unilateral Vocal Cord Paralysis

The unilateral loss of innervation to the intrinsic musculature of the larynx will result in a vocal cord that is paralyzed in either the paramedian or lateral position. This has a significant impact on the patient's ability to phonate, swallow without aspiration, and generate a strong cough. These latter two put the patient at significant risk for pulmonary complications. For this reason, it has been an accepted technique to medialize the vocal cord that is paralyzed so that the vocal cord is fixed in midline. This allows the contralateral normal vocal cord, which maintains normal mobility, to close the glottis on phonation, swallowing, and when generating a cough or Valsalva.

There are several techniques available that medialize the paralyzed vocal cord. When it is felt that the vocal cord paralysis may be short term, and is of reversible causes, it is acceptable to inject a Gelfoam solution into the paralyzed vocal cord (Schramm, Max, & Lavorato, 1978). This is done under local anesthesia using direct laryngoscopy. By injecting the Gelfoam solution, the surgeon is able to add volume and bulk to the vocal cord and bring its medial edge to midline. This is a reversible procedure in that over the course of several weeks the body will resorb the injected Gelfoam and the vocal cord will return to its original position. If the paralysis is from a reversible cause, it may have resolved by that time.

Another injection technique, which was very popular from the 1960s through the 1980s, is the injection of Teflon into the paralyzed vocal cord. The principle is the same as that previously discussed. The Teflon is in-jected into the paralyzed vocal cord and creates extra volume to the cord, which allows medialization of the medial edge of the vocal cord to mid-line. This procedure results in improvement in glottic competence of pa-tients with vocal cord paralysis 60% of the time (Montgomery, Blaugrund, & Varvares, 1993). This technique, however, has recently fallen out of favor as it has been replaced by more precise techniques and because of the possibility of formation of a Teflon granuloma (Varvares, Montgomery, & Hillman, 1995).

The techniques most frequently used today to medialize the paralyzed vocal cord are medialization laryngoplasty (thyroplasty) and arytenoid adduction. These procedures may be used separately or in combination to close the unilaterally incompetent glottis. Medialization laryngoplasty is performed under local anesthesia. The larynx is exposed externally and a window is removed from the thyroid cartilage at the level that corresponds to the paralyzed vocal cord. At this point, silicone prosthesis is placed into the window to medialize the paralyzed vocal cord. As the prosthesis is being placed, by using a combination of fiberoptic nasopharyngoscopy and changes in the patient's vocal characteristics, the prosthesis is adjusted to the most appropriate size that results in the optimal degree of medialization. Criticisms of this technique are that it does not allow medialization of the most posterior aspect of the glottis. The technique described by Montgomery et al. (1993), however, has consistently illustrated a complete medialization of the entire vocal cord, including the vocal process of the arytenoid. The Montgomery prosthesis results in a consistent closure of the posterior glottis (Figure 11–1a–e).

Arytenoid adduction is a procedure used by laryngologists who feel that thyroplasty techniques do not adequately close the posterior aspect of the glottis (Netterville, Stone, Luken, Civantos, & Ossnoff, 1993). This procedure is done with the patient in a sedated but awake state, using local anesthesia. The posterior aspect of the thyroid cartilage is identified. By either disarticulating the cricothyroid joint, or by removing a small portion of the posterior aspect of the thyroid cartilage, the arytenoid cartilage is identified. The muscular process of the ipsilateral arytenoid is identified and a suture is placed through the muscular process. The suture is directed out through the thyroid ala to the anterolateral aspect of the larynx. By tightening this nonabsorbable suture, the muscular process is brought anteriorly, causing the vocal process to pass medially, and close the posterior glottis.

Management of Severe Aspiration of Multifactorial Cause

In patients with severe and life-threatening aspiration, a rigorous approach is necessary. The goal of treatment of patients with severe aspiration should be protection of the pulmonary system from food and saliva, yet at the same time preservation of as normal a voice, respiration, and deglutition as possible. In most cases of severe aspiration, it is impossible to achieve this goal without loss of normal vocalization and respiration.

A simple yet imperfect way to aid the patient with severe aspiration from a neurogenic cause is to place a cuffed tracheotomy tube and a feeding tube. The presence of a cuffed tracheotomy tube will not prevent aspiration

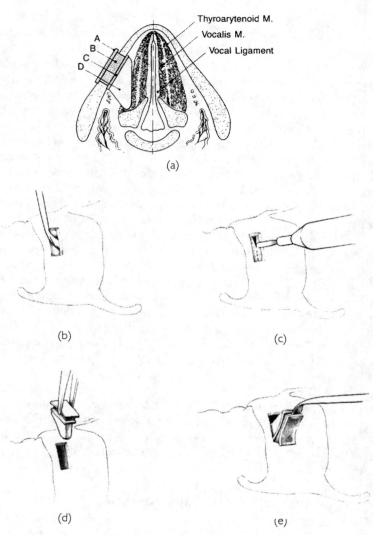

Figure 11–1. (a) Cross-sectional view of an implanted larynx at the level of the midvocal cord. Note that the implant pushes the vocal cord to midline and medializes the vocal process of the arytenoid cartilage, closing the posterior glottis. (b) A window has been made in the thyroid cartilage at the level of the vocal cord. The perichondrium is elevated from the inner aspect of the thyroid cartilage. (c) The perichondrium is carefully divided. (d) Implant is inserted by placing the posterior portion in first. (e) After engaging the posterior portion of the implant in the cartilage window, the anterior portion is inserted. (From "Thyroplasty: A new approach," by W. W. Montgomery, S. M. Blaugrund, and M. A. Varvares, 1993, *Annals of Otology, Rhinology, & Laryngology*, 102(8), 572, 576, 577.

completely. Saliva and food can make their way around the cuffed tracheotomy tube and into the upper airway. In addition, the potential for long-term complications related to a chronically inflated tracheotomy tube cuff are significant. Tracheal stenosis and tracheomalacia are very problematic, particularly in patients with severe neurologic deficits. The presence of the tracheotomy tube will also inhibit laryngeal elevation and further compromise the airway during swallowing.

For patients with severe aspiration who are felt either to have a potentially reversible cause of their aspiration or who may not have an extended period of life remaining, aspiration can be adequately controlled by placing a conforming laryngeal stent into the larynx and performing a tracheotomy (Weisberger, 1991). When the procedure is completed, the larynx is obturated with a silicone "cork." The tracheotomy tube maintains the patient's airway. Although this results in a very high degree of control of the aspiration, this does leave the patient without the ability to voice with lung-powered speech. Placement of the laryngeal stent can be done either with a laryngofissure where the larynx is opened, or endoscopically (Figure 11–2). It does have a potential advantage of reversibility, should the patient recover function of the laryngopharynx.

Other techniques that prevent aspiration in patients with severe neurologic dysfunction result in laryngeal closure. There are a variety of techniques available to close the larynx. Montgomery's (1975) technique involves opening the larynx by laryngofissure, removing the mucosa of the vocal cords, ventricles, and false cords, and suturing of the vocal cords together. Sasaki modified this technique by employing a superiorly based sternohyoid muscle flap that passes through the thyroid notch, and is sutured into the interarytenoid muscle. This was designed to help prevent aspiration posteriorly, which was felt to be the most frequent source of failure following the Montgomery technique (Sasaki, Milmoe, Yanagisawa, Berry, & Kirchner, 1980). Other techniques of laryngeal closure involve epiglottoplasty, whereby the epiglottis and aryepiglottic folds are sutured onto themselves, either to obliterate or to leave a very narrow supraglottic inlet (Biller, Lawson, & Baek, 1983; Habal & Murray, 1972).

For patients who are severely neurologically devastated and have life-threatening aspiration, the definitive surgical approach is one that anatomically separates the digestive and respiratory systems. The most frequently used technique of airway and digestive system separation is that described by Lindeman (1975) (Lindeman, Yarington, & Sutton, 1976). This technique involves the creation of a permanent tracheostomy by transecting the cervical trachea and suturing the distal stump to the skin. The proximal tracheal end is either sewn onto itself to create a blind pouch, or sewn end-to-side into the cervical esophagus (Figure 11–3a–c). One disadvantage

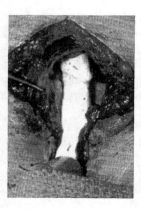

Figure 11–2. The larynx has been opened by laryngofissure and the conforming laryngeal stent placed. The stent will be sewn into position by sutures that are tied in the subcutaneous tissues. These may be exposed and cut, allowing the stent to be removed transorally without laryngofissure should the patient's neurologic status improve.

of this technique is that the patient is unable to phonate. However, by placing a tracheoesophageal shunt prosthesis through the posterior wall of the tracheostomy and into the esophagus, these patients could develop tracheoesophageal speech. Unfortunately, most patients with a neurologic insult severe enough to require a Lindeman procedure probably would be unable to perform the manual tasks needed to use a tracheoesophageal voice prosthesis. By completely diverting the airway from the digestive system, there is absolutely no possibility of aspiration and the cure rate of aspiration is 100% following this procedure. This procedure is theoretically reversible and has been successfully reversed clinically (Snyderman & Johnson, 1988).

As a final means of controlling aspiration, a total laryngectomy may be performed. This technique, however, has no advantage over the Lindeman procedure and puts the patient at greater risk for perioperative complications. The Lindeman procedures are simple, require little operative time, and have a minimal risk of major operative complications.

The Management of Sialorrhea

The problem of sialorrhea is not infrequent in patients with significant neurologic pathology. In this population, drooling is felt to be related to a buildup of saliva in the mouth because of an inability to initiate the oral phase of swallowing and due to a lack or incoordination of oromotor tone,

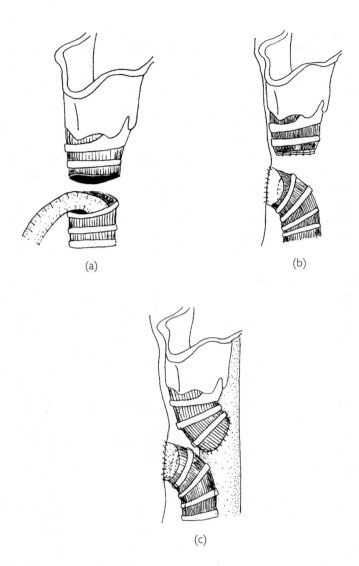

(a)

(b)

(c)

Figure 11–3. (a). Trachea is transected between the second and third tracheal rings. (b). The second tracheal ring is removed and the underlying mucosa is inverted and sutured to close the subglottic trachea. The inferior trachea is sewn to the skin for creation of a tracheostome. (c). Procedure as initially described by Lindeman, consisting of a proximal end to side tracheoesophageal anastomosis and distal tracheostomy. (From "Laryngotracheal separation for intractable aspiration," by C. H. Snyderman and J. T. Johnson, 1988, *Annals of Otology, Rhinology, & Laryngology*, 97(5), 467. Reprinted with permission.)

head position, and posture that leads to oral incompetence. The three major pairs of salivary glands-the parotid, sublingual, and submandibular glands-produce approximately 1.5 liters of saliva a day. The majority (70%) is contributed by the submandibular glands while the parotid glands add 25% and the sublingual glands, 5%.

Surgical approaches to the management of sialorrhea aim primarily at rerouting the flow of saliva, or interrupting it completely.

Bilateral tympanic neurectomy, with section of the chorda tympani nerve, will result in disruption of the parasympathetic preganglionic fibers from the seventh cranial nerve that innervate the submandibular and sublingual glands and the ninth cranial nerve that innervates the parotid gland (Parisier, Blitzer, Binder, Friedman, & Marovitz, 1978). This is a simple procedure that can be done on an ambulatory basis. It has a very high success rate with minimal morbidity. It does result in an alteration in the sense of taste. It is contraindicated in patients with significant sensorineural hearing loss.

Techniques that reroute the salivary glands will either address the parotid or submandibular glands. The Wilke procedure relocates the parotid duct orifice high into the tonsillar fossa by mobilization of the parotid duct through a submucosal tunnel (Rosen, Komisar, Ophir, & Marshak, 1990). When combined with submandibular gland excision, this technique has an 89% control of sialorrhea. The excision of submandibular glands eliminates 70% of the normal salivary volume, and relocating the parotid ducts results in release of 25% of the remaining saliva into the pharynx, where it can be swallowed. There is slightly increased morbidity related to the submandibular gland excision.

Another approach to control drooling is to perform bilateral submandibular gland excisions with parotid duct ligation. Although this is a more simplified procedure than the Wilke procedure, it does result in a high rate of success without significant morbidity and increased hospitalization (Shott, Myer, & Cotton, 1989).

Bilateral submandibular duct relocation into the tonsillar fossa has been reported to have high success rates for the control of drooling (Crysdale & White, 1989). As with parotid duct relocation (Wilkie procedure), the submandibular ducts are routed posteriorly into the tonsillar fossa through a submucosal tunnel. The submandibular gland is responsible for the majority of saliva in the oral cavity, and by relocating its duct into the posterior pharynx, the potential for drooling is significantly diminished without the loss of saliva. Although this technique does enjoy a high success rate, there are significant complications, which include edema of the floor of mouth, sialadenitis, and ranula formation.

CONCLUSION

Dysphagia and aspiration continue to be a difficult problem in the management of patients with neurogenic dysphagia. Although surgery does have a significant role in the management of these patients, decisions regarding therapy must be made in a multidisciplinary setting. By excellent coordination among the speech pathologist, neurologist, internist, and surgeon, appropriate patient selection can be made and the appropriate surgical intervention used.

12

Legal and Reimbursement Issues of Documentation

Although most clinicians receive training on how to write clinical goals in dysphagia, few are trained to document their services with respect to the legal and reimbursement aspects of their care. This chapter discusses how to document dysphagia services to meet the rigorous standards set for reimbursement and to provide legal protection to the clinician. Specific suggestions are given regarding how to document dysphagia services to reduce the risk of being accused of fraud, malpractice, or unethical practice.

This chapter is not intended to replace legal counsel or specific recommendations from reimbursement agencies, but serves to highlight the major aspects of legal and reimbursement documentation required of clinicians.

DOCUMENTATION ISSUES IN DYSPHAGIA

Medical documentation in dysphagia provides a record of the clinical services rendered and simultaneously serves as a legal and business document. This documentation may be used in litigation, and it often is used for reimbursement of dysphagia services. A well-written medical record of dysphagia services will provide a clinician with the legal protection and peace of mind sought by many.

Most clinicians recognize the importance of the clinical component of documentation. They usually receive extensive training regarding how to write diagnostic reports, long- and short-term goals, treatment progress notes, and discharge summaries. The focus of training commonly is specific to the development of clinical skills and use of professional terminology, so that a clinical supervisor in speech-language pathology can evaluate a clinician's level of competence in providing dysphagia services.

Clinical documentation of dysphagia services must always reflect sound clinical judgment and have a rationale that meets at least a minimum standard of clinical practice. It does not have to be based on what is considered the majority viewpoint of dysphagia practice, but it should reflect current theory and evidence-based practices. It is hoped that the theories and evidence presented in this text regarding current dysphagia treatment will help clinicians make sound decisions regarding their intervention(s).

However, it is apparent that clinicians also must recognize the importance of documenting their services as a legal and business document. Legal documentation will serve as the best protection against malpractice litigation for clinicians if they follow the suggestions put forth in this chapter. Documentation requirements for reimbursement will vary according to setting, with some settings imposing strict timelines and content requirements for payment to be made.

Clinicians who provide dysphagia services are frequently concerned that they could be accused of committing fraud, professional malpractice, or an ethical violation. There are ways to reduce the risk of being accused of these serious allegations significantly, but there is no way to completely prevent it. Someone can always accuse a clinician of these violations or crimes, with or without merit. However, clinicians can learn how to document their services to reduce their risk of being accused, and provide clinical accountability that their services were appropriate and reimbursable.

What Constitutes Fraud and Larceny by Fraud?

Scott (1994), an attorney and physical therapist, gives the legal definition of fraud as "a false representation of material (decisional) fact, made with the intent to deceive, which causes another person to take some action, detrimental to his or her own (or the public's) interest" (p. 218). When a clinician submits documentation for reimbursement of services not provided or when excessive use of treatment services are paid for by third party payers, this is an example of larceny by fraud. The legal definition of larceny by fraud is when a theft occurs by deception of money, goods, services, or property (Scott, 1994). Administrative, criminal, or civil legal action may be taken against clinicians who commit fraud, with severe penalties. Civil fines and liability, criminal convictions with monetary fines, and revocation of their license and/or certification to practice speech-language pathology from ASHA or their state board/association could occur.

Clinicians are often worried about being accused of committing larceny by fraud when employers encourage them to maximize reimbursement for their patients. Some employers educate clinicians how to document and provide dysphagia services that result in the highest reimbursement rates possible for a given patient. Although all clinicians obviously wish to provide the highest quality of services possible, it is important to provide treatment on clinical need, not reimbursement potential. To do otherwise may place a clinician at risk for conviction of committing larceny by fraud.

What Constitutes Professional Malpractice?

Scott (1994) explains that the definition of professional malpractice traditionally was narrowly defined as "professional negligence only," but the trend recently has expanded the definition to include more parameters that can apply to clinicians providing health care services. The legal definition of professional negligence is the "delivery of patient care that falls below the standard expected of ordinary reasonable practitioners of the same profession acting under the same or similar circumstances" (Scott, 1994, p. 220). In addition, the broader definition of professional malpractice now includes the potential for liability if there is a breach of a patient-clinician contractual promise, liability for defective treatment-related products that cause harm to a patient, and/or liability for abnormally dangerous treatment activities.

Clinicians may be accused of civil malpractice by a patient, and be required to pay compensatory money for damages if found guilty. Criminal action may also be taken if the clinician is accused of performing gross negligence, reckless conduct, or intentional misconduct, with the penalties ranging from incarceration to probation to a fine. Since the possible penalties are different and potentially more severe in a criminal case against a clinician, the standard of proof required for conviction is different. In a civil malpractice lawsuit, a patient's attorney needs to provide only a "preponderance of evidence" to gain possible conviction, which means the judge or jury believes the patient's evidence to be true "more likely than not" over the clinician's evidence. In a criminal trial, a state or federal prosecutor brings legal action against a clinician and must prove evidence "beyond a reasonable doubt" (Scott, 1994).

There are four criteria that *all* must be met to be found guilty of professional malpractice (Ohliger, 1996). If even one of these criteria is not met during the legal proceedings, a clinician will not be convicted. Ohliger explains that the four elements necessary to prove professional malpractice are

1. Existence of a Duty of Care—an agreement by the clinician to enter a patient/provider relationship. Clinicians are not bound to provide care to every patient, but once the clinician accepts a patient for care, this creates a duty on the clinician to protect the patient from foreseeable harm.
2. A Failure to Exercise a Standard (Duty) of Care—clinicians must provide care that is similar to the care that is provided by members of the same profession, using "recognized and approved methods of treatment" (Ohliger, 1996, p. 79). This does not mean clinicians must provide treatment according to what the majority of clinicians provide, only that the care rendered was approved as appropriate by selected, respected colleagues. Traditionally, clinicians were compared to peers in their same community, but recently changes have been noted whereby they may be compared to colleagues in similar communities, or even to state or national peers acting in the same or similar circumstances (Scott, 1994). Once the "standard of care" is defined, the clinician is evaluated based on the evidence of whether another reasonable clinician would have acted in a similar manner in the same or similar circumstances. Alternatively, did the clinician fail to act appropriately in this circumstance? (Ohliger, 1996.)
3. Foreseeable Harm—clinicians must act in some manner to cause actual harm or injury to a patient, and that harm must be foreseeable or anticipated. A clinician may be shown to have provided an inappropriate standard of care, but if no harm or injury was caused to patient, or the harm was not foreseeable, a clinician will not be found liable.
4. Causation—clinicians must be found guilty of actions that actually caused or contributed to a foreseeable harm to the patient. In other words, the harm occurred directly as a result of a clinician's actions, and if the clinician did not act this way, the harm would not have occurred. This is called "cause in fact." In addition, clinicians must be found to be

guilty of "proximate cause," a complex legal term that refers to the manner in which an injury occurred, and may limit the liability of a clinician if it would seem "unjust."

The law is unclear as to whether a clinician may be liable under "proximate cause," given a variety of common clinical scenarios. For example, one common scenario may involve a nurse's aide. The aide is instructed by the clinician not to give a patient thin water and to provide constant supervision during all meals. However, the aide leaves the patient unattended, and an unexpected visiting family member arrives and gives the patient thin water, which is subsequently aspirated. The question becomes whether the actions that caused harm were foreseeable by the clinician. Since this is a gray area of the law, it is not known how these actions may be interpreted in a court of law. However, in a similar scenario described by Ohliger (1996, p. 82), she concluded that it would seem that actions of this type are not foreseeable, even though the harm caused by these actions was foreseeable.

There are many clinical scenarios that may place a clinician at risk of being accused of professional malpractice. Although it is impossible to provide a comprehensive list of do's and dont's regarding how a clinician provides dysphagia services, it behooves every clinician to document all aspects of the care they render to patients carefully, and be prepared to defend it.

The Importance of Informed Consent to Treat

The legal definition of informed consent is "providing a patient with sufficient information about a proposed treatment and its reasonable alternatives to allow the patient to make a knowing, intelligent, and unequivocal decision regarding whether to accept or reject the proposed treatment" (Scott, 1994, p. 219). According to Scott, the legally correct form for documenting a patient's informed consent for treatment varies from state to state. It is recommended that all clinicians check with the legal counsel available in their facility regarding their state's requirements.

Obtaining informed consent is a *process* that ensures patients truly understand the parameters of the proposed treatment and agree to it, not just the completion of a checklist of information provided (Scott, 1994). Failure to obtain a patient's informed consent before initiating treatment constitutes professional negligence. Exceptions to the need for informed consent do exist, such as in a medical emergency or when it is believed that disclosing the information regarding treatment may be detrimental to the mental health of the patient, such as in the diagnosis of a life-threatening disease.

The use of preprepared forms of informed consent that patients sign may meet this legal obligation, but clinicians are encouraged to check with their facility and their legal counsel about what form(s) can be used to fulfill this requirement. Scott (1994) includes the following essential points.

1. A description of the patient's diagnosis and evaluation findings, and proposed treatment, presented to the patient in layperson's terms.
2. A discussion of what "material" risks could occur with the proposed treatment, including foreseeable complications associated with the treatment or precautions that would cause an ordinary person to think about whether he or she wishes to have the treatment or not.
3. A discussion of reasonable alternatives to the proposed treatment, which would be acceptable substitutes under legal standards of practice, including a discussion of what the clinician believes are the risks and prognosis associated with the alternative treatment(s).
4. A discussion of the expected benefits and prognosis associated with the proposed treatment.
5. Questions regarding the proposed treatment plan must be solicited from the patient, and answered to the patient's satisfaction.

Documentation of this critical process of securing informed consent to treat must occur in the medical record. It is required by law, and even by some accreditation organizations such as the Joint Commission on the Accreditation of Healthcare Organizations (JCAHO) and the American Hospital Association's *Patient Bill of Rights* (1992). If a patient is cognitively or physically unable to give consent, then the legal guardian or person able to make medical decisions regarding a patient must sign.

While this requirement may appear burdensome, it actually is not very difficult to meet. Most clinicians can rely on an "abbreviated document of consent in patient treatment records" when the facility where treatment will occur has established standard operating procedures for consent for specific procedures, or consent forms are used that the clinicians, not patients, sign and date to verify that informed consent was obtained (Scott, 1994, p. 137). It is not necessary to obtain informed consent repeatedly throughout the course of treatment, unless the original treatment plan is substantially changed. In addition, this process is not necessary in a large facility when a substitute clinician may treat a patient during a staff clinician's vacation or illness, since patients cannot expect exclusive treatment by only one provider in this type of settings. However, it may be advisable to obtain another informed consent in small private practices for substitute clinicians, but this is a gray area of the law, with few reported cases (Scott, 1994).

A clinician may be held liable for failure to obtain informed consent to treat if "an undisclosed risk materializes, resulting in injury to the patient, and the patient establishes (proves) that he or she would not have consented to treatment had the risk been disclosed" (Scott, 1994, p. 122). This should never occur since it is a legal prerequisite that informed consent be obtained prior to initiating any treatment. This process should become an integral part of every initial evaluation.

What Constitutes a Violation of Professional Ethics?

Adherence to a professional code of ethics is mandated by the American Speech-Language-Hearing Association (ASHA) for clinicians who are certified and/or members, and by many state or professional associations in which clinicians hold membership. The Principles of Ethics, as described by the American Speech-Language-Hearing Association (1994), provide the "underlying moral basis for the Code of Ethics" (Appendix A). Interestingly, many of the Rules of Ethics described in this document provide a code of conduct for clinicians to follow that would minimize the risk of being found guilty of professional malpractice, according to legal criteria.

Procedures and Sanctions of an ASHA Ethical Violation

Specific procedures are followed when a clinician is reported for unethical behavior (Appendix B). While ASHA and various organizations, such as state associations, may have different procedures to conduct an investigation of unethical behavior, all require written documentation of the alleged violation. The term used by the Board of Ethics to identify the clinician being accused of a violation is *Respondent*, while the person(s) alleging that a violation has occurred is called *Complainant*. ASHA requires a waiver be signed by the Complainant to allow the Board of Ethics to send a copy of the complaint to the Respondent for the Respondent's response. In this manner, clinicians brought before ASHA for an unethical violation will know who has accused them of a violation. The Complainant must provide all documentation and evidence against the Respondent to the Board of Ethics for review.

After an Initial Determination from the Board of Ethics is decided, the Respondent is notified of its decision, including what sanctions are to be imposed and who will be notified of the decision other than the respondent. This is called disclosure, and may involve any state agency that licenses or credentials speech-language pathologists, or any professional organization that has a Code of Ethics in which the respondent holds a membership. Several levels of sanctions can be handed down, such as reprimand, withhold, suspend, or revoke membership and/or certification or other measures determined at the discretion of the Board of Ethics. Clinicians may apply for reinstatement after the period of revocation is completed, but it is at the discretion of the Board of Ethics to allow reinstatement, based on whether it is in the best interest of ASHA and the individuals served and the fulfillment of current certification standards and/ or membership criteria.

A Respondent may request Further Consideration to the Initial Determination, if desired. A Respondent is responsible for all personal fees incurred in connection to the Board of Ethics Further Consideration proceedings, such as travel, lodging, witnesses, and/or legal counsel. However, it is not required that a Respondent be physically present at the proceedings or even that he or she hire counsel.

Common Ethical Questions in Dysphagia

Although a variety of behaviors may constitute unethical behavior according to ASHA, clinicians are often worried about upholding the most central element of professional ethics. The ASHA Code of Ethics (1994) states "individuals shall honor their responsibility to hold paramount the welfare of persons they serve professionally" when providing any speech-language pathology or audiology services. This causes anxiety in many clinicians since deciding what treatment is best to uphold the welfare of a patient is not always clear or agreed on among the clinician, the patient and family, and medical treatment team. For example, clinicians may struggle with their decision regarding whether to treat advanced oropharyngeal dysphagia in a patient with progressive and profound cognitive loss, and how that treatment should be administered, if at all. If nonoral treatment is offered and declined, or the treatment desired by the patient, family, or physician may increase a patient's health risk in the clinician's opinion, what is the best professional action to take? How do clinicians provide services that maintain a patient's welfare?

Most difficult situations arise regarding appropriate ethical behavior when there is a difference in opinion regarding treatment or the need for further testing. While clinicians worry about unethical professional actions, they are also concerned about legal repercussions. While ASHA and state associations may invoke ethical sanctions, anyone may bring legal action against a clinician, with legal sanctions and punishments. Specifically, clinicians often are unsure how to handle clinical issues such as refusal for treatment after initial evaluation, a lack of compliance or poor progress, or how to handle differences in opinion regarding dysphagia management with a patient, family, physician, and/or the third-party payer. Careful documentation of the actions taken by a clinician is crucial to minimize the risk of professional malpractice or ethical violation.

When a Patient Refuses Treatment

If a patient or guardian decides to refuse initial treatment, as discussed during the informed consent process, the clinician must explain the expected consequences of refusing treatment, in an objective manner (Scott, 1994). Often, clinicians are concerned that they may be liable, if harm occurs after a patient's refusal for treatment. However, if clinicians discuss all possible treatment options, including the expected consequences due to no treatment, this is all reasonable clinicians can be expected to do in a similar situation and they would probably not be liable (Ohliger, 1996). All the information discussed during the informed consent process, including the explanation of expected consequences of refusing treatment, should be carefully and completely documented in the medical record. This comprehensive documentation by the clinician would constitute legally "informed refusal" of treatment (Scott, 1994, p.125).

How to Terminate Services with a Patient

Terminating services with a patient involves breaking the patient-provider "duty of care" contract. This may occur when a personality conflict occurs, or when the patient is not compliant or progressing in the treatment goals. Although clinicians can decline to treat almost any patient, there are specific legal rules that must be followed to stop providing treatment, once a patient has been accepted for treatment. If these rules are not followed, a clinician may be sued for abandonment (Scott, 1994).

It is suggested that every facility have a written policy regarding patient compliance in treatment, to be reviewed during the initial evaluation. In addition, a written policy should be in place regarding the steps clinicians need to take to terminate services with patients by either discharging or transferring them from therapy (Scott, 1994):

1. Give advance notice to the patient of a pending discharge or transfer, including notification to the referred clinician, if any.
2. Provide a reasonable time for the patient to find a new clinician, if continuing care is needed.
3. Carefully draft and send a disengagement letter to the patient, coordinated through the facility or personal legal advisor.
4. Document the patient's status at the time of discharge carefully in the medical record.

5. Attempt to contact the new clinician as quickly as possible after discharge to provide all pertinent clinical information, including copies of the patient's treatment records.

How to Handle Differences in Opinion Regarding Dysphagia Management

The most difficult situation clinicians face is the dilemma of what to do when the recommendations they propose are not accepted by either the patients, their family or caregivers, their physician, or perhaps the third-party payer. If a difference in opinion arises between a clinician and a patient or family member regarding a dysphagia management recommendation, the clinician's first obligation is to keep the patient safe (Ohliger, 1996). Clinicians should not succumb to pressure from a patient or family to provide treatment that the clinician believes to be unsafe or inappropriate. However, as discussed previously, patients or their surrogates may legally refuse treatment. Clinicians do not need to pressure or force a patient or family to follow their recommendations.

If a treatment is provided based on pressure from the family that the clinician believes not to be "optimally safe," the clinician must still ensure the patient and environment are "as safe as reasonably possible under the circumstances" (Ohliger, 1996, p. 84). In these cases, clear and comprehensive documentation of all discussions with the family is imperative to minimize a clinician's malpractice liability. Ohliger suggests clinicians take the following steps to provide full information.

1. Document family discussions regarding all treatment options, the risks and safety concerns of each option, clinical opinions and recommendations of treatment options, and the consequences of declining treatment. Document the family's reactions and level of understanding as perceived by the clinician, to this information, in an objective manner.
2. Document the written instructions given to the family, including any specific safety precautions, and their response and level of understanding regarding this information.
3. Document physician conferences, the physician's response to the family's requests, and what treatment option the physician favors. If a treating physician holds a different opinion from the clinician regarding treatment, regardless of whether a patient or family concur, it is imperative to document clearly the difference of opinion with the physician, the physician's stated reasons for this opinion, the clinician's safety concerns regarding the physician's proposed treatment, and what specific recommendations were made to the physician and why.

When differences of opinion occur regarding how best to manage a patient's dysphagia, clinicians should follow two important guidelines to minimize their malpractice liability. They should take every step to ensure safety for their patient with any treatment provided and they need to document their actions very clearly and completely (Ohliger, 1996). A court of law could find a clinician liable if the clinician knowingly provided a treatment judged to be completely unsafe to the patient, even if the physician ordered it. Safety must come first. In these cases, clinicians may have a responsibility to refuse to administer a physician ordered treatment that is judged absolutely unsafe for the patient.

The withholding or withdrawal of life-sustaining treatments, such as the removal of a feeding tube for nutrition, involves a complicated area of the law and ethics. Legal judgments in this area fall under the Patient Self-Determination Act, a law signed into effect by President Bush in 1990 that allows patients the common-law right to control treatment decisions, both routine and extraordinary (Scott, 1994). A key concept to this act was to ensure patient education regarding informed consent to their treatment and the right to make "advance directives" (Scott, 1994, p. 181). Advance directives involve such documents as living wills and "durable power of attorney" for health care, which provide information regarding what life-sustaining measures should occur if patients become unable to communicate their wishes.

How to Handle Differences in Opinion with Third-Party Payers

With all of the changes in health care reimbursement, clinicians increasingly are confronted with the dilemma of what to do when a payer denies authorization for treatment the clinician believes to be medically necessary. In these situations, courts have ruled that a clinician cannot relinquish the obligation to provide appropriate treatment to a patient based merely on whether the services will be paid by a payer. The clinician "retains the right and the *legal and ethical obligation* to provide appropriate treatment for the patient," regardless of coverage (Ohliger, 1996, p. 86).

In one legal case, a physician was found negligent for the harm caused to a patient that occurred after the payer refused to extend the hospital stay (*Wickline v. California*, 1986). Although the physician had initially requested an extended hospital stay, the court found the physician solely responsible because no contest to the discharge was filed by the physician. In other words, clinicians may be held liable if their actions fall below what is considered a standard level of care, even when that care was denied reimbursement by the payer.

Ohliger (1996) suggests 10 specific actions clinicians should take when payers refuse to authorize treatment recommended for a patient (Table 12–1).

Table 12–1. How to decrease liability when authorization for treatment is denied by payers.

1. The speech pathologist should provide all relevant information to the payer, whether requested or not.

2. The speech pathologist should verify the exact basis for the utilization review denial.

3. The speech pathologist should articulate to the payer the risks and dangers of failing to provide the requested treatment.

4. The speech pathologist should insist on review of the decision by another speech pathologist.

5. The speech pathologist should inform the patient of the speech pathologist's recommendations, the payer's response, and the risks of not providing treatment.

6. The speech pathologist should request the payer to reconsider the denial, and use any available formal appeals process.

7. The speech pathologist should submit updated patient information to the payer.

8. The speech pathologist should consider expedited court relief.

9. The speech pathologist should resolve all doubts in favor of patient safety.

10. The speech pathologist should remember the "golden rule"—document, document, document.

Source: Reprinted with permission from "Legal implications in dysphagia practice" by Paula C. Ohliger in *Dysphagia: A continuum of care* (p. 87), by Barbara C. Sonies, Gaithersburg, MD: Aspen Publishers, Inc. © 1997 Aspen Publishers, Inc..

She reminds clinicians that courts will not absolve them from liability if their actions fall below a standard level of care, even if a payer refused to authorize the treatment.

COMPONENTS OF REIMBURSEMENT DOCUMENTATION

The components of reimbursement documentation vary according to setting and third-party payers. Nursing homes have federally mandated documentation requirements for reimbursement, which may be modified within each state. Hospitals, home health agencies, and free-standing clinics have different documentation requirements to complete for payment. Eligibility and payment for dysphagia services can vary between state Medicaid regulations, insurance companies, health management organizations, and

Medicare. All of these different documentation criteria can overwhelm a clinician, young or old. It is beyond the scope of this chapter to provide a comprehensive summary of all reimbursement documentation requirements for every clinical situation, but all settings require clinicians to provide information that does not misrepresent services provided or attempt to deceive the payer. This would constitute larceny by fraud.

Examples of larceny by fraud would include claims for services not actually rendered, such as "no shows," excessive use of treatment sessions not required to achieve the stated objectives, collection of monies for referrals ("kickback") or self-referrals, and routine waiver of patient copayments and deductibles required under Medicare Part B (Scott, 1994). Clinicians must carefully record and claim only what is legally billable, according to the third-party payer and specific setting.

Documentation for Medicare dysphagia claims (Appendix C) must follow very specific documentation criteria. Documentation of a medical workup by a physician must be present, and specific information regarding a patient's level of alertness, motivation, cognition, and deglutition must be given. In addition, at least one of seven listed conditions must be present and documented to show the presence of dysphagia, which are:

1. History of aspiration problems, or aspiration pneumonia, or definite risk for aspiration, reverse aspiration, chronic aspiration, nocturnal aspiration, or aspiration pneumonia. Nasal regurgitation, choking, frequent coughing up food during swallowing, wet or gurgly voice quality after swallowing liquids or delayed or slow swallow reflex.
2. Presence of oral motor disorders such as drooling, oral food retention, leakage of food or liquids placed into the mouth.
3. Impaired salivary gland performance and/or presence of local structural lesions in the pharynx resulting in marked oropharyngeal swallowing difficulties.
4. Incoordination, sensation loss, (postural difficulties) or other neuromotor disturbances affecting oropharyngeal abilities necessary to close the buccal cavity and/or bite, chew, suck, shape, and squeeze the food bolus into the upper esophagus while protecting the airway.
5. Postsurgical reaction affecting ability to use oropharyngeal structures used in swallowing adequately.
6. Significant weight loss directly related to nonoral nutritional intake (g-tube feeding) and reaction to textures and consistencies.
7. Existence of other conditions such as presence of tracheostomy tube, reduced or inadequate laryngeal elevation, labial closure, velopharyngeal closure, laryngeal closure, or pharyngeal peristalsis, and cricopharyngeal dysfunction. (Health Care Financing Administration, 1990, p. 10-155)

The presence of esophageal dysphagia (lower two-thirds of the esophagus) is also documented, if applicable. Assessment to determine this diagnosis may be approved, however, even if direct intervention is not appropriate. However, the Health Care Financing Administration (HCFA) does state the following regarding reimbursement for intervention of esophageal dysphagia:

> Inefficient functioning of the esophagus during the esophageal phase of swallowing is a common problem in the geriatric patient. Swallowing disorders occurring only in the lower two thirds of the esophageal stage of the swallow have not generally been shown to be amenable to swallowing therapy techniques and may not be approved. (HCFA, 1990, p. 10-156.)

The assessment of oropharyngeal dysphagia must document a patient's history, current eating status, and specific clinical observations during the clinical bedside dysphagia evaluation to determine the necessity for further instrumental medical testing. HCFA lists videofluoroscopy (modified barium swallow), upper GI series, and endoscopy as approved tests. Videofluoroscopy is approved when "the exact diagnosis of the swallowing disorder cannot be substantiated through oral exam and there is a question as to whether aspiration is occurring" (HCFA, 1990, p. 10-156).

Claims from speech-language pathology for videofluoroscopy may be submitted as a separate line-item charge, and the final analysis and interpretation of results of this test occur in consultation with a radiologist and input from the physician. There is one billing code for swallowing evaluation, that includes the clinical bedside evaluation and videofluoroscopy (CPT Code 92525). If FEES is performed, the speech-language pathologist may additionally bill CPT Code 31575 or 92511.

What constitutes appropriate treatment for dysphagia, and how to document these services for Medicare reimbursement, is a lengthy, complex topic. While there are many suggestions offered to clinicians to enhance payment and decrease Medicare payment denials, there are specific documentation guidelines provided by Medicare to demonstrate that their treatment services are reimbursable (Appendix C).

Clinicians must document goals and treatment procedures that specifically address the problems identified in the assessment, and "there must be a reasonable expectation that the patient will make material improvement within a reasonable period of time." In addition, ongoing dysphagia treatment must require the "highly specialized" services of the professional providing the care to be paid. Documentation of

> routine, repetitive observation or cuing may not qualify as skilled rehabilitation. For example, repeated visits in which the caregiver appears only to

be observing the patient eating a meal, reporting on the amount of food consumed, providing verbal reminders (e.g., slow down or cough) in the absence of other skilled assistance or observation suggests a nonskilled or maintenance level of care. Maintenance programs are covered for a brief period and are usually included during the final visits of the professional. (Health Care Financing Administration, 1990, pp. 10-158–10-159).

The plan of care for Medicare reimbursement must have the following components (Colmar, Oliver, & Wilcox, 1997):

1. Specific information regarding the type and nature of the care to be provided.
2. Estimate of the frequency of the therapy to be rendered, such as 3 times/week, and medical documentation to justify the intensity of the services rendered. This is crucial when the amount of therapy is more than 3 times/week billed to Medicare Part B.
3. Estimate duration of the need for therapy to meet the stated goals, expressed as days, weeks, or months. A range such as 4 to 6 weeks is not acceptable.
4. Diagnosis—document the speech-language pathology diagnosis of dysphagia and medical diagnoses. (Remember that dysphagia is *not* a medical diagnosis. It is a symptom.)
5. Rehabilitation Potential—what is the prognosis in the clinician's opinion regarding the patient's ability to meet the stated initial therapy goals? Need to update the care plan if any changes occur, and document changes in the progress notes.
6. Functional Goals—document what the patient is expected to achieve as a result of the highly specialized dysphagia treatment provided. A functional goal may reflect a small, but meaningful change that enables the patient to function more independently in a reasonable amount of time. Goals must be measurable, objective, and behavioral, with long- and short-term goals listed.

What constitutes a functional goal is vague and not specifically defined by many third-party payers, but clinicians may need to keep in mind that physiologic improvement that is not recognized by the patient and others as an improvement in their swallowing or eating skills will probably not be reimbursed.

Documentation of updated progress reports must be specific to be paid by any payer. It must include detailed information regarding what progress has been attained, what factors may influence progress, and why continued specialized services are needed. General descriptions of progress may be denied if this information is not supplied. There are no Medicare regulations that state how frequently progress must be documented. Some facilities require daily progress notes, while others may require them weekly, biweekly, or even monthly.

In the long-term care setting, physicians must certify the need for specialized speech-language pathology services no later than the 14th day after admission, followed by intervals not to exceed 30 days for Medicare Part A reimbursement. For Medicare Part B reimbursement, the physician must certify the need for continuing rehabilitation services at least every 30 days. Every year, HCFA updates a public information publication called *Your Medicare Handbook* (HCFA, 1997) to describe eligibility, reimbursement allowances, and patient rights for all Medicare programs. This handbook is available on the Internet (http://www.hcfa.gov) and is for sale by the U.S. Government Printing Office. Since the benefits may change each year, it is not possible to list all eligibility criteria and reimbursement allowances for Medicare programs. However, in general, Medicare Part A will help to pay for hospitalization costs, skilled nursing facility following a hospital stay (including rehabilitation services), home health and hospice care, and blood. Medicare Part B will help to pay for medical and rehabilitation expenses, inpatient and outpatient, clinical laboratory services, blood, and home health care. Many of these services have specified criteria and exceptions that patients and clinicians should be aware of to avoid any misunderstandings.

Although all settings and payers follow these general guidelines, nursing homes have specific documentation requirements unique to their setting. Since many clinicians provide dysphagia services in nursing homes, a brief synopsis of the documentation requirements mandated in nursing homes is presented.

NURSING HOME DOCUMENTATION REQUIREMENTS

All nursing homes that participate in Medicare or Medicaid programs must complete a special assessment form for every resident admitted, according to specific timelines and criteria, to develop an individualized plan of care. The information collected in this form is used not only to document timely assessments and appropriate care planning of residents, but to determine how much money a facility can receive daily to cover all the services required to care for this resident, including dysphagia services. The more services necessary, the more money the nursing home can collect. This assessment instrument is still being studied and revised by HCFA, with the final version to be published in the future. Based on the information derived from this assessment tool, the final version will provide payment classification and quality monitoring systems. This information will provide one part of the criteria used to develop the reimbursement rates for the prospective payment system (PPS), due to be implemented in January, 1999. Since this instrument will obviously have direct impact on the reimbursement of dysphagia services, as well as all speech-language pathology services in the nursing home setting, it may help clinicians to understand the history of why this monumental task was undertaken by HCFA and what information is currently being collected.

History of Omnibus Budget Reconciliation Act of 1987

As early as 1959, a Senate subcommittee found the quality of care in some nursing homes to be inadequate and inconsistent (HCFA, 1992). Further investigations in the 1970s and 1980s by HCFA resulted in regulations aimed at improving the quality of care provided to nursing home residents. However, they were not fully implemented, and the need for reform was becoming clear. In 1984, a pivotal court case found the Department of Health and Human Services responsible for assuring the quality of care of nursing home residents (HCFA, 1992). In addition, the U.S. Congress in the early 1980s called for a study into what current regulations existed and what recommendations would help nursing homes provide satisfactory care for residents. Both of these important events led HCFA to contract with the Institute of Medicine of the National Academy of Sciences to conduct a study. The results of that study were submitted to Congress in 1986 by the Institute, and Congress incorporated many of its recommendations in its Omnibus Budget Reconciliation Act of 1987, known as OBRA '87. This act outlined new federal requirements for the training of nursing home assistants, minimum staffing by licensed and registered nursing, and specific systems for ensuring that all residents receive quality care while maintaining a quality of life and respecting their rights.

Development of the Resident Assessment Instrument

One of the major requirements mandated by OBRA '87 was the development of a national uniform system called the Resident Assessment Instrument (RAI), to assess every resident's ability to perform daily life functions and to identify significant impairments in a resident's functional capacity (HCFA, 1992). The Secretary of the Department of Health and Human Services was charged with the task of developing this instrument, and implementing it within all nursing homes participating in Medicare or Medicaid programs by 1990. HCFA contracted with the Research Triangle Institute (North Carolina) to develop the RAI and collaborated with the nursing home industry in general, including many experts from a variety of professional disciplines who provided care to nursing home residents and the residents themselves.

HCFA (1992) explains that the Resident Assessment Instrument (RAI) consists of three basic components called the Minimum Data Set (MDS), Resident Assessment Protocols (RAPs) and a State Operations Manual (SOM). The MDS provides basic information regarding a resident's strengths, needs, and preferences, and the RAPs "trigger" or flag conditions present that may require specific care plan intervention. The SOM describes the utilization guidelines for facilities to implement the RAI.

The MDS has sections that deal with communication, cognition, and nutrition. The professional registered nurse is instructed to complete the MDS according to the documentation provided in the medical record, so speech-language pathology issues and proposed treatment plans can be integrated into the MDS when appropriately documented. Facilities can change this procedure, and ask various professionals to participate in the completion of the MDS. Speech-language pathologists may be asked to complete and sign certain sections of the MDS that are within their professional scope of practice in some facilities.

The MDS is still evolving since the information obtained from it has many different uses. It allows facilities to assess specific information about a resident regarding physical health, functional status, nutritional status, cognition, communication skills, vision, hearing, pyschosocial well-being, mood, behavior problems, dental status, activity preferences, use of medications and restraints, potential for self-care improvement, and indicators for quality of life. The identification of a resident's problems as determined by the MDS must then be directly addressed in the care plan.

In addition, the information obtained by the MDS is used by HCFA to determine payment classification and quality monitoring systems. Certain states (Maine, New York, South Dakota, Kansas, Texas, and Louisiana) are currently involved in what is called the Multistate Nursing Home Case Mix and Quality Demonstration Project. The current "Demonstration Project," as it is commonly referred to, is scheduled to end December 1998, but extensions have occurred in the past. Additional items are placed in the MDS in those facilities participating in the project to provide extra data that HCFA will use to develop national payment classifications and quality monitoring systems. Although no one knows what items the final version of the MDS will include, it is certain that payment for dysphagia services, and all speech-language pathology services, will be directly linked to it. The latest version is called MDS 2.0.

Among the information collected in the MDS, documentation is required regarding the number of minutes treatment was provided, not including evaluation, by speech-language pathology, occupational therapy, and physical therapy over designated 7-day periods, periodically assessed over 1 year. This information is linked directly to the daily reimbursement rate from Medicare to the nursing home.

It is important to remember that clinicians must first decide how much treatment is clinically necessary, and then allow the nursing home to bill for their services accordingly. It is illegal to determine initially how to maximize billing for speech-language pathology services, such as determining how many minutes of therapy per week are necessary for the highest reimbursement rate, and then document that treatment is required at that intensity solely to meet that billing criteria. That would be larceny by fraud.

Timing Requirements of the Resident Assessment Instrument

The RAI requires nursing homes to assess residents comprehensively within 21 days of admission and have an individualized care plan documented in the medical record, with signatures of all those who developed the care plan. Repeat assessments are conducted every 3 months, at times using a partial assessment if no significant changes have occurred, to assure that the care plan is accurately meeting the resident's needs. Interestingly, JCAHO requires long-term care facilities to complete an individualized care plan within 5 days of admission, making facilities and clinicians follow a different timeline than what is required by the RAI.

A comprehensive reassessment must occur immediately if a "significant change" occurs. There are many reasons a significant change could "trigger" a reassessment, including a decline or improvement in physical functioning or a sudden change in medical status. The intense monitoring and documentation requirements for the RAI often require facilities to hire additional staff to help all providers meet the regulations within the specified time periods. Speech-language pathologists must maintain careful records of the actual time spent directly with each resident (not including evaluation, documentation, or conference time), date(s) of service, what type of session was conducted (evaluation or treatment), and thorough documentation of progress in treatment goals.

PUTTING IT ALL TOGETHER: DOCUMENTING DYSPHAGIA SERVICES

How can clinicians document dysphagia services and meet all the different clinical, legal, reimbursement, and ethical requirements? Given all the information described thus far in this chapter, clinicians may feel this is an impossible task. However, all requirements can be met, given adherence to the following simple suggestions.

The First Draft is the Last Draft

Medical chart entries are meant to be written correctly the first time, with no changes or mistakes. This is one reason black, indelible ink is required for entries so that they cannot be easily erased or smeared. Do not use erasable ink pens, pencils, or felt-tipped pens. For computerized patient care entries, make sure the entry is saved on the computer before logging off. Preferably, all facilities that require computerized charting will provide a secure backup system that will save all entries automatically, and not allow changes to occur after the initial entry is saved.

A very serious legal charge to be avoided is called "spoliation," an illegal alteration of a patient medical record. To avoid being accused of spoliation, write on every line, with no spacing between entries. Draw a line to the end of the line or through page lines, to inhibit the temptation to add information later on and, thereby, alter the original record. Do not write over an entry a second time for any reason, even if it is to increase readability because of light pen ink. Do not try to hide a mistake by scratching it out, erasing it, or using correction liquid. Trial experts and judges can become suspicious of spoliation when reviewing the record at a later date, and wonder if an illegal entry alteration has occurred. If a pen does run out of ink, use a short parenthetical phrase stating the first pen ran out of ink at that point and initial the entry.

If an error is accidentally written, draw a single line through the error written in the record, and initial and date the correction. Some authorities suggest writing the word "error" above the correction, while others suggest "mistake" so as not to imply a clinical negligence by using the word "error." Others suggest the initials "M.E." be written to stand for "mistaken entry," while some suggest making a brief note in the margin adjacent to the correction indicating why it was made. Clinicians should refer to their facility policy regarding how to document corrections to a patient medical chart entry.

Use a SOAP Format

Many facilities use a format for documenting all health care services in a medical chart called SOAP, an acronym that stands for subjective information, objective information, assessment, and plan. It is important that effective communication between all members of a medical and rehabilitation team occur so that no confusion occurs regarding the recommended treatment, or where important information can be found within the chart. Therefore, the same documentation format as used by others in the facility should be followed.

Subjective information contains actual verbatim quotes from the patient regarding their status. A description of the patient age, sex, diagnosis, pertinent medical history, and medication list should be listed in the initial entry. If this information is provided on an initial evaluation form or elsewhere in the chart, documentation should tell where this information can be found in the chart.

Objective information contains data and facts only regarding what dysphagia services were rendered and whether is was a diagnostic or treatment session. Specific information regarding conferences held with the patient, family, caregivers, and/or physician is also reported in an objective fashion in this section.

The assessment section is a summary of the clinical findings and impressions of the data collected during the session. If the session was a diagnostic session, the diagnosis of dysphagia, type, and severity, must be clearly written along with any information that needs to be conveyed to the medical team. Clinical impressions regarding the response to treatment are given, along with any changes in dysphagia diagnosis, type, and severity. If a lack of progress is noted, the hypothesized reasons are written, with suggestions to improve progress.

The plan section contains the proposed treatment plan, including all pertinent recommendations, referrals and intensity of dysphagia services recommended. These are usually numbered and bulleted for quick reference and clarity. The number of sessions recommended per week, length of the session, and estimated length of time services will be required are written in this section. It is in this section that documentation of the patient's informed consent to the proposed treatment occurs. If or when no further speech-language pathology services are indicated, a discharge from these services must be clearly written. Any recommendations or referrals after discharge must be documented in this section.

Other Documentation Do's and Don'ts

It is important to write legibly as this provides legal protection. Illegible writing can lead to a lawsuit if others in the medical team are unable to read a clinician's note and patient injury occurs. Sign the entry legibly, too, along with the appropriate professional credentials and license number, if applicable. State or federal law will dictate whether a rubber stamp impression or computer-generated signature constitutes a "legal signature."

Clinicians are encouraged to check with the legal counsel in their facility about the use of stamps or computer-generated signatures.

Be sure to identify the patient being treated, using the patient's full name, on every page written in the medical chart. Include any other pertinent identifying information as well, such as patient medical record number and room number. It is the clinician's responsibility to make sure the patient is clearly identified on every piece of paper that documents patient care information.

Use only authorized abbreviations so that others will understand what information is being conveyed. Facilities can develop their own list of approved abbreviations but it must be widely disseminated and understood by all staff. When in doubt, write out the entire word or phrase if the intended meaning may not be clear within the context of the entry or there is a chance for misunderstanding or confusion. There are lists available of typical medical abbreviations used widely in medical documentation, and clinicians are encouraged to learn to use them.

Make sure the physician's orders are written prior to seeing a patient, since reimbursement may be denied without it. Check facility policy regarding how referrals are to occur, and what time frame clinicians must adhere to see the patient after the initial physician's order for an evaluation. Often, clinicians are required to see the patient within 24 or 48 hours after the physician gives the initial order for a speech-language pathology evaluation.

Document all services in a timely manner, which means as soon as possible after the service occurred. Failure to record important information regarding patient care in a timely fashion may constitute professional negligence if harm occurred to a patient because vital information was not recorded.

Be careful not to document observations or concerns perceived by another clinician or health care provider as your own observations. Otherwise, you may be legally responsible for the information recorded. Eliminate all unnecessary verbiage not affecting patient care, taking care to use proper spelling and grammar. Do not blame or disparage another provider or express personal feelings about the patient. Document with specificity, avoiding generalizations such as "within normal limits." Be specific regarding what was observed and assessed. Do not document "hearsay" as fact. Hearsay is a statement made by a person and adopted by another as fact. It is secondhand speech. If hearsay is documented, place it in quotation marks, identifying who made the statement.

Thoroughly document a patient's informed consent to treatment, and, on discharge, all home care and follow-up instructions issued to the patient and/or caregivers and family. Written, personalized discharge instructions given to the patient should routinely be documented as being provided in the discharge documentation. This is typically customary practice at most facilities.

Carefully document a patients' or family/caregivers' actions that increase the risk for harm, despite specific education regarding the risk of these actions. This would protect a clinician from possibly being sued for malpractice since the patient has acted with contributory negligence. A clinician cannot be held responsible for patients' or caregivers' actions if they fail to conform to the standards required by law for their own safety, and it is documented that they were educated about the risk.

With regard to writing treatment goals, there are many components that must be met. The goal(s) must be functional, yet the definition of what constitutes "functional" is not clearly defined by reimbursement agencies to date. It clearly must be directed toward a patient's usual eating practices, and be measurable, objective, and behavioral. It must specify the intensity of treatment necessary to meet the stated goals, and the estimated time period and prognosis to meet the goals. Excessive use of treatment will be scrutinized by payers, and clinicians should be able to justify the need for intensive treatment and its duration based on individual need and standard clinical practices. In addition, JCAHO mandates that a specific goal be written to educate the patient and caregivers regarding the results and recommendations of the evaluation, and involve them in the development and implementation of the treatment plan for all facilities receiving accreditation. This is quite similar to the process of documenting informed consent for treatment, but is addressed and documented via an education goal in the care plan.

Coaching Tips

▶ To decrease your risk of being accused or convicted of any legal or ethical impropriety, ask yourself: "Could I sit in a court of law and justify my actions?" On what basis could you defend your actions? If you have any doubts you couldn't defend your actions professionally and legally, don't do it.

▶ Consult the billing office of your facility to determine the specific eligibility and documentation requirements required for dysphagia services, so you can inform the patient and provide the appropriate information for payment. If an authorization to treat is denied and you believe that treatment is essential for the safety of the patient, fight the denial and document, document, document.

▶ Consult the legal counsel in your facility to determine specific documentation protocols desired and how to document appropriately within that facility.

▶ If you have a legal question, consult the legal counsel for the facility. A nurse, administrator, or medical records director cannot provide the legal information you need.

CONCLUSION

Medical documentation of dysphagia services requires clinicians to become aware of the legal, ethical, and reimbursement requirements of documenting their dysphagia services. Different practice settings (such as nursing homes) may require different documentation, but all documentation can serve to protect the clinician if it is performed appropriately.

The medical record serves as both a legal and business document. There are many specific suggestions that clinicians can implement when documenting their dysphagia services that will help them defend themselves if ever accused of fraud, professional malpractice, or an ethical violation. The art of medically documenting dysphagia services is not yet typically taught within universities, but surely that is only a matter of time. Beginning clinicians must not only develop their own clinical competence in providing dysphagia services, but they must learn how to document those services to establish an appropriate legal and reimbursement medical record.

CHAPTER

13

The Patient's Perspective

Deborah Dwyer Batjer

Knowing the patient's point of view is critical to modern practice in dysphagia. That point of view can motivate the clinician to act quickly and decisively, or more cautiously, depending on what a patient wants, needs, and values. Equally important, the patient's perspective can be a rich source of ideas about what to do. Few indeed are the patients who do not go to work to manage their own problems. What patients do can be as rich a source of techniques as a textbook. We are indebted to Deborah for sharing her experience with dysphagia.

Like the mother who forgets her labor pains after she holds her newborn child, I have willfully forgotten some of the details of my inability to swallow for 2 years. Thanks to my ever-patient, loving family who helped jog my memory, I can tell the story of dysphagia from a patient's point of view.

271

On March 11, 1993, when I was 48 years old, a benign meningioma was surgically removed from the right side of my brain stem. To remove the tumor, several nerves and vessels were severed, resulting in a stroke. Shortly after I awakened from surgery, I had a respiratory arrest and was moved into the ICU. Two days later, another stroke necessitated a tracheostomy. When I was finally moved out of the ICU, I was receiving nutrition and hydration through a nasogastric tube, had a mechanical suction device to "vacuum" out my trach tube periodically, and had a lot of physical problems. Swallowing was not then a high priority. I was mechanically supported and had other, more consuming physical difficulties, like double vision and nystagmus, right-sided weakness, and an inability to speak, sit up, or move independently in the hospital bed. In short, I was a mess!

Gradually, I learned to sit up without keeling over and to communicate with a magic marker and a reader board. I gradually regained some speech, although garbled and largely unintelligible. I became aware that the nasogastric tube and aspirator were still plugged in because I was not swallowing and, since I equated living with the ability to swallow, I thought I was just marking time until I died. I remember vividly "mumbling" to my sister that I understood that my survival depended on regaining my swallow reflex soon. I was moved to a rehab center in the area and began three weeks of grueling physical and occupational rehab. The speech therapist there gave my husband and I lots of material to read about the swallowing process, and somewhere I gleaned that the function would likely return naturally. She gave me exercises and ice chips to stimulate swallowing, and I wondered what I was doing wrong for them not to work. I continued to be linked to life through my nasogastric tube.

Just before discharge, a percutaneous endoscopic gastrostomy (PEG) tube was inserted into my stomach and I happily got rid of the nasogastric tube. There was again the oft-repeated professional belief that my swallowing reflex would eventually return on its own and the PEG, I was told, was merely an interim measure to sustain me. I returned home equipped with a suction device, feeder pole, feedbags, a home-delivery plan to receive monthly shipments of Jevity,® and an expectation that the swallowing would just magically return. Dysphagia was a nuisance, to be sure, but it was only one of many challenges I faced. Besides I had learned that survival without swallowing was indeed possible. In the meantime, I focused on the problems associated with stroke-related vertigo, vision, speech, and mobility.

I continued home rehab for a month, visited often by physical, occupational, and speech therapists, the latter of whom continued spooning me ice chips and mostly concentrated on articulation difficulties. To mark my progress, I had the suction device and pole for my feed bag, among the other accoutrements that defined me as unhealthy, reclaimed by the home health care delivery folks. Their nutritionist began monthly visits to weigh me and check for skin turgor, growing concerned at my continuous weight loss. She advised me to add whatever fattening calories I could to the Jevity,® and substituted three cans per day of Ensure Plus® for their added calories/volume.

Though I was unable to taste anything, the smell of canned "food" became offensive. I added chocolate weight-gainer powder, peanut butter, yogurt, and a variety of juices as a supplement to, and to mask the smell of, the 48 oz of protein food I needed daily. Eventually, my weight stabilized. Throughout the period of time I had the PEG, my guiding rule was simply that whatever would pass through the tube was worth a try.

"Cheating the tube" became a game throughout the next 2 years. Once, I melted ice cream and ground up some homemade pie, shoving the mixture through my tube and feeling satisfied that somehow my pie a la mode had won. Another time, a friend ground up zucchini casserole, mixed it with tomato juice, and I successfully pushed that through my tube. It was exhausting, though. Too many times to recount, the tube became clogged with my crazy concoctions, and milking it to clear the bolus took incredible time and energy.

Unilateral facial pain and high blood pressure necessitated daily medications. In addition, there were others I periodically needed. None was available in liquid form. To ingest pills, then, I ground them up and mixed them with water.

But I get ahead of myself. In June 1993, when I began 4 months of outpatient therapy locally, the speech pathologist identified two areas to focus on: swallowing and articulation. My tracheostomy tube was subsequently removed, helping articulation immensely. Articulation became the predominant area of work, as there was also the professional belief that my swallowing would, if it was ever going to, come back naturally. One vocal chord was paralyzed in the midline position, so my speech was labored, monotonous, and breathy. To evacuate the constant secretions that pooled in my mouth and precluded speaking clearly, I began "spitting" often into tissues, which we bought in bulk, easily using more than one box per day. No matter what mobility I recovered over the next many months, the tissue and "spit bag" always accompanied me.

It was embarrassing. At theaters, restaurants, or other public places, people with forbidding glares would move away from us after hearing me "clear." Many a salesperson commented on my "terrible cold," and I always felt dirty. Strangers did not know that I could not swallow.

Typically reflective of the common lack of understanding, a room maid at a hotel we visited 10 months after my surgery was asking about "my condition"as she cleaned around cans of Jevity and Ensure, 60-cc syringes, and an overflowing tissue-filled waste basket. After I explained that I was unable to swallow anything, she advised me to be sure to try the hotel's special quiche at lunch!

Since so much of our culture and entertainment are built around food, I was determined not to let my dysphagia preclude my family's enjoyment of life. We frequently went to friends' homes for meals or to restaurants and we had lots of company in. I began reading cookbooks for the first time, used my imagination, smell, and appearance to "taste" food, and prepared, so I am told, some creative, attractive, and delicious meals. I rarely chewed-and-spit food even though my taste buds were intact, because the increased salivation was hardly worth the trouble. We went on many trips during the 2 years post-op, either carting my cans with us or buying them along the way. I dreamed of things I would like to eat and played mental games in my head about what I would"eat" first, if able.

Socially, the tube feedings became simply a matter of juggling. Either I had my tube feeding before meeting others, or I had it simultaneously with their eating. Bless my family's and friends' souls, they never acted offended when I pulled my tube from beneath a waistband, removed the cap, inserted a 60-cc syringe (without the plunger), and proceeded to pour into it a foul-smelling mixture of Jevity, Ensure Plus, and water.

Periodically, I would overflow the syringe, remove the cap without pinching the tube closed, or fail to put the cap back on the tube securely after feedings. In any case, there were too many"accidents" to count. My family and friends were quick to clean up after me and a change of clothes always seemed to make things "right" again. I lived in fear that I would have such an accident in some public place, but that did not keep us home. I cannot begin to describe how important to my perception of normalcy were the love and patience of those around me, particularly on the part of my husband, our kids, extended family and our friends. They were always supportive, never acted embarrassed, and rejoiced with me over so many "little" firsts.

About 4 months postop, the physiatrist and speech therapists recommended a modified barium swallow test to see what was causing my prolonged dysphagia. It revealed a hang-up in my hypopharyngeal area. Again, I was advised to hope for a natural return of function. The gastroenterologist who had inserted the PEG assured us that he had never implanted a tube permanently.

A year later as other functions improved, we repeated the swallow test. There was no change. I was advised then that I probably would never swallow again. That was a low day for me, though it hardly compared with the other stroke-related challenges I had faced. Craving hope, I immediately telephoned a 70-year-old woman we had heard about, whose swallowing ability had returned 2 years following a brainstem stroke. In our conversation it became readily apparent that, while she had not been able to swallow solids for 2 years, she had never lost the ability to swallow liquids. Shattered, I then called the Stoke Association in Seattle. Although that organization has lots of worthwhile programs for stroke survivors and caregivers, I was only interested in tapping into their national database to ascertain the incidence of permanent dysphagia and getting other dysphagic contacts. Always being tied to a tube and bunch of cans kept me from being as independent as possible. Finding someone else who had confronted a similar problem and had dealt with it became very important in my ability to move forward. There was unfortunately no such database. Moreover, the person at the other end of telephone assured me, there were not many brain stem stroke survivors who were functionally able to handle routine tasks. On the one hand, I felt very blessed to be an exception. On the other hand, I felt very isolated.

As so often happened during this and subsequent periods, out of my despair something happened to turn things around. A friend across the country phoned to tell me about her 42-year-old cousin here in Seattle who had been initially unable to swallow following a brain stem stroke. I immediately called this person and learned that she, too, had been discharged from the hospital with a PEG and had been unable to swallow for 6 months poststroke. She was eating normally now. She gave me hints about using a straw to "spit" into a lidded cup for social unobtrusiveness, and related how she had not allowed herself to prepare meals or eat with others during her 6 months of tube feedings. For the first time, I wondered if I was somehow delaying the return of swallowing function because I was adapting so well to my tube! I tried the straw technique, but had difficulty getting my lips to hug the straw. My drooling was more often outside than inside the straw, and I abandoned the technique.

On the recommendation of a friend, I scheduled two appointments with an acupuncturist to see if that treatment would trigger some swallowing response. To his credit, he made no guarantees. Nothing happened, though. Other friends, with the best of intentions, gave me clippings of this "cure" or that one, told of incantations over my body, of prayers that I should say, or of mental visualizations of swallowing. There was an unmistakable implication by many of them that if I did not subscribe to these interventions, I chose not to overcome my dysphagia. Despite nagging self-doubts that usually followed, I resolved not to be emotionally influenced by the promises of alternative therapies. My husband, a physician, had a firm belief in the scientific method rather than anecdotal testimony, and I, too, subscribed to this.

The rest of my body seemed to be making progress. After 18 months of having either family, friends, the disability van, or a taxi transport me, having groceries and pharmaceuticals delivered, and catalogue shopping, I returned to driving. The day I was approved for driving is still a precious memory! The joy! To this day, I try to do a daily errand, just to put a few miles on the car and to remind myself that I am gradually, but definitely, improving.

Interestingly, as other functions returned, the inability to swallow became a bigger issue. I could not receive Eucharist at church. While my husband and I could attend benefit dinners, I could never eat the food. Thanksgiving and Christmas were sheer agony as food-filled memories of past holidays tormented me. Always, I had to think about the availability of Jevity and Ensure Plus. On a family trip to Hawaii, I called ahead to a drugstore to order my "food." If my husband and I were going anywhere for a few days, I always packed the requisite number of cans. On several trips with friends and relatives, while they were anxious to try various restaurants, I always had to consume my "dinners" differently. A small price to pay on the road to wellness, to be sure. But a price I was increasingly feeling frustrated paying.

During the $2\frac{1}{2}$ years that I had the tube, there was always a smelly discharge from around the PEG site in my stomach. I would keep this from staining my clothes with twice/daily applications of gauze and daily swabbing with hydrogen peroxide. The gastroenterologist who had put it in had told me it would probably need replacing yearly, but at each examination he confirmed that it was in good condition. I did replace the caps twice because of breaking or leakage.

In early 1995, I telephoned Ross Laboratories, makers of Jevity and Ensure Plus, to ask if they had another product that was less bulky than their canned or powdered versions. Motivated by my husband's and my desire to travel overseas "or wherever," we were stopped in our planning by my cumbersome daily requirements of 48 oz of protein diet. We assumed we could always buy bottled water and, if need be, I could subsist for a time on purchased baby food and formula. But we wondered if there was something better, less bulky on the market; there apparently was not. The fact that we were even discussing such a venture gave us tremendous encouragement, though.

I also put the word "dysphagia" out over the Internet and got plugged into the StrokeNet bulletin board. I was unable to find anyone who had a permanent inability to swallow, though I found many stroke survivors who are a wonderful, continuing source of support.

In February 1995, the speech pathologist who had done the previous swallow test, called to tell me about a treatment program using instrumental biofeedback modalities in dysphagia therapy. She and her colleagues thought I might be a good candidate for this type of program. Because it was noninvasive, plausible, and relatively straightforward, my husband and I were anxious for more information.

Before starting treatment, another barium swallow test was conducted. It continued to show a profound dysphagia problem. Although the clinician was candidly unsure if biofeedback would improve it, we were not to be dissuaded, and the clinician agreed to give the treatment a try. We left for the therapy program at the end of March, guardedly hopeful. Five days and nine sessions later, another modified barium swallow test confirmed that I could swallow again! The biofeedback technique had taught me to use other muscles to replicate a "swallow." At first, we were thrilled with 2 teaspoons per half hour, for they gave legitimacy to the promise of eventually swallowing everything again. This promise was a gift that I will forever be thankful for.

My husband and I returned to Seattle and told my story to anyone who would listen. As a result, several area hospitals have now established dysphagia programs utilizing biofeedback as a treatment tool.

Initially, the volume I could swallow was minute. Even the texture of tapioca pudding or applesauce was problematic. I would gag and choke, spit, and wonder if anything had "gone down." Sometimes, food, especially jello, came out my nose, a terribly unattractive state of affairs! My online network of stroke survivors was remarkably helpful in cautioning patience and keeping me firmly grounded. Accounts by them of resting their faces on the table, using a mirror, or eating only pureed foods made me realize that I might never eat steak and potatoes, or salad and seafood again. That I was in for a long process became painfully clear. And that I might never eat the dreamed-about dishes was a real, but unacceptable, possibility. I resolved to regain all eating function again and to have my tube removed eventually. Thankfully, my body thankfully permitted it.

Initially, I ate baby food, yogurt, puddings, ice cream, cottage cheese, cream of wheat, soups thickened with instant potatoes, and the like, adding new textures gradually. My volume increased over time, as did the repertoire of foods. Early on, my teeth throbbed with pain from their unaccustomed use and I wondered if perhaps I was in for a lot of dental work. This eventually disappeared on its own, but it is of note. By August, I was taking all solid foods orally-everything-and using my tube only for medications and supplementary hydration. Liquids, especially water, remained difficult to control.

My tube was removed in mid-September 1995, $2\frac{1}{2}$ years after my operation/stroke. To celebrate, my husband and I went to Europe in October for 2 weeks to see friends in Germany and France and to spend time absorbing sun on Italy's Amalfi Coast. We did not take any cans. The wonderful richness of native foods with flavors that literally burst in our mouths was an unbeatable experience! Breads, tart flambé, salami, cheeses, seafood, pastas, olives marinated in oil and garlic, seaweed and radicchio, citrus, artichokes, antipasto, wines, and liqueurs: I tried them all!

Before concluding, there are a few spinoffs that merit mentioning. My cough reflex is strong, having been developed over the past 2 years by constant clearing. This is essential, because often when food gets "stuck," my cough eventually expels it. Also, remaining calm and bending from the waist to let gravity help dislodge "plugs" are important techniques. The ability to swallow has also significantly reduced my dependence on tissue and spitting, though I am always prepared with tissues ready to cover my mouth or receive a mouthful.

I am still cautious about what food and the amount I eat in public now. And I am often nervous about eating with others. I am reluctant to drink anything in front of others, because liquids are still my nemesis. Despite everyone's protestations that it's no bother to them, a coughing jag can be sudden, surprising, and discomfiting for everyone. I make lots of noise, eat slowly, chew everything ridiculously well, and then swallow it over several attempts. Eating requires concentration on each bite to the exclusion of all else, including mealtime chatter. In short, it is not pretty and it is slow, but it continues to improve dramatically and I will continue to push the limits. Mostly, swallowing is, oh, so wonderful a gift, I will never take it for granted again!

APPENDIX

American Speech-Language-Hearing Association Code of Ethics*

PREAMBLE

The preservation of the highest standards of integrity and ethical principles is vital to the responsible discharge of obligations in the professions of speech-language pathology and audiology. This Code of Ethics sets forth the fundamental principles and rules considered essential to this purpose.

Every individual who is (a) a member of the American Speech-Language-Hearing Association, whether certified or not, (b) a nonmember holding the Certificate of Clinical Competence from the Association, (c) an applicant for membership or certification, or (d) a Clinical Fellow seeking to fulfill standards for certification shall abide by this Code of Ethics.

Any action that violates the spirit and purpose of this Code shall be considered unethical. Failure to specify any particular responsibility or practice in this Code of Ethics shall not be construed as denial of the existence of such responsibilities or practices.

*Last Revised January 1, 1994. Reprinted with permission from ASHA.
Source: American Speech-Language-Hearing Association (1994). Code of ethics, *ASHA*, *36*, (3, Suppl. 13), 1–2.

The fundamentals of ethical conduct are described by Principles of Ethics and by Rules of Ethics as they relate to responsibility to persons served, to the public, and to the professions of speech-language pathology and audiology.

Principles of Ethics, aspirational and inspirational in nature, form the underlying moral basis for the Code of Ethics. Individuals shall observe these principles as affirmative obligations under all conditions of professional activity.

Rules of Ethics are specific statements of minimally acceptable professional conduct or of prohibitions and are applicable to all individuals.

Principle of Ethics I

Individuals shall honor their responsiblity to hold paramount the welfare of persons they serve professionally.

Rules of Ethics

A. Individuals shall provide all services competently.
B. Individuals shall use every resource, including referral when appropriate, to ensure that high-quality service is provided.
C. Individuals shall not discriminate in the delivery of professional services on the basis of race or ethnicity, gender, age, religion, national origin, sexual orientation, or disability.
D. Individuals shall fully inform the persons they serve of the nature and possible effects of services rendered and products dispensed.
E. Individuals shall evaluate the effectiveness of services rendered and of products dispensed and shall provide services or dispense products only when benefit can reasonably be expected.
F. Individuals shall not guarantee the results of any treatment or procedure, directly or by implication; however, they may make a reasonable statement of prognosis.
G. Individuals shall not evaluate or treat speech, language, or hearing disorders solely by correspondence.
H. Individuals shall maintain adequate records of professional services rendered and products dispensed and shall allow access to these records when appropriately authorized.
I. Individuals shall not reveal, without authorization, any professional or personal information about the person served professionally, unless required by law to do so, or unless doing so is necessary to protect the welfare of the person or of the community.

J. Individuals shall not charge for services not rendered, nor shall they misrepresent,* in any fashion, services rendered or products dispensed.
K. Individuals shall use persons in research or as subjects of teaching demonstrations only with their informed consent.
L. Individuals whose professional services are adversely affected by substance or other health-related conditions shall seek professional assistance and, where appropriate, withdraw from the affected areas of practice.

Principle of Ethics II

Individuals shall honor their responsibility to achieve and maintain the highest level of professional competence.

Rules of Ethics

A. Individuals shall engage in the provision of clinical services only when they hold the appropriate Certificate of Clinical Competence or when they are in the certification process and are supervised by an individual who holds the appropriate Certificate of Clinical Competence.
B. Individuals shall engage in only those aspects of the professions that are within the scope of their competence, considering their level of education, training, and experience.
C. Individuals shall continue their professional development throughout their careers.
D. Individuals shall delegate the provision of clinical services only to persons who are certified or to persons in the education or certification process who are appropriately supervised. The provision of support services may be delegated to persons who are neither certified nor in the certification process only when a certificate holder provides appropriate supervision.
E. Individuals shall prohibit any of their professional staff from providing services that exceed the staff member's competence, considering the staff member's level of education, training, and experience.
F. Individuals shall ensure that all equipment used in the provision of services is in proper working order and is properly calibrated.

---

*For purposes of this Code of Ethics, misrepresentation includes any untrue statements or statements that are likely to mislead. Misrepresentation also includes the failure to state any information that is material and that ought, in fairness, to be considered.

Principle of Ethics III

Individuals shall honor their responsibility to the public by promoting public understanding of the professions, by supporting the development of services designed to fulfill the unmet needs of the public, and by providing accurate information in all communications involving any aspect of the professions.

Rules of Ethics

A. Individuals shall not misrepresent their credentials, competence, education, training, or experience.
B. Individuals shall not participate in professional activities that constitute a conflict of interest.
C. Individuals shall not misrepresent diagnostic information, services, rendered, or products dispensed or engage in any scheme or artifice to defraud in connection with obtaining payment or reimbursement for such services or products.
D. Individuals' statements to the public shall provide accurate information about the nature and management of communication disorders, about the professions, and about professional services.
E. Individuals' statements to the public—advertising, announcing, and marketing their professional services, reporting research results, and promoting products—shall adhere to prevailing professional standards and shall not contain misrepresentations.

Principle of Ethics IV

Individuals shall honor their responsibilities to the professions and their relationships with colleagues, students, and members of allied professions. Individuals shall uphold the dignity and autonomy of the professions, maintain harmonious interprofessional and intraprofessional relationships, and accept the professions' self-imposed standards.

Rules of Ethics

A. Individuals shall prohibit anyone under their supervision from engaging in any practice that violates the Code of Ethics.
B. Individuals shall not engage in dishonesty, fraud, deceit, misrepresentation, or any form of conduct that adversely reflects on the professions or on the individual's fitness to serve persons professionally.

C. Individuals shall assign credit only to those who have contributed to a publication, presentation, or product. Credit shall be assigned in proportion to the contribution and only with the contributor's consent.

D. Individuals' statements to colleagues about professional services, research results, and products shall adhere to prevailing professional standards and shall contain no misrepresentations.

E. Individuals shall not provide professional services without exercising independent professional judgment, regardless of referral source or prescription.

F. Individuals shall not discriminate in their relationships with colleagues, students, and members of allied professions on the basis of race or ethnicity, gender, age, religion, national origin, sexual orientation, or disability.

G. Individuals who have reason to believe that the Code of Ethics has been violated shall inform the Ethical Practice Board.

H. Individuals shall cooperate fully with the Ethical Practice Board in its investigation and adjudication of matters related to this Code of Ethics.

APPENDIX

B

American Speech-Language-Hearing Association Statement of Practices and Procedures of the Board of Ethics*

The Board of Ethics (BE) is charged by the Bylaws of the American Speech-Language-Hearing Association with the responsibility to interpret, administer, and enforce the Code of Ethics of the Association. Accordingly, the BE hereby adopts the following practices and procedures to be followed in administering and enforcing that Code.

A fundamental precept that guides the BE in the discharge of its responsibility is that an effective Code of Ethics requires an orderly and fair administration and enforcement of its terms and requires full compliance by all members of the Association and all holders of Certificates of Clinical Competence. The BE recognizes that each case must be judged on an individual basis, and that no two cases are likely to be identical. Thus, the BE

*Effective February 8, 1998; revised 1993; revised 1997; revised 1998. Reprinted with permission from ASHA.
Source: American Speech-Language-Hearing Association (1998, Spring). Statement of practices and procedures of the board of ethics. *American Speech-Language-Hearing Association*, 40, (2), (Suppl. 18), 46–49.

has the responsibility to exercise its judgment on the merits of each case and on its interpretation of the Code.

A. DEFINITION OF TERMS

1. BE: Board of Ethics
2. Association: American Speech-Language-Hearing Association
3. Code: Code of Ethics of the Association
4. Certificate(s): Certificate(s) of Clinical Competence
5. Respondent: The alleged offender
6. Complainant(s): The person(s) alleging that a violation occurred
7. Initial Determination: Initial Determination by the BE, subject to Further Consideration and appeal, of the (a) finding, (b), proposed sanction, (c) extent of disclosure
8. Sanction(s); Penalties imposed by the BE
9. Disclosure: Announcement of the final BE Decision to other than Respondent
10. Further Consideration: Further consideration by the BE of its Initial Determination
11. BE Decision: Final decision of the BE after: (a) Further Consideration; or (b) 30 days from the date of notice of the Initial Determination by the BE if no request for Further Consideration is received.
12. Appeal: Written request from Respondent to BE alleging error in the BE Decision and asking that it be reversed in whole or in part by the Executive Board.

B. CASE REVIEW PROCEDURES

1. Alleged violations shall be reviewed by the BE in such manner as the BE may, in its discretion, deem necessary and proper. If the BE determines that it has jurisdiction over the person(s) and subject matter of the allegation, the BE shall notify Respondent of the alleged offense in writing and shall advise Respondent that Respondent's answer to the allegation shall be in writing and must be received by the BE no later than 45 days after the date of the BE notice to Respondent. Voluntary resignation of membership and/or voluntary surrender of the Certificate(s) of Clinical Competence shall not preclude the BE from continuing to process the alleged violation to conclusion, and the notice from the BE to Respondent requesting an answer shall so advise Respondent.

2. At the discretion of the BE, the appropriate staff of the Association's National Office may be informed that Respondent is the subject of an alleged violation of the Code and may be instructed that no changes in membership and/or certification status shall be permitted without approval of the BE.
3. The BE shall consider all information provided by the Complainant(s), Respondent, or any other relevant source, and shall base its Initial Determination on that information.
4. If the BE finds that there is not sufficient evidence to warrant further proceedings, Respondent and Complainant(s) shall be so advised and the case shall be closed.
5. Except when the complainant is the BE, the Complainant(s) shall submit a signed waiver to the BE consenting to allow the BE to send a copy of the complaint to the Respondent for the Respondent's response. In cases where the BE issues a sanction of Censure, or the Withholding, suspension, or Revocation of Membership and/or Certificate(s) of Clinical Competence, the waiver shall also consent to allow the BE to send its Final Decision and any relevant case information provided by the Complainant(s) to:
   (a) any state agency that licenses or credentials speech-language pathologists or audiologists, and which the Respondent is licensed or credentialed by, or is an applicant for licensure or credentialing.
   (b) any other professional organization that enforces a Code of Ethics or a Code of Professional Conduct of which the Respondent is a member or is an applicant for membership.
6. When a Respondent is initially contacted regarding a complaint filed against him/her, the Respondent shall be advised that in cases where the BE issues a sanction of either Censure, or the Withholding, Suspension, or Revocation of Membership and/or Certificate(s) of Clinical Competence, any Final Decision of the BE and any relevant case information provided by the Complainant(s) and/or the Respondent, may be sent to:
   (a) any state agency that licenses or credentials speech-language pathologists or audiologists, and which the Respondent is licensed or credentialed by, or is an applicant for licensure or credentialing.
   (b) any other professional organization that enforces a Code of Ethics or a Code of Professional Conduct of which the Respondent is a member or is an applicant for membership.
7. If the BE finds that there is sufficient evidence to warrant further proceedings, the BE shall make an Initial Determination, which includes

(a) the finding of violation, (b) the proposed sanction, and (c) the proposed extent of disclosure. In this regard, the final decision of any state, federal, regulatory, or judicial body may be considered sufficient evidence that the Code was violated.

8. The BE may, as part of its Initial Determination, order that the Respondent cases and desist from any practice found to be violation of the Code. Failure to comply with such a Cease and Desist Order is, itself, a violation of the code, and shall normally result in Revocation of Membership and/or Revocation of the Certificate(s) of Clinical Competence. The BE may require the Respondent to attest in writing that s/he has complied with the Cease and Desist Order.

9. The BE shall give Respondent notice of its Initial Determination. The notice shall also advise Respondent of the right to request Further consideration by the BE and of the right, after Further consideration, to request an appeal to the Executive Board. The procedures to be followed in exercising those rights are described in Sections F and G of the statement.

C. NOTICES AND ANSWERS

All notices and answers shall be in writing and considered to be given or furnished (a) to Respondent when sent—Certified Mail, Addressee Only, Return Receipt Requested—to the address then listed in the ASHA membership records, and (b) to the BE when received by the BE.

D. SANCTIONS

Sanctions shall consist of one or more of the following: Reprimand; Censure; Withhold, Suspend, or Revoke Membership and/or the Certificate(s) of Clinical Competence; or other measures determined by the BE at its discretion. A Cease and Desist Order may become part of any sanction.

E. DISCLOSURE

1. The BE Decision, upon becoming final, shall be published in an ASHA publication distributed to all of the membership, and shall be provided to any person or entity requesting a copy of the Decision, if the sanction is Censure, or the Withholding, Suspension, or Revocation of Membership and/or Certificate(s) of Clinical Competence. In the case of

Reprimand, the BE Decision shall be disclosed only to Respondent, Respondent's counsel, Complainant(s), witnesses at the BE Further Consideration hearing, staff, and Association counsel, each of whom shall be advised that the decision is strictly confidential and that any breach of that confidentiality by any party who is a member and/or certificate holder of the Association is, itself, a violation of the Code.

2. In cases where the sanction is Censure, or the Withholding, Suspension, or Revocation of Membership and/or Certificate(s) of Clinical Competence, the BE may provide its Final Decision and relevant case information to:

    (a) any state agency that licenses or credentials speech-language pathologists or audiologists, and which the Respondent is licensed or credentialed by, or is an applicant for licensure or credentialing.

    (b) any other professional organization that enforces a Code of Ethics or a Code of Professional Conduct of which the Respondent is a member or is an applicant for membership.

F. FURTHER CONSIDERATION BY THE BE OF THE INITIAL DETERMINATION

1. When the notice of Initial Determination from the BE states that Respondent has violated the Code and announces a proposed sanction and extent of disclosure, Respondent may request that the BE give Further consideration to the Initial Determination.

2. Respondent's request for Further consideration shall be in writing and must be received by the BE no later than 30 days after the date of notice of Initial Determination. In the absence of a timely request for Further Consideration, the initial Determination shall be the BE Decision, which decision shall be final. There shall be no further right of appeal to the Executive Board.

3. If Respondent submits a timely request for Further Consideration by the BE, the BE shall schedule a hearing and notify Respondent. Respondent shall be entitled to submit a written brief, which must be received at least 30 days prior to the hearing. Respondent may choose to appear pesonally before the BE to present evidence and to be accompanied by counsel. The proceedings shall be informal; strict adherence to the rules of evidence shall not be observed, but all evidence shall be accorded such weight as it deserves. As an alternative to personal appearance at the hearing, the BE shall afford Respondent the opportunity to make a presentation to the BE and to respond to questions

from the BE via a conference telephone call placed to Respondent by the BE. All personal costs in connection with the further consideration, including travel and lodging costs incurred by the Respondent, and Respondent's counsel and witnesses, and counsel and other fees, shall be Respondent's sole responsibility. At the Respondent's request, a copy of the hearing transcribed in full shall be made available to Respondent at Respondent's expense. The request by Respondent must be received by BE within 30 days after Further Consideration Decision has been received by the Respondent.

4. After the Further Consideration Hearing, the BE shall render its decision and notify Respondent. If evidence present at the hearing warrants, the BE may modify the finding, increase or decrease the severity of the sanction, and/or modify the extent of disclosure that was announced to Respondent in the notice of Initial Determination. This decision shall be the BE Decision, an , in the absence of a timely appeal to the Executive Board, the BE Decision shall be final.

G. APPEAL OF BE DECISION TO EXECUTIVE BOARD

1. Respondent may appeal the BE Further Consideration Decision to the Executive Board. The request for appeal shall be in writing and must be received by the BE no later than 30 days after the date of notice of the BE Further Consideration Decision. Respondent may only appeal a Further consideration Decision if the claim is based on a showing that the BE did not adhere to procedural requirements, or that the decision of the BE was arbitrary and capricious and without any evidentiary basis. The Executive Board Appeals Panel may not receive or consider any evidentiary matters not included in the official record of the Further Consideration Decision.

2. The procedures for a hearing before the Executive Board as described in the Statement of Practices and Procedures for Appeals of Decisions of the Board of Ethics.

H. REINSTATEMENT

Persons whose membership or certification has been revoked may apply for reinstatement at the completion of the revocation period. Reinstatement requires a two-thirds vote of the BE. The BE may set any conditions or requirements it deems necessary for the protection and benefit of the public and the professions in the issuance of any order for reinstatement. The applicant for reinstatement must meet all certification standards and/ or membership requirements that are in effect at the time of the Reinstatement Order.

In all cases, the applicant bears the burden of demonstrating with appropriate documentation that conditions that led to revocation have been rectified and that, upon reinstatement, the applicant will abide by the Code. The BE's deliberation will be guided by the premise that reinstatement must be in the best interests of the Association and of persons served professionally.

I. AMENDMENT

This Statement of Practices and Procedures may be amended on recommendation of the BE and a vote of the Executive Board. All such changes will be given appropriate publicity.

APPENDIX

C

Medicare Intermediary Manual Part 3— Claims Process

NEW PROCEDURES—EFFECTIVE DATE: 9/24/90

Section 3910, Special Instructions for Medical Review of Dysphagia Claims—
This initiates MR [Medical Review] instructions unique to one or more therapy
types. It provides specific guidance for the type of documentation you
need in reviewing claims for dysphagia treatment by providers of speech-
language pathology, occupational therapy, and physical therapy services.

3910. Special Instructions for MR of Dysphagia Claims

For your MR of dysphagia claims for speech-language pathology (SLP),
occupational therapy (OT), and physical therapy (PT) services follow these
procedures:

A. *Medical Workup*—Documentation by the physician must establish a preliminary diagnosis and form the basis of estimates of progress. Patients

must be selected for therapy after a proper medical diagnostic evaluation by a physician. The medical workups must document whether the
difficulty involves the oral, pharyngeal, or esophageal phase of swallowing. This may involve collaboration with therapist or speech-language pathologist.

B. *Dysphagia Criteria—Oral, Pharyngeal, or Esophageal (Upper One Third)
Phase of Swallowing*—Documentation must indicate the patient's level
of alertness, motivation, cognition, and deglutition. In addition, at least
one of the following conditions must be present:

▶ History of aspiration problems or aspiration pneumonia, or definite risk for aspiration, reverse aspiration, chronic aspiration, nocturnal aspiration, or aspiration pneumonia. Nasal regurgitation,
choking, frequent coughing up food during swallowing, wet or
gurgly voice quality after swallowing liquids or delayed or slow
swallow reflex.

▶ Presence of oral motor disorders such as drooling, oral food retention, leakage of food or liquids placed into the mouth.

▶ Impaired salivary gland performance and/or presence of local structural lesions in the pharynx resulting in marked oropharyngeal swallowing difficulties.

▶ Incoordination, sensation loss, (postural difficulties) or other neuromotor disturbances affecting oropharyngeal abilities necessary to
close the buccal cavity and/or bite, chew, suck, shape and squeeze
the food bolus into the upper esophagus while protecting the airway.

▶ Postsurgical reaction affecting ability to adequately use oropharyngeal structures used in swallowing.

▶ Significant weight loss directly related to nonoral nutritional intake
(g-tube feeding) and reaction to textures and consistencies.

▶ Existence of other conditions such as presence of tracheostomy tube,
reduced or inadequate laryngeal elevation, labial closure, velopharyngeal closure, laryngeal closure, or pharyngeal peristalsis, and
cricopharyngeal dysfunction.

C. *Esophageal (Lower Two Thirds) Phase of Swallow*—Esophageal dysphagia
(lower two thirds of esophagus) is difficulty in passing food from the
esophagus to the stomach. If peristalsis is inefficient, patients may complain of food getting stuck or of having more difficulty swallowing solids than liquids. Sometimes patients experience esophageal reflux or
regurgitation if they lie down too soon after meals.

Inefficient functioning of the esophagus during the esophageal phase
of swallowing is a common problem in the geriatric patient. Swallowing

disorders occurring only in the lower two thirds of the esophageal stage of the swallow have not generally been shown to be amenable to swallowing therapy techniques and may not be approved. An exception might be when discomfort from reflux results in food refusal. A therapeutic feeding program in conjunction with medical management may be indicated and constitute reasonable and necessary care. A reasonable and necessary assessment of function, prior to a conclusion that difficulties exist in the lower two thirds of the esophageal phase, may be approved, even when the assessment determines that skilled intervention is not appropriate.

D. *Assessment*—Medical workup and professional assessments must document history, current eating status, and clinical observations *such as:*

  ▶ Presence of a feeding tube;
  ▶ Paralysis;
  ▶ Coughing or choking;
  ▶ Oral motor structure and function;
  ▶ Oral sensitivity;
  ▶ Muscle tone;
  ▶ Cognition;
  ▶ Positioning;
  ▶ Laryngeal function;
  ▶ Oropharyngeal reflexes; and
  ▶ Swallowing function.

This information is used to determine necessity for further medical testing, e. g., videofluoroscopy, upper GI series, endoscopy. If videofluoroscopic assessment is conducted (modified barium swallow), documentation must establish that the exact diagnosis of the swallowing disorder cannot be substantiated through oral exam and there is a question as to whether aspiration is occurring. The videofluoroscopy assessment is conducted and interpreted by a radiologist with assistance and input from the physician and/or individual disciplines. The assessment and final analysis and interpretation should include a definitive diagnosis, identification of the swallowing phase(s) affected, and a recommended treatment plan. An analysis by an individual discipline may be submitted as a separate line item charge.

E. *Care Planning*—Documentation must delineate goals and type of care planned which specifically addresses each problem identified in the assessment, such as:

  ▶ Patient caregiver training in feeding and swallowing techniques;
  ▶ Proper head and body positioning;

▶ Amount of intake per swallow;
▶ Appropriate diet;
▶ Means of facilitating the swallow;
▶ Feeding techniques and need for self-help eating/feeding devices;
▶ Food consistencies (texture and size);
▶ Facilitation of more normal tone or oral facilitation techniques;
▶ Oromotor motor and neuromuscular facilitation exercises to improve oromotor control;
▶ Training in laryngeal and vocal cord adduction exercises;
▶ Compensatory swallowing techniques; and
▶ Oral sensitivity training.

As with all rehabilitation services, there must be a reasonable expectation that the patient will make material improvement within a reasonable period of time.

F. *Professional Services*—Services are sometimes performed by speech-language pathologists, occupational therapists and physical therapists in concert with other health professionals. Services are often performed as a team with each member performing unique roles which do not duplicate services of others. Services may include, but are not limited to, the following example:

EXAMPLE: One professional assisting with positioning, adaptive self-help devices, inhibiting abnormal oromotor and/or postural reflexes, while another professional is addressing specific exercises to improve oromotor control, determining appropriate food consistency form, assisting the patient in difficulty with muscular movements necessary to close the buccal cavity or shape food in the mouth in preparation for swallowing. Another professional might be addressing a different role, such as increasing muscle strength, sitting balance and head control. Medically review in accordance with general principles for coverage in SS3101ff. and documentation in SS3904ff., SS3905ff., and 3906ff.

G. *Chronic Progressive Diseases*—Patients with progressive disorders, such as Parkinson's disease, Huntington's disease, Wilson's disease, multiple sclerosis, or Alzheimer's disease and related dementias, do not typically show improvement in swallowing function, but will often be helped through short-term assistance/instruction in positioning, diet, feeding modifications, and in the use of self-help devices. Medically review documentation in support of short-term assistance/teaching and establishment of a safe and effective maintenance dysphagia program.

Chronic diseases such as cerebral palsy, status post-head trauma or stroke (old) may require monitoring of swallowing function with short-term intervention for safety and/or swallowing effectiveness. Documentation should relate to either loss of function, or potential for change.

As with other conditions/disorders, the reasonableness and necessity of services must be documented. Documentation should include:

▶ Changes in condition or functional status;
▶ History and outcome of previous treatment for the same condition; and
▶ Other information which justifies the start of care.

H. *Nasogastric Tube or Gastrostomy Tube*—The presence of a nasogastric or gastrostomy tube does not preclude need for treatment. Removal of a nasogastric or gastrostomy tube may be an appropriate treatment goal.

I. *Safety*—Although the documentation must indicate appropriate treatment goals to improve a patient's swallowing function, it must also indicate that the treatment is designed to ensure that it is safe for the patient to swallow during oral feedings. Improving the patient's safety and quality of life by reduction or elimination of alternative nutritional support systems and advancement of dietary level, with improved nutritional intake should be the primary emphasis and goal of treatment. The documentation must be consistent with these goals and indicate the reasonableness and need for skilled intervention.

J. *Skilled Level of Care*—Documentation of ongoing dysphagia treatment should support the need for skilled services such as observation, treatment, and diet modification. Documentation which is reflective of routine, repetitive observation or cuing may not qualify as skilled rehabilitation.

For example, repeated visits in which the caregiver appears only to be observing the patient eating a meal, reporting on the amount of food consumed, providing verbal reminders (e.g., slow down or cough) in the absence of other skilled assistance or observation suggests a nonskilled or maintenance level of care. Maintenance programs are covered for a brief period and are usually included during the final visits of the professional.

K. *Professional Qualifications*—Swallowing rehabilitation is a highly specialized service. Assume that the professionals rendering care have the necessary specialized training and experience. Refer to the RO any suspected patterns of poor quality.

L. *Consultation*—You are encouraged to seek consultation/advice from the American Speech-Language-Hearing Association, American Occupational Therapy Association, and American Physical Therapy Association as these claims often require MR by therapy or speech-language pathology consultants.

References

Abrams, W. B., Beers, M. H., & Berkow, R. (Eds.). (1995). *The Merck manual of geriatrics* (2nd ed.). Whitehouse Station, NJ: Merck Research Publishers.

Ackerman, T. F. (1996). The moral implications of medical uncertainty: tube feeding demented patients. *Journal of the American Geriatrics Society, 44*(10), 1265–1267.

Adrian, E. D., & Bonk, D. W. (1929). The discharge of impulses in motor nerve fibres. Part II. The frequency of discharge in reflex and voluntary contractions. *Journal of Physiology, 67,* 119–151.

Alexander, C. M., Teller, L. E., & Gross, J. B. (1989). Principles of pulse oximetry: Theoretical and practical considerations. *Anesthesia and Analgesia, 68,* 368–376.

Alfonzo, M. Ferdjallah, M. Shaker, R., & Wertsch, J. (1998). *Electrophysiologic validation of deglutitive UES opening head lift exercise.* Unpublished research submitted for presentation at American Gastroenterological Association meeting.

Ali, G., Lundl, T., Wallace, K., deCarle, D., & Cook, I. (1996). Influence of cold stimulation on the normal pharyngeal swallow response. *Dysphagia, 11,* 2–8.

American Dietetic Association. (1996). Position of the American Dietetic Association: Nutrition, aging, and the continuum of care. *Journal of the American Dietetic Association, 96*(10), 1048–1052.

American Gastroenterological Association. (1995). American gastroenterological association technical review on tube feeding for enteral nutrition. *Gastroenterology, 108*(4), 1282–1301.

American Hospital Association. (1992). *Patient Bill of Rights.*

American Speech-Language-Hearing Association. (1998, Spring). Statement of practices and procedures of the Board of Ethics. *American Speech-Language-Hearing Association, 40* (2), (Suppl. 18), 46–49.

299

American Speech-Language-Hearing Association (1994). Code of ethics. *ASHA, 36* (3, Suppl.13), 1–2.

American Speech-Language-Hearing Association, Task Force on Treatment Outcomes/Cost Effectiveness. (1996). National report cards; numbers 1–8; adults in health care settings. *National treatment outcome data project.* Rockville, MD.

Ardran, G. M., & Kemp, F. H. (1952). The protection of the laryngeal airway during swallowing. *British Journal of Radiology, 25,* 406–416.

Arney, W. K., & Pinnock, C. B. (1993). The milk mucus belief: Sensations associated with the belief and characteristics of believers. *Appetite, 20*(1), 53–60.

Athlin, E., Norberg, A., Axelsson, K., Moller, A., & Nordstrom, G. (1989). Aberrant eating behavior in elderly parkinsonian patients with and without dementia: analysis of video-recorded meals. *Research in Nursing & Health, 12*(1), 41–51.

Atkinson, J. C., & Fox, P. C. (1992). Salivary gland dysfunction. *Clinics in Geriatric Medicine, 8,* 499–511.

Aviv, J. E., Hecht, C., Weinberg, H., Dalton, J. F., & Urken, M.L. (1992). Surface sensibility of the floor of the mouth and tongue in healthy controls and in radiated patients. *Otolaryngology-Head and Neck Surgery, 107,* 418–423.

Aviv, J. E., Kim, T., Thomson, J. E., Sunshine, S., Kaplan, S., & Close, L. G. (1998). Fiberoptic endoscopic evaluation of swallowing with sensory testing (FEESST) in healthy controls. *Dysphagia, 13,* 87–92.

Aviv, J. E., Martin, J. H., Jones, M. E., Wee, T. A., Diamond, B., Keen, M. S., & Blitzer, A. (1994). Age-related changes in pharyngeal and supraglottic sensation. *Annals of Otology, Rhinology and Laryngology, 103* (10), 749–752.

Aviv, J. E., Martin, J. H., Keen, M. S., Debell, M., & Blitzer, A. (1993). Air pulse quantification of supraglottic and pharyngeal sensation: A new technique. *Annals of Otology, Rhinology and Laryngology, 102* (10), 777–780.

Aviv, J. E., Martin, J. H., Sacco, R. L., Zagar, D., Diamond, B., Keen, M. S., & Blitzer, A. (1996). Supraglottic and pharyngeal sensory abnormalities in stroke patients with dysphagia. *Annals of Otology, Rhinology and Laryngology, 105,* 92–97.

Backstrom, A., Norberg, A., & Norberg, B. (1987). Feeding difficulties in long-stay patients at nursing homes: Caregiver turnover and caregivers' assessments of duration and difficulty of assisted feeding and amount of food received by the patient. *International Journal of Nursing Studies, 24,* 69–76.

Baines, Z.V., & Morris, E. R. (1987). Flavor/taste perception in thickened systems: the effect of quar gum above and below c*. *Food Hydrocolloids, 1,* 197–205.

Barrocas, A., Chernoff, R., Cope, K., Jastram, C., Laurant, A., Lipschitz, D., & Morley, R. (1995, January). *Nutritional management of the elderly.* Postgraduate course #10 presented at the American Society for Parenteral and Enteral Nutrition 19th Clinical Congress, Miami, FL.

Bartelome, G., & Neumann, S. (1993). Swallowing therapy in patients with neurological disorders causing cricopharyngeal dysfunction. *Dysphagia, 8, 146–149.*

Batchelor, B., Neilsen, S., & Sexton, K. (1996). *Journal of Medical Speech-Language Pathology, 4*(3), 217–221.

Bednarek, K., Tucker, F., & Conlin, P. (1994, November) *Use of electromyography in investigating the normal swallow*. Poster presented at the annual meeting of the American Speech-Language-Hearing Association, New Orleans, LA.

Bennet, J. (1992, October 10). Hidden malnutrition worsens health of elderly. *New York Times*, 1p.

Berg, H. M., Persky, M. S., Jacobs, J. B., & Cohen, N. L. (1985). Cricopharyngeal myotomy: A review of surgical results in patients with cricopharyngeal achalasia of neurogenic origin. *Laryngoscope, 95,* 1337–1340.

Bergstrom, L. R., Larson, D. E., Zinsmeitster, A. R., Sarr, M. G., & Silverstein, M. D. (1995). Utilization and outcomes of surgical gastrostomies and jejunostomies in an era of percutaneous endoscopic gastrostomy: A population-based study. *Mayo Clinic Proceedings, 70*(9), 829–836.

Berman, L., Boczko, F., & Licht, B. (1995, November). *Is electromyography an effective therapeutic tool with dysphagic geriatric patients?* Poster presented at the annual meeting of the American-Speech-Language-Hearing Association, Orlando, FL.

Bernstein, L. H., & Jordan, L. (1995). Protein energy malnutrition: A potential financial burden for nursing homes. *Nursing Home Medicine, 3*(4), 72–78.

Biller, H. F., Lawson, W., & Baek, S. (1983). Total glossectomy. A technique of reconstruction eliminating laryngectomy. *Archives of Otolaryngology, 109,* 69–73.

Bistrian, B. R., Blackburn, G. L., Vitale, J., Cochroan, D., & Naylor, J. (1976). Prevalence of malnutrition in general medical patients. *Journal of the American Medical Association, 235*(3), 1567–1570.

Blakeley, W. R., Garety, E. J., & Smith, D. E. (1968). Section of the cricopharyngeus muscle for dysphagia. *Archives of Surgery, 96,* 745–762.

Boiron, M., Rouleau, Pl, Metman, E. H., (1997). Exploration of pharyngeal swallowing by audiosignal recording. *Dysphagia, 12,* 86–92.

Bonanno, P. C. (1970). Swallowing dysfunction after tracheostomy. *Annals of Surgery, 174,* 29–33.

Bourne, M.C. (1982). *Food texture and viscosity: concept and measurement*. New York: Academic Press.

Bowes, W. A., Corke, B. C., & Hulka, J. (1989). Pulse oximetry: A review of the theory, accuracy, and clinical applications. *Obstetrics and Gynecology, 74,* 541–546.

Bryant, M. (1991). Biofeedback in the treatment of a selected dysphagic patient. *Dysphagia, 6,* 140–144.

Buchholz, D. W., & Robbins, J. (1997). Neurologic diseases affecting oropharyngeal swallowing. In A. L. Perlman & K. S. Schulze-Delrieu (Eds.), *Deglutition and its disorders: Anatomy, physiology, clinical diagnosis, and management* (pp. 319–342). San Diego: Singular Publishing Group.

Buckwalter, J. A., & Sasaki, C. T. (1984). Effects of tracheostomy on laryngeal function. *Otolaryngologic Clinics of North America, 17,* 41–48.

Burtch, G. D., & Shatney, C. H. (1985). Feeding gastrostomy: Assistance or assassin? *American Journal of Surgery, 51*(4), 204–207.

Calcaterra, T. C. (1971). Laryngeal suspension after supraglottic laryngectomy. *Archives of Otolaryngology, 94,* 306–309.

Calhoun, K. H., Gibson, B., Hartley, L., Minton, J., & Hokanson, J. A. (1992). Age-related changes in oral sensation. *Laryngoscope, 102*, 109–116.

Cameron, A. M. (Ed.). (1997). *Nursing care ready reference: Resident assessment protocols.* Columbus, OH: Ross Products Division, Abbott Laboratories.

Cameron, J. L., & Zuidema, G. D. (1972). Aspiration pneumonia: Magnitude and frequency of the problem. *Journal of the American Medical Association, 219*(9), 1194–1196.

Campbell, J. R., & Sasaki, T. M. (1974). Gastrostomy in infants and children: An analysis of complications and techniques. *American Journal of Surgery, 40*, 505–508.

Carman G., & Ryan, G. (1989). Electromyographic biofeedback and the treatment of communication disorders. In J. V. Basmajian (Ed.), *Biofeedback: Principles and practice for clinicians* (pp. 287–297). Baltimore: Williams & Wilkins.

Carroll, P. (1997, February). Pulse oximetry—at your fingertips. *RN*, pp. 22–27.

Casper, M. L., Tobochnik, A. M., Brown, J. A., & Mills, R. H. (1996, November). *Issues forum: thickened liquids in the dysphagia diet.* Seminar presented at the Annual Convention of the American Speech-Language-Hearing Association, Seattle, WA.

Castell, J. A., Castell, D. O., Schultz, A. R., & Georgeson, S. (1993). Effect of head position on the dynamics of the upper esophageal sphincter and pharynx. *Dysphagia, 8*, 1–6.

Cataldi-Betcher, E. L., Seltzer, M. H., Slocum, B. A., & Jones, K.W. (1983). Complications occurring during enteral nutrition support: A prospective study. *Journal of Parenteral and Enteral Nutrition, 7*(6), 546–552.

Cherney, L. R., Cantieri, C. A., & Pannell, J. J. (1986). *Clinical evaluation of dysphagia.* Rockville, MD: Aspen Systems.

Chicero, J. A., & Murdoch, B. E. (1998) The physiologic cause of swallowing sounds: Answers from heart sounds and vocal tract acoustics. *Dysphagia 13*(1), 39–52.

Chidester, J. C., & Spangler, A. A. (1997). Fluid intake in the institutionalized elderly. *Journal of the American Dietetic Association, 97*(1), 23–28.

Ciocon, J. O. , Silverstone, F. A., Graver, L. M., & Foley, C. J. (1988). Tube feedings in elderly patients: Indications, benefits, and complications. *Archives of Internal Medicine, 148*(2), 429–443.

Clark, N. (1989, June). Dairy tales. *Runner's World*, pp. 44–50.

Clark, N. (1990). Milk: Destroying the myths. *The Physician and Sportsmedicine, 18*(2), 133–135.

Clark, R. C. (1990). Flavor and texture factors in model gel systems. In A. Turner (Ed.), *Food Technology International Europe 1990* (pp. 271–277). London: Sterling Publications International, Ltd.

Cluskey, M. M. (1989).The use of pureed diets among the elderly. *Dietetic Currents, 16*, 17–20.

Colmar, M., Oliver, L., & Wilcox, D. (1997, September). *Plan of treatment for OT/ PT/SLP.* Paper presented at seminar, The Clinical and Reimbursement Issues for the Provision of Rehab Services in Long Term Care. Syracuse, NY.

Cooper D. S., & Perlman A. L., (1997) Electromyography in the functional and diagnostic testing of deglutition. In A. L. Perlman & K. S. Shulze-Delrieu

(Eds.) *Degluition and its disorders: Anatomy, physiology, clinical diagnosis, and management* (pp. 255–284). San Diego: Singular Publishing Group.

Coats, K. G., Morgan, S. L., Bartolucci, A. A., & Weinsier, R. L. (1993). Hospital associated malnutrition: A reevaluation 12 years later. *Journal of the American Dietetic Association, 93*(4), 27–33.

Coben, R. M.,Weintraub, A., DiMarino, A. J., Jr., & Cohen, S. (1994). Gastroesophageal reflux during gastrostomy feeding. *Gastroenterology, 106*(1), 13–18.

Codispoti, C. L., & Bartlett, B. J. (1994). Food and nutrition for life: Malnutrition and older Americans. *Report by the Assistant Secretary for Aging.* Washington, DC: Department of Health and Human Services.

Cooper, J. W., & Cobb, H. H. (1988). Patient nutritional correlates and changes in a geriatric nursing home. *Nutritional Support Services, 8,* 5–7.

Cooper, R. M., Bikash, I., & Zubek, J. P. (1959). The effect of age on taste sensitivity. *Journal of Gerontology, 14,* 56–58.

Cope, K. (1996). *Malnutrition in the elderly: A national crisis.* Washington, DC: U. S. Government Printing Office.

Cordaro, M. M., & Sonies, B. C. (1993). An image processing scheme to quantitatively extract and validate hyoid bone motion based on real-time ultrasound recordings of swallowing. *IEEE Transactions on Biomedical Engineering, 40*(8), 941–944.

Cote, C. J., Goldstein, E. A., Cote, M. A., Hoaglin, D. C., & Ryan, J. F. (1988). A single blind study of pulse oximetry in children. *Anesthesiology, 68,* 184–188.

Crary M. A. (1995). A direct intervention program for chronic neurogenic dysphagia secondary to brainstem stroke. *Dysphagia, 10,* 6–18.

Crary, M. A., & Baldwin, B.O. (1997).Surface electromygraphic characteristics of swallowing in dysphagia secondary to brainstem stroke. *Dysphagia 12*(4), 180–187.

Crossley, K. B., & Thurn, J. R. (1989). Nursing home-acquired pneumonia. *Seminars in Respiratory Infections, 4,* 64–72.

Crysdale, W. S., & White, A. (1989). Submandibular duct relocation for drooling: A 10 year experience with 194 patients. *Otolaryngology—Head and Neck Surgery,101,* 87–92.

Curran, J., & Groher, M. E. (1990). Development and dissemination of an aspiration risk reduction diet. *Dysphagia, 5,* 6–12.

DePaso, W. J. (1991). Aspiration pneumonia. *Clinics in Chest Medicine, 12*(2), 269–284.

DePippo, M.Y., Holas, M., Reding, M., Mandel, F., & Lesser, M. (1994). Dysphagia therapy following stroke: A controlled trial. *Neurology, 44,* 1655–1660.

DeVita, M. A., & Spierer-Rundback, L. (1990). Swallowing disorders in patients with prolonged orotracheal intubation or tracheostomy tubes. *Critical Care Medicine, 18,* 1328–1330.

Denk, D. M., & Kaider, A. (1997).Videoendoscopic biofeedback: A simple method to improve the efficacy of swallowing rehabilitation of patients after head and neck surgery. *Annals of Otology, Rhinology and Laryngology, 59,*100–105.

Dettelbach, M. A., Gross, R. D., Mahlmann, J., & Eibling, D. E., (1995). Effect of the Passy-MuirValve on aspiration in patients with tracheostomy. *Head and Neck, 17,* 297–302.

Dikeman, K. J., & Kazandjian, M. S. (1995). *Communication and swallowing management of tracheostomized and ventilator dependent adults.* San Diego: Singular Publishing Group.

Dohlman, G., & Mattsson, O. (1960). The endoscopic operation for hypopharyngeal diverticula. *Archives of Otololaryngology, 71,* 744–752.

Dooley, J. M., Goulden, K. J., Gatien, J. G., Gibson, E. J, & Brown, B. S. (1986). Topical therapy for oropharyngeal symptoms of myasthenia gravis. *Annals of Neurology, 19(2),* 192–194.

Drazier, A. (1986). Clinical EMG feedback in motor speech disorders. *Archives of Physical Medicine and Rehabilitation, 65,* 691–696.

Dworkin, J. P., & Nadal, J. C. (1991). Nonsurgical treatment of drooling in a patient with closed head injury and severe dysarthria. *Dysphagia, 6,* 40–49.

Dwyer, J. T., Coleman, K. A., Krall, E., Yang, G. A., Scanlan, M., Galper, L., Winthrop, E., & Sullivan, P. (1987). Changes in relative weight among institutionalized elderly adults. *Journal of Gerontology, 42,* 246–251.

Eibling D. E., & Gross, R. D. (1996). Subglottic air pressure: A key component of swallowing efficiency. *Annals of Otology, Rhinology and Laryngology 105(4),* 253–8.

Ekberg, O. (1986). Posture of the head and pharyngeal swallow. *Acta Radiologica Diagnosis, 27,* 691–696.

Empey, G., Kiyak, A., & Milgrom, P. (1983). Oral health in nursing homes. *Special Care in Dentistry, 3,* 65–68.

Feinberg, M. (1996). The effects of medications on swallowing. In B. Sonies (Ed.), *Dysphagia: A continuum of care* (pp. 107–120). Gaithersburg, MD: Aspen Publishers.

Feinberg, M. J., Knebl, J., Tully, J., & Segall, L. (1990). Aspiration and the elderly. *Dysphagia, 4,* 61–71.

Finestone, H. M., Greene-Finestone, L. S., Wilson, E. S., & Teasell, R. W. (1995). Malnutrition in stroke patients on the rehabilitation service and at follow-up: Prevalence and predictors. *Archives of Physical Medicine and Rehabilitation, 76(4),* 310–316.

Fischer, J. (1983). Central hyperalimentation. In J. E. Fischer (Ed.), *Surgical nutrition* (pp. 663–702). Boston: Little, Brown & Company.

Fischer, M., Adkins, W., Hall, L., Scaman, P., Hsi, S., & Martlett, J. (1985). The effect of dietary fiber in a liquid diet on bowel function of mentally retarded individuals. *Journal of Mental Deficiency Research, 29(4),* 373–381.

Frank, H. A., & Green, L. C. (1979). Successful use of a bulk laxative to control the diarrhea of tube feeding. *Journal of Plastic and Reconstructive Surgical Nursing, 13,* 193–194.

Frankenfield, D. C., & Beyer, P. L. (1989). Soy-polysaccharide effect on diarrhea in tube-fed, head-injured patients. *American Journal of Clinical Nutrition, 50(3),* 553–558.

Fujiu, M., Logemann, & J. A., Pauloski, B. (1995). Post-operative posterior pharyngeal wall movement in patients with anterior oral cancer: Preliminary findings and possible implications for treatment. *American Journal of Speech-Language Pathology, 4,* 24–30.

Fujui, M., & Logemann, J. A. (1996). Effect of tongue-holding maneuver on posterior pharyngeal wall movement during deglutition. *American Journal of Speech-Language Pathology, 5*(1), 23–30.

Gallagher, M. W., Tyson, K. R. & Ashcraft, K. W. (1973). Gastrostomy in pediatric patients: An analysis of complications and techniques. *Surgery, 74,* 536–539.

Ganger, D., & Craig, R. M. (1990). Swallowing disorders and nutritional support. *Dysphagia, 4,* 213–219.

Garon, B. R., Engle, M., & Ormiston, C. (1997). A randomized control study to determine the effects of unlimited oral intake of water in patients with identified aspiration. *Journal of Neurologic Rehabilitation, 11,* 139–148.

Godshall, M. A., & Solms, J. (1992, June). Flavor and sweetener interactions with starch. *Food Technology,* pp. 140–144.

Goode, R. L. (1976). Laryngeal suspension in head and neck surgery. *Laryngoscope, 86,* 349–55.

Granieri, E. (1990). Nutrition and the older adult. *Dysphagia, 4,* 196–201.

Groher, M. E. (1987). Bolus management and aspiration pneumonia in patients with pseudobulbar dysphagia. *Dysphagia, 1,* 215–216.

Groher, M. E. (1990). Managing dysphagia in a chronic care setting: An introduction. *Dysphagia, 5,* 59–60.

Groher, M. E. (Ed.). (1992). *Dysphagia: diagnosis and management.* Boston: Butterworth-Heinemann.

Groher, M., & Bukatman, R. (1986). The prevalence of swallowing disorders in two teaching hospitals. *Dysphagia, 1,* 3–6.

Groher, M. E., & McKaig, T. N. (1995). Dysphagia and dietary levels in skilled nursing facilities. *Journal of the American Geriatrics Society, 43*(5), 528–532.

Guinard, J. X., & Marty, C. (1995). Time-intensity of flavor release from a model gel system: Effect of gelling agent type and concentration. *Journal of Food Science, 60* (4), 727–730.

Guenter, P. A., Settle, G., Perlmutter, S., Marino, P. L., DeSimone, G. A., & Rolandelli, R. H. (1991). Tube feeding-related diarrhea in acutely ill patients. *Journal of Parenteral and Enteral Nutrition, 15*(3), 277–280.

Gupta, V., Reddy, N., & Canilang, E. (1996). Surface EMG measurements at the throat during dry and wet swallow. *Dysphagia, 11,* 173–179.

Habal, M. B., & Murray, J. E. (1972). Surgical treatment of life-endangering chronic aspiration pneumonia. Use of an epiglottic flap to the arytenoids. *Plastic and Reconstructive Surgury, 49,* 305–311.

Hageman, C. F., & Crow, J. (1996, October). *A concurrent study of the computerized laryngeal analyzer and the modified barium swallow.* Poster presented at the annual meeting of the Dysphagia Research Society, Aspen, CO.

Hamlet, S., Nelson, R. J., & Patterson, R. L. (1990). Interpreting the sounds of swallowing: Fluid flow through the cricopharyngeus. *Annals of Otology, Rhinology and Laryngology, 99,* 749–752.

Hart, P. D., & Associates. (1993). *National survey on nutrition screening and treatment for the elderly.* Washington, DC: Nutrition Screening Initiative.

Hartlage, C., & Panther, K. (1992). New directions in dysphagia. *Network Newsletter, 2*(4), 2–3.

Haws, E. B., Sieber, W. K., & Kiesewetter, W. B. (1966). Complications of tube gastrostomy in infants and children. *Annals of Surgery, 164*(2), 284–290.

Health Care Financing Administration. (1990). *Medicare intermediary manual, part 3—claims process.* Section 3910, 10-154-10-159.

Health Care Financing Administration. (1992). *The multistate nursing home case mix and quality demonstration training manual.* Natick, MA: Eliot Press.

Health Care Financing Adminstration. (1997). *Your Medicare Handbook 1997.* Washington, DC: U. S. Government Printing Office.

Henderson, C. T. (1991). Safe and effective tube feeding of bedridden elderly. *Geriatrics, 48*(8), 56–66.

Herod, E. L. (1994). The use of milk as a saliva substitute. *Journal of Public Health Dentistry, 54*(3), 184–189.

Heymsfield, S. B., Horowitz, J., & Lawson, D. (1980). Enteral hyperalimentation. In J. E. Birk (Ed.), *Developments in digestive diseases* (pp. 59–83). Philadelphia: Lea and Febiger.

Hillel, A. D., Miller, R. M., Yorkston, K., McDonald, E., Norris, R. H., & Konikow, N. (1989). Amyotrophic lateral sclerosis severity scale. *Neuroepidemiology, 8,* 142–150.

Hinsdale, J. G., Lipkowitz, G. S. , Pollock, T. W., Hoover, E. L., & Jaffe, B. M. (1985). Prolonged enteral nutrition in malnourished patients with nonelemental feeding. *American Journal of Surgery, 149,* 334–338.

Hoffman, N. B. (1991). Dehydration in the elderly: Insidious and manageable. *Geriatrics, 46*(6), 35–38.

Hogan, R. B., DeMarco, D. C., Hamilton, J. K., Walker, C. O., & Polter, D. E. (1986). Percutaneous endoscopic gastrostomy—to push or pull. *Gastrointestinal Endoscopy, 32*(4), 253–258.

Holder, T. M., & Gross, R. E. (1960). Temporary gastrostomy in pediatric surgery: Experience with 187 cases. *Pediatrics, 26,* 36–41.

Holder, T. M., Leape, L. L., & Ashcraft, K. W. (1972). Gastrostomy: its use and dangers in pediatric patients. *New England Journal of Medicine, 286,* 1345–1347.

Horner, J., & Massey, W. (1988). Silent aspiration following stroke. *Neurology, 38,* 317–319.

Horner, J., Massey, E. W., Riski, J. E., Lathrop, D., & Chase, K. N. (1988). Aspiration following stroke: Clinical correlates and outcomes. *Neurology, 38*(9), 1359–1362.

Hotaling, D. L. (1990). Adapting the mealtime environment: Setting the stage for eating. *Dysphagia, 5,* 77–83. Hotaling, D. L. (1992). Nutritional considerations for the pureed diet texture in dysphagic elderly. *Dysphagia, 7,* 81–85.

Hu, T., Huang, L., & Cartwright, W. S. (1986). Evaluation of the cost of caring for the senile demented elderly: A pilot study. *Gerontologist, 26,* 158–163.

Huckabee, M. L. (1997). The risks of good intentions: Neuromuscular electrical stimulation. *American Speech-Language-Hearing Association Special Interest Division 13 (Dysphagia), 6*(1), 10–13.

Huckabee, M., & Cannito, M. (1998). Outcomes of swallowing rehabilitation in chronic brain stem dysphagia: A retrospective evaluation. Manuscript submitted for publication.

Huckabee, M. L., Cannito, M. P. & Kahane, J. C. (1996, November). *Outcomes of swallowing treatment after brain stem infarct.* Miniseminar presented at the annual meeting of the American Speech-Language-Hearing Association, Seattle, WA.

Huckabee, M. L., Garcia, M., & Barofsky, I. (1995, October). *SEMG measurements of the head and neck: Applications to dysphagia rehabilitation.* Poster presented at the annual meeting of the Dysphagia Research Society, McLean, VA.

Ibanez, J., Penafiel, A., Raurich, J. M., Marse, P., Jorda, R., & Mata, F. (1992). Gastroesophageal reflux in intubated patients receiving enteral nutrition: Effect of supine and semirecumbent positions. *Journal of Parenteral and Enteral Nutrition, 16*(5), 419–422.

Iskowitz, M. (1997, May 5). Pulse oximetry: new pathway for evaluating PPD. ADVANCE for Speech-Language Pathologists & Audiologists, pp. 11, 15.

Jacobson, E. (1933). Electrical measurements concerning muscular contraction (tonus) and the cultivation of relaxation in man: Studies on arm flexors. *American Journal of Physiology, 107* 230–48.

Jaime, I., Mela, D. J., & Bratchell, N. (1993). A study of texture-flavor interactions using free-choice profiling. *Journal of Sensory Studies, 8,* 177–188.

Joint Commission on Accreditation of Healthcare Organizations. (1996). *1996 accreditation manual for long term care.* Oakbrook Terrace, IL.

Jones, M., Santanello, S. A., & Falcone, R. E. (1990). Percutaneous endoscopic vs. surgical gastrostomy. *Journal of Parenteral and Enteral Nutrition, 14,* 533–534.

Jurell, K. C. (1996) Spectral analysis to evaluate superhyoid muscle involvement in neck exercise. *Muscle and Nerve, 19,* 1224.

Kaatze-McDonald, M., Post, E., Davis, P. (1996). The effects of cold, touch, and chemical stimulation of the anterior faucial pillars on human swallowing. *Dysphagia, 11,* 198–206.

Kagle, D. M., Alexander, C. M., Berko, R. S., Gruffre, M., & Gross, J. B. (1987). Evaluation of the Ohmeda 3700 pulse oximeter: Steady state and transient response characteristics. *Anesthesiology, 66,* 376–380.

Kahrilas, P. J., Logemann, J. A., & Gibbons, M.S. (1992). Food intake by maneuver: An extreme compensation for impaired swallowing. *Dysphagia, 7,* 155–159.

Kahrilas, P. J., Logemann, J. A., Krugler, C., & Flanagan, E. (1991). Volitional augmentation of upper esophageal sphincter opening during swallowing. *American Journal of Physiologoy, 260,* G450–G456.

Kahrilas, P. H., Logemann, J. A., Lin, S., & Ergun G. A. (1991). Pharyngeal clearance during swallow: A combined manometric and videofluoroscopic study. *Gastroenterology 103,* 128–136.

Kahrilas, P. J., Logemann, J., Lin S, Ergun G & Facchini, R. (1993). Deglutitive tongue action: Volume accommodation and bolus propulsion. *Gastroenterology, 104*(1), 152–162.

Kamath, S. K., Lawler, J., Smith, A. E., Kalat, T., & Olson, R. (1986). Hospital malnutrition: A 33 hospital screening study. *Journal of the American Dietetic Association, 86*(2), 203–206.

Kandil, H. E., Opper, F. H., Switzer, B. R., & Heiser, W. D. (1993). Marked resistance to tube-feeding-induced diarrhea: the role of magnesium. *American Journal of Clinical Nutrition, 57*(1), 73–80.

Kaplan, M. D., & Baum, B. J. (1993). The functions of saliva. *Dysphagia, 8,* 225–229.

Kasarskis, E. J., Berryman, S., Vanderleest, J. G., Schneider, A. R., & McClain, C. J., (1996). Nutritional status of patients with amyotrophic lateral sclerosis: Relation to the proximity of death. *American Journal of Clinical Nutrition, 63*(1), 130–137.

Kasman, G. (1994). Surface EMG and biofeedback in physical therapy. Instructional course handouts (11/21-22/1994).

Kaw, M., & Sekas, G. (1994). Long-term follow-up consequences of percutaneous endoscopic gastrostomy (PEG) tubes in nursing home patients. *Digestive Diseases and Sciences, 39*(4), 738–743.

Kazdin, A. E. (1982). *Single-case research designs.* New York: Oxford University Press.

Keller, H. H. (1993). Malnutrition in institutionalized elderly: How and why? *Journal of the American Geriatrics Society, 41*(11), 1212–1218.

Kelly, J. H., & Buchholz, D. W. (1996). Nutritional management of the patient with a neurologic disorder. *Ear, Nose & Throat Journal, 75*(5), 293–300.

Kelly, T. W., Patrick, M. R., & Hillman, K. M. (1983). Study of diarrhea in critically ill patients. *Critical Care Medicine, 11*(1), 7–9.

Kerstetter, J. E., Holthausen, B. A., & Fitz, P. A. (1993). Nutrition and nutritional requirements for the older adult. *Dysphagia, 8,* 51–58.

Kleinfeld, M., Casimir, M, & Borra, S. (1979). Hyponatremia as observed in a chronic disease facility. *Journal of the American Geriatrics Society, 27*(4), 156–161.

Kolasa, K. M., Schmidt, C., & Bartlett, J. A. (1989). Feeding Alzheimer's patients. *American Journal of Alzheimer's Care and Related Disorders and Research, 4,* 17.

Koltin, S. E., & Rosen, H. S. (1996). Hemiplegia and feeding: An occupational therapy approach to upper extremity management. In Topics in stroke rehabilitation: Clinical management of dysphagia (pp. 69–86). Frederick, MD: Aspen Publishers.

Kozarek, R. A., Ball, T. J., & Ryan, J. A. (1986). When push comes to shove: A comparison between two methods of percutaneous endoscopic gastrostomy. *American Journal of Gastroenterology, 81*(8), 642–664.

Kummer, B. A., Tiszenkel, H. I., Kotler, D. P., & Miller, R. E. (1985). Percutaneous endoscopic gastrostomy: Procedure of choice. *Gastrointestinal Endoscopy, 31*(2), 156–157. Laclede Research Laboratories. *Biotene.*™ Gardena, CA.

Langley, J. (1989). *Working with swallowing disorders.* Southampton, UK: Hobbs The Printers.

Langmore, S. E. (1998). Laryngeal sensation: A touchy subject. *Dysphagia, 13* (2), 93–94.

Langmore, S. E., & McCulloch, T. M. (1997). Examination of the pharynx and larynx and endoscopic examination of pharyngeal swallowing. In A. L. Perlman & K. S. Schulze-Delrieu (Eds.), *Deglutition and its disorders* (pp. 201–226). San Diego: Singular Publishing Group.

Langmore, S. E., & Miller, R. M. (1994). Behavioral treatment for adults with oropharyngeal dysphagia. *Archives of Physical Medicine and Rehabilitation, 75*(10), 1154–1162.

Langmore, S. E., Schatz, K., & Olsen, N. (1988). Fiberoptic endoscopic examination of swallowing safety: A new procedure. *Dysphagia, 2,* 216–219.

Langmore, S. E., Terpenning, M. S., Schork, A., Chen, Y., Murray, J. T., Lopatin, D., & Loesche, W. J. (1998). Predictors of aspiration pneumonia: How important is dysphagia? *Dysphagia, 13* (2), 69–81.

Larsen, G. (1973). Conservative management for incomplete dysphagia paralytica. *Archives of Physical Medicine and Rehabilitation, 54,* 180–185.

Larson, D. E., Burton, D. D., Schroeder, K. W. & DiMagno, E. P. (1987). Percutaneous endsocsopic gastrostomy: Indications, success, complications, and mortality in 314 consecutive patients. *Gastroenterology, 93,* 48–52.

Larson, D. E. , Fleming, C. R., Ott, B. J., & Schroeder, K. W., (1983). Percutaneous endoscopic gastrostomy : Simplified access for enteral nutrition. *Mayo Clinic Proceedings, 58,* 103–107.

Lavizzo-Mourey, R. J. (1987). Dehydration in the elderly: A short review. *Journal of the National Medical Association, 79*(10), 1033–1038.

Lavizzo-Mourey, R., Johnson, J., & Stolley, P. (1988). Risk factors for dehydration among elderly nursing home residents. *Journal of the American Geriatrics Society, 36*(3), 213–218.

Layne, K. A. (1990). Feeding strategies for the dysphagic patient: A nursing perspective. *Dysphagia, 5,* 84–88.

Lazarra, G., Lazarus, C., Logemann, J. A. (1986). Impact of thermal stimulation on the triggering of the swallowing reflex. *Dysphagia, 1,* 73–77.

Lazarus, B. A., Murphy, J. B., & Culpepper, L. (1990). Aspiration associated with long-term gastric versus jejunal feeding: A critical analysis of the literature. *Archives of Physical Medicine and Rehabilitation, 71*(1), 46–53.

Leaf, A. (1984). Dehydration in the elderly. *New England Journal of Medicine, 113*(12), 791–792.

Leder, S. B., Ross, D. A., Briskin, K. B., & Sasaki, C. T. (1997). A prospective, double-blind, randomized study on the use of a topical anesthetic, vasoconstrictor, and placebo during transnasal flexible fiberoptic endoscopy. *Journal of Speech, Language, and Hearing Research, 40* (6), 1352–1357.

Levinsky, N. G. (1987). Fluids and electrolytes. In E. Braunwald, K. J. Isselbacher, R. G. Petersdorf, J. D. Wilson, J. B. Martin, & A. S. Fauci (Eds.). *Harrison's principles of internal medicine* (pp. 198–204). New York: McGraw-Hill.

Levy, L. (1993). Model of human occupation frame of reference. In H. L. Hopkins & H. D. Smith (Eds.), *Willard & Spackman's occupational therapy* (8th ed.). Philadelphia: J. B. Lippincott.

Li, M., Brasseur, J. G., Kern, M. K., & Dodds, W. J. (1992). Viscosity measurements of barium sulfate mixtures for use in motility studies of the pharynx and esophagus. *Dysphagia, 7,* 17–30.

Lindeman, R. C. (1975). Diverting the paralyzed larynx: A reversible procedure for intractable aspiration. *Laryngoscope, 85,* 157–180.

Lindeman, R. C., Yarington, C. T., Jr., & Sutton, D. (1976). Clinical experience with the tracheoesophageal anastomosis for intractable aspiration. *Annals of Otology, Rhinology and Laryngology, 85,* 609–612.

Linden-Castelli, P. (1991). Treatment for adult dysphagia. *Seminars in Speech and Language 12*, 255–261.

Lindsley, D. B. (1935). Electrical activity of human motor units during voluntary contraction. *American Journal of Physiology, 114*, 90–99.

Lipner, H. S., Bosler, J., & Giles, G. (1990). Volunteer participation in feeding residents: Training and supervision in a long-term care facility. *Dysphagia, 5,* 89–95.

Liss, L. & Gomez, F. (1958). The nature of senile changes of the human olfactory bulb and tract. *Archives of Otolaryngology 67*, 167.

Lo, B., & Dornbrand, L. (1992). Understanding the benefits and burdens of tube feedings. *Archives of Internal Medicine, 149*(9), 1925–1926.

Logemann, J. A. (1997). *Evaluation and treatment of swallowing disorders.* Austin, TX: Pro-Ed.

Logemann, J. A. (1986). Treatment for aspiration related to dysphagia: An overview. *Dysphagia, 1,* 34–38.

Logemann, J. A. (1989a). Evaluation and treatment planning for the head-injured patient with oral intake disorders. *Journal of Head Trauma Rehabilitation, 4*(4), 24–33.

Logemann, J. A. (Ed.). (1989b). Swallowing disorders and rehabilitation. *Journal of Head Trauma Rehabilitation, 4*(4), Frederick, MD: Aspen.

Logemann, J. A. (1993a). The dysphagia diagnostic procedure as a treatment efficacy trial. *Clinics in Communication Disorders, 3*(4), 1–10.

Logemann, J. A. (1993b). *A manual for the videofluoroscopic evaluation of swallowing* (2nd ed.). Austin, TX: Pro-Ed.

Logemann, J. A. (1997). Therapy for oropharyngeal swallowing disorders. In A. L. Perlman & K. S. Schulze-Delrieu (Eds.), *Deglutition and its disorders: Anatomy, physiology, clinical diagnosis, and management* (pp. 449–461). San Diego: Singular Publishing Group.

Logemann, J. A., Kahrilas, P. J. (1990). Relearning to swallow after stroke—application of maneuvers and indirect biofeedback: A case study. *Neurology, 40,* 1136–1138.

Logemann, J. A., Kahrilas, P., Kobaraa, M, & Vakil, N. (1989b). The benefit of head rotation on pharyngoesophageal dysphagia. *Archives of Physical Medicine and Rehabilitation, 70*(10), 767–771.

Logemann, J. A., Pauloski, B. R., Colangelo L., Lazarus C., Fujui M., & Kahrilas, P. J. (1995). Efects of sour bolus on oropharyngeal swallowing measures in patients with neurogenic dysphagia. *Journal of Speech and Hearing Research, 38,* 556–563.

Logemann, J. A., Rademaker, A. W., Pauloski, B. R., & Kahrilas, P. J. (1994). Effects of postural change on aspiration in head and neck surgical patients. *Otolaryngology-Head and Neck Surgery, 110*(2), 222–227.

Mann, L. L. & Wong, K. (1996). Development of an objective method for assessing viscosity of formulated foods and beverages for the dysphagic diet. *Journal of the American Dietetic Association, 96*(6), 585–588.

Mansson, I., & Sandberg, N. (1975). Oral-pharyngeal sensitivity and elicitation of swallow in man. *Acta Otolaryngology, 79,* 140–145.

Martens, L., Cameron, T., & Simonsen, M. (1990). Effects of a multidisciplinary management program on neurologically impaired patients with dysphagia. *Dysphagia, 5,* 147–151.

Martin, B. J., & Corlew, M. (1990). The incidence of communication disorders in dysphagic patients. *Journal of Speech and Hearing Disorders, 55,* 28–32.

Martin, B. J. W., Corlew, M. M., Wood, H., Olson, D., Golopol, L. A., Wongo, M., & Kirmani, N. (1994). The association of swallowing dysfunction and aspiration pneumonia. *Dysphagia, 9,* 1–6.

Martin-Harris, B. J. & Cherney, L. R. (1996). Treating swallowing disorders following stroke. In L. R. Cherney & A. S. Halper (Eds.) *Topics in Stroke Rehabilitation, 3(3),* 27–40.

Martin, B. J. W., Logemann, J. A., Shaker, R., & Dodds, W. J. (1993). Normal laryngeal valving patterns during three breath-holding maneuvers: A pilot investigation. *Dysphagia, 8,* 11–20.

Mazzini, L., Corra, T., Zaccala, M., Mora, G., DelPiano, M., & Galante, M. (1995). Percutaneous endoscopic gastrostomy and enteral nutrition in amyotrophic lateral sclerosis. *Journal of Neurology, 242(10),* 695–698.

McHorney, C. A., & Rosenbek, J. C. (1998). Outcome assessment of adults with oropharyngeal dysphagia. In C. Frattali (Issue Ed.), *Seminars in speech and language, topic: functional outcome assessment of neurogenic populations.* New York: Thieme Medical Publishers.

McKaig, N. (1995, October). Miniseminar presented at the Annual Symposium on Cervical Auscultation, McLean, VA.

McReynolds, L. V. & Kearns, K. P. (1983). *Single-subject experimental designs in communicative disorders.* Baltimore: University Park Press.

Miller, J. L., & Watkin, K. L. (1996) *Color flow doppler ultrasonography of lingual vascularization in post-operative oral cancer subjects.* Poster presented at the annual meeting of the Dysphagia Research Society, Aspen, CO.

Miller, J. L., & Watkin, K. L. (1997). Lateral pharyngeal wall motion during swallowing using real time ultrasound. *Dysphagia, 12(3),* 125–32.

Miller, R. E., Kummer, G. A., Kotler, D. P., & Tiszenkel, H. I. (1986). Percutaneous endoscopic gastrostomy: procedure of choice. *Annals of Surgery, 204(5),* 543–545.

Miller, R. M., & Groher, M. E. (1982). The management of neuromuscular and mechanical swallowing disorders. In *Dysarthria, dysphonia, dysphagia, 1* (pp. 50–70). Chicago: Biolinguistics Clinical Institutes.

Miller, R. M. & Langmore, S. E. (1994). Treatment efficacy for adults with oropharyngeal dysphagia. *Archives of Physical Medicine and Rehabilitation, 75,* 1256–1262.

Mills, R. H., Stewman, D., Smith, N., Berman, M. S., Howard, J., & Hubbard, B. (1992, November). *The importance of viscosity control in dysphagia management.* Seminar presented at the Annual Convention of the American Speech-Language-Hearing Association, San Antonio, TX.

Mitchell, S. L., Kiely, D. K., & Lipsitz, L. A. (1997). The risk factors and impact on survival of feeding tube placement in nursing home residents with severe cognitive impairment. *Archives of Internal Medicine, 157(3),* 327–332.

Mittal, R. K., Stewart, W. R., & Schirmer, B. D. (1992). Effect of a catheter in the pharynx on the frequency of transient lower esophageal sphincter relaxations. *Gastroenterology, 103*(4), 1236–1240.

Mohr, J. P. (1986). Vertebrobasilar occlusive disease. In H. J. M. Barnett, J. P. Mohr, B. M. Stein & F. M. Yatsu (Eds.), *Stroke* (2nd ed, pp. 475–496). New York: Churchill Livingstone

Montgomery, W. W. (1975). Surgery to prevent aspiration. *Archives of Otolaryngology, 101*, 679–682.

Montgomery, W. W. (1989). *Surgery of the cervical esophagus in surgery of the upper respiratory system (2nd ed.), Vol. II.* (pp. 310–330)., Philadelphia: Lea & Febiger.

Montgomery, W. W., Blaugrund, S. M., & Varvares, M. A. (1993). Thyroplasty, a new approach. *Annals of Otology, Rhinology and Laryngology, 102*, 571–579.

Montgomery, W. W., Hillman, R. E., & Varvares, M.A. (1994). Combined thyroplasty type I and inferior constrictor myotomy. *Annals of Otology, Rhinology and Laryngology, 103*, 858–862.

Montgomery, W. W., & Lynch, J. P. (1971). Oculopharyngeal muscular dystrophy treated by inferior constrictor myotomy. *Transactions of the American Academy of Opthalmology and Otolaryngology, 75*, 986–993.

Moore, J. P., Curreri, P. W., & Rodning, C. B. (1986). Percutaneous endoscopic gastrostomy. *American Journal of Surgery, 52*, 495–499.

Moqhissi, K., & Teasdale, P. (1980). Parenteral feeding in patients with carcinoma of esophagus treated surgery: Energy and nitrogen requirements. *Journal of Parenteral and Enteral Nutrition, 4*(4), 371–375.

Mosby's medical, nursing & allied health dictionary (4th ed.). (1994). St. Louis: Mosby-Yearbook, Inc.

Mowe, M., & Behmer, T. (1991). The prevalence of undiagnosed protein-calorie undernutrition in a population of hospitalized elderly patients. *Journal of the American Geriatrics Society, 39*(11), 1089–1092.

Mullan, H., Roubenoff, R. A., & Roubenoff, R. (1992). Risk of pulmonary aspiration among patients receiving enteral nutrition support. *Journal of Parenteral and Enteral Nutrition, 16*(2), 160–164.

Musson, N. D., Kincaid, J., Ryan, P., Glussman, B., Varone, L., Gamarra, N., Wilson, R., Reefe, W., & Silverman, M. (1990). Nature, nurture, nutrition: Interdisciplinary programs to address the prevention of malnutrition and dehydration. *Dysphagia, 5*, 96–101.

Muz, J., Hamlet, S., Mathog, R., & Farris, R. (1994). Scintigraphic assessment of aspiration in head and neck cancer patients with tracheostomy. *Head and Neck, 16*, 17–20.

Muz, J., Mathog, R. H., Nelson, R., & Jones, L. A. (1989). Aspiration in patients with head and neck cancer and tracheostomy. *American Journal of Otolaryngology, 10*, 282–286.

Napierski, G., & Danner, M. (1982). Oral hygiene for the edentulous total care patient. *Special Care in Dentistry, 2*, 257–259.

Nash, M., (1988). Swallowing problems in the tracheostomized patient. *Otolaryngologic Clinics of North America, 21*, 701–709.

National Dairy Council. (1991). *Food Power* (2nd ed.) Rosemont, IL: National Dairy Council.

National Dysphagia Diet Task Force. (1997, October). *The national dysphagia diet: The science behind the practice.* Paper presented at the Annual Meeting and Exhibit of the American Dietetic Association, Boston, MA.

National Research Council. (1989). *Improving risk communication.* Washington, DC: National Academy Press.

Nelson, J. K., Moxness, K. E., Jensen, M. D., & Gastineau, C. F. (1994). *Mayo clinic diet manual: A handbook of nutrition practices* (7th ed.). St. Louis: Mosby-Year Book.

Netterville, J. L., Stone, R. E., Luken, E. S., Civantos, F. U., & Ossoff, R. H. (1993). Silastic medialization and arytenoid adduction: The Vanderbilt experience. *Annals of Otology, Rhinology and Laryngology, 102,* 413–424.

New, W. (1985). Pulse oximetry. *Journal of Clinical Monitoring, 1,* 126–129.

North Carolina Department of Human Resources, S. R. Vandak. (1993). *National nutrition screening initiative survey results and follow-up survey.* Raleigh, NC.

Nutrition Screening Initiative. (1992). *The nutrition screening manual for professionals caring for older americans.* Washington, DC: Greer, Margolis, Mitchell, Grunwald & Associates, Inc.

Nutrition Screening Initiative. (1994). *Incorporating nutrition screening and interventions into medical practice.* Washington, DC: Greer, Margolis, Mitchell, Grunwald & Associates, Inc.

Ohliger, P.C. (1996). Legal implications in dysphagia practice. In B. C. Sonies (Ed.), *Dysphagia: A continuum of care* (pp. 77–89). Gaithersburg, MD: Aspen Publishers.

O'Gara, J. A. (1990), Dietary adjustments and nutritional therapy during treatment for oral-pharyngeal dysphagia. *Dysphagia, 4,* 209–212.

Overbosch, P., Afterof, W. G. M., & Haring, P. G. M. (1991). Flavor release in the mouth. *Food Reviews. International, 7,* 137–184.

Pardoe, E. M. (1993). Development of a multistage diet for dysphagia. *Journal of the American Dietetic Association, 93,* 568–571.

Parisier, S. C., Blitzer, A, Binder, W. J., Friedman, W. F., & Marovitz, W. T. (1978). Tympanic neurectomy and chorda tympanectomy for the control of drooling. *Archives of Otolaryngology—Head and Surgery, 104,* 273–277.

Parrish, R. A., & Cohen, J. (1972). Temporary tube gastrostomy. *American Journal of Surgery,38,* 168.

Pedretti, L. W. (Ed.). (1996). *Occupational therapy: Practice skills for physical dysfunction* (4th ed, p. 474). St. Louis: Mosby-Year Book.

Pelletier, C. A. (1997). A comparison of consistency and taste of five commercial thickeners. *Dysphagia, 12,* 74–78.

Pelletier, C. A., & Huckabee, M. H. (1997, October). *A practical method to standardize dietary viscosity.* Poster presented at the 6th Annual Dysphagia Research Society Meeting, Toronto, Canada.

Perlman, A., Luschei, E., Dumond, C. (1989). Electrical activity from the superior pharyngeal constrictor during reflexive and nonreflexive tasks. *Journal of Speech and Hearing Research, 32 (4),* 749–754.

Perlman, A. L., & Schulze-Delrieu, K. (1997). *Deglutition and its disorders: Anatomy, physiology, clinical diagnosis, and management.* San Diego: Singular Publishing Group, Inc.

Pinnock, C. B., & Arney, W. K. (1991). Sensory analysis and randomized, controlled trial of the milk-mucus belief. *Proceedings of the Nutrition Society of Australia, 16,* 59.

Pinnock, C. B., Graham, N. M., Mylvaganam, A., & Douglas, R. M. (1990). Relationship between milk intake and mucus production in adult volunteers challenged with rhinovirus-2. *American Review of Respiratory Disease, 141(2),* 352–356.

Pinnock, C. B., Martin, A. J., & Mylvaganam, A. (1989). Cross-over trial of a high milk diet in asthmatic children. *Proceedings of the Nutrition Society of Australia, 14,* 131.

Plezia, P. M., Thornley, S. M., Kramer, T. H., & Armstrong, E. P. (1990). The influence of enteral feedings on sustained release theophylline absorption. *Pharmacotherapy, 10(5),* 356–361.

Ponsky, J. L., Gauderer, M. W. L., Stellato, T. A., & Aszodi, A. (1985). Percutaneous approaches to enteral alimentation. *American Journal of Surgery, 149,* 334–338.

Quill, T. E. (1992). Utilization of nasogastric feeding tubes in a group of chronically ill, elderly patients in a community hospital. *Dysphagia, 7,* 64–70.

Randall, H. R. (1984). Enteral nutrition: tube feeding in acute and chronic illness. *Journal of Parenteral and Enteral Nutrition, 8(2),* 113–136.

Rasley, A., Logemann, J. A., Kahrilas, P. J., Rademaker, A. W., Pauloski, B. R., & Dodds, W. J. (1993). Prevention of barium aspiration during videofluoroscopic swallowing studies: Value of change in posture. *American Journal of Roentgenology, 160,* 1005–1009.

Reddy, N. P., Gupta, V. Simcox, D., Motta, G., & Coppenger, J. (1997, October). *A computerized bio-feedback system for treating patients with poor laryngeal elevation.* Poster presented at the annual meeting of the Dysphagia Research Society, Toronto, CA.

Reiff, T. R. (1989). Body composition with special reference to water. In A. Horowicz, D. M. Macfadyen, H. Munro, N. S. Scrimshaw, B. Steen, & T. F. Williams (Eds.), *Nutrition in the elderly* (pp. 115–122). Oxford: Oxford University Press.

Reilly, J. J., Jr., Hull, S. F., Albert, N., Waller, A., & Bringardener, S. (1988). Economic impact of malnutrition: A model system for hospitalized patients, *Journal of Parental and Enteral Nutrition, 12(4),* 371–376.

Robbins J. & Levine, R: (1988) Swallowing after unilateral stroke of the cerebral cortex. Preliminary experience. *Dysphagia, 3,* 11–17.

Rogers, B., Msall, M., & Shucard, D. (1993). Hypoxemia during oral feedings in adults with dysphagia and severe neurological disabilities. *Dysphagia, 8,* 43–48.

Rogers, D. A., & Bowden, T. A., Jr. (1992). Gastrostomy: operative or nonoperative? *Surgical Clinics of North America, 72(2),* 515–524.

Rolls, B. J. (1989) Regulation of food and fluid intake in the elderly. In *Nutrition and the chemical senses in aging: recent advances and current research needs: Vol. 561* (pp. 217–225). New York: The New York Academy of Sciences.

Rolls, B. J., & Phillips, P. A. (1990). Aging and disturbances of thirst and fluid balance. *Nutrition Reviews, 1(4),* 137–144.

Rontal, E., Rontal, M., Morse, G, & Brown, E. M. (1976) Vocal cord injection in the treatment of acute and chronic aspiration. *Laryngoscope, 86(5),* 625–34.

Rosen A., Komisar A., Ophir D., & Marshak, G. (1990). Experience with the Wilkie procedure for sialorrhea. *Annals of Otology, Rhinology and Laryngology, 99*, 730–732.

Rosenbek, J. C. (1995). Efficacy in dysphagia: The need for data. *American Speech-Language-Hearing Association Special Interest Division 13.*

Rosenbek, J. C., Robbins, J., Fishback, B., Levine, R. L. (1991). Effects of thermal application on dysphagia after stroke. *Journal of Speech and Hearing Research, 34*, 1257–1268.

Rosenbek, J. C., Robbins, J., Willford, W. O., Kirk, G., Shiltz, A., Sowell, T. W., Deutsch, S. E., Milanti, F. J., Ashford, J., Gramigna, G. D., Fogerty, A., Dong, K., Rau, M. T., Prescott, T. E., Lloyd, A. M., Sterkel, M. T., & Hansen, J. E. (1998) Comparing treatment intensities of tactile-thermal application. *Dysphagia, 13(1)*, 1–9.

Rosenbek, J. C., Roecker, E. B., Wood, J. L., Robbins, J. (1996). Thermal application reduces the duration of stage transition in dysphagia after stroke. *Dysphagia, 11(4)*, 225–233.

Roubenoff, R., Preto, J., & Balke, C. W. (1987). Malnutrition among hospitalized patients: A problem of physician awareness. *Archives of Internal Medicine, 147(8)*, 1462–1465.

Rouse, J. (1994). *Dietary intake guide.* Columbus, OH: Ross Products Division, Abbott Laboratories.

Rubow, R. (1984). Role of biofeedback, reinforcement, and compliance on training and transfer in biofeedback based rehabilitation of motor speech disorders. In M. McNeil, J. Rosenbek, & A. Aronson (Eds.) *The Dysarthrias: Physiology, acoustics, perception and management* (pp. 207–229). San Diego: College-Hill Press.

Ruge, J., & Vazquez, R. M. (1986). An analysis of the advantages of Stamm and percutaneous endoscopic gastrostomy. *Surgery, Gynecology and Obstetrics, 162*, 13–16.

Russell, C. M. (1997). Practice points: Translating research into practice. *Journal of the American Dietetic Association, 97(1)*, 28.

Russell, T. R., Brotman, M., & Norris, F. (1984). Percutaneous gastrostomy: A new simplified and cost-effective technique. *American Journal of Surgery, 184*, 132–137.

Salassa, J. R. (1997). A functional outcomes swallowing scale (FOSS) for staging dysphagia. Paper presented at the 39th Meeting of the American Society for Head and Neck Surgery, Scottsdale, AZ.

Samii, A. M., & Suguitan, E. A. (1990). Comparison of operative gastrostomy with percutaneous endoscopic gastrostomy. *Military Medicine, 155(11)*, 534–535.

Sanders, H. N., Hoffman, S. B., & Lund, C. A. (1992). Feeding strategy for dependent eaters. *Journal of the American Dietetic Association, 92(11)*, 1389–1390.

Sandman, P., Adolfsson, R., Nygren, C., Hallmans, G., & Winblad, B. (1987). Nutritional status and dietary intake in Alzheimer's disease and multiinfarct dementia. *Journal of the American Geriatrics Society, 35*, 31–38.

Sasaki, C. T., Milmoe, G., Yanagisawa, E., Berry, K., & Kirchner, J. (1980). Surgical closure of the larynx for intractable aspiration. *Archives of Otolaryngology, 106*, 422–423.

Sasaki, C. T., Suzki, M., Horiuchi, M., & Kirchner, J. (1977). The effect of tracheostomy on the laryngeal closure reflex. *Laryngoscope, 87,* 1428–1433.

Schiffman, S. S. (1973). *The dietary rehabilitation clinic and a multi-aspect, dietary, and behavioral approach to the treatment of obesity: taste and smell of foods.* Paper presented at the meeting of the Association of Adverse Behavioral Therapists. Miami Beach, FL.

Schmidt, J., Holas, M., Halvorson, K., & Reding, M. (1994). Videofluoroscopic evidence of aspiration predicts pneumonia and death but not dehydration following stroke. *Dysphagia, 9,* 7–11.

Schoeller, D. A. (1989). Changes in total body water with age. *American Journal of Clinical Nutrition, 50*(5), 1176–1181.

Schramm, V. L., Max, M., & Lavorato, A. S. (1978). Gelfoam paste injection for vocal cord paralysis. Temporary rehabilitation of glottic incompetence. *Laryngoscope, 88,* 1268–1273.

Scott, R.W. (1994). *Legal aspects of documenting patient care.* Gaithersburg, MD: Aspen Publishers.

Sellars, C., Dunnet, C., & Carter, R. (1998). A preliminary comparison of videofluoroscopy of swallow and pulse oximetry in the identification of aspiration in dysphagic patients. *Dysphagia, 13,* 82–86.

Senac, M. O., & Lee, F. A. (1983). Small-bowel volvulus as a complication of gastrostomy. *Radiology, 149,* 136.

Shaker, R., Kern, M., Bardan, E., Taylor, A., Stewart, E., Hoffmann, R., Arndorfer, R., Hofmann, C., & Bonnevier, J. (1997). Augmentation of deglutitive upper esophageal sphincter opening in the elderly by exercise. *American Journal of Physiology, 272*(6, Pt. 1), G1518–1522.

Shanahan, T. K., Logemann, J. A., Rademaker, A. W., Pauloski, B. R., & Kahrilas, P. J. (1993). Chin-down posture effect on aspiration in dysphagic patients. *Archives of Physical Medicine and Rehabilitation, 74*(7), 736–739.

Shapiro, J. & Martin, S. (1995). In M. P. Fried (Ed.). *Disorders of the upper esophageal sphincter.* The larynx: A multidisciplinary approach (2nd ed., pp. 337–355). St. Louis, MO: Mosby-Year Book.

Shawker, T. H., & Sonies, B. C. (1985). Ultrasound biofeedback for speech training. *Investigative Radiology, 20,* 90–93.

Shawker, T. H., Sonies, B. Hall, T.E. & Baum, B. F. (1984) Ultrasound analysis of tongue, hyoid and larynx activity during swallowing. *Investigative Radiology 19*(2), 82–86.

Shawker, T. H., Sonies, B. C., & Sonte, M. (1984). *Sonography of speech and swallowing: Ultrasound annual.* New York: Raven Press.

Shawker, T. H., Sonies, B. C., Stone, M., & Baum, B. J. (1983). Real-time ultrasound visualization of tongue movement during swallowing. *Journal of Clinical Ultrasound, 11,* 485–490.

Sheiman, S. L. (1996). Tube feeding the demented nursing home resident. *Journal of the American Geriatrics Society, 44*(10), 1268–1270.

Shellito, P. C., & Malt, R. A. (1985). Tube gastrostomy: Techniques and complications. *Annals of Surgery, 201*(2), 180–185.

Shoemaker, A. (1997, March 10). Religious and cultural issues in dysphagia treatment. In *ADVANCE for Speech-Language Pathologists & Audiologists* pp. 10, 19.

Shott, S. R., Myer, C. M., & Cotton, R. T. (1989). Surgical management of sialorrhea. *Otolaryngology—Head and Neck Surgery, 101,* 47–50.

Siebens, H., Trupe, E., Siebens, A., Cook, F., Anshen, S., Hanauer, R., & Oster, G. (1986). Correlates and consequences of eating dependency in institutionalized elderly. *Journal of the American Geriatrics Society, 34(3),* 192–198.

Silver, A. J., Morley, J. E., Strome, S., Jones, D., & Vickers, L. (1988). Nutritional status in an academic nursing home. *Journal of the American Geriatrics Society, 36,* 487–491.

Sitzmann, J. V. (1990). Nutritional support of the dysphagic patient: Methods, risks, and complications of therapy. *Journal of Parenteral and Enteral Nutrition, 14(1),* 60–63.

Sitzmann, J. V., Townsend, T. R., Siler, M. C., & Bartlett, J. G. (1985). Septic and technical complications of central venous catheterization. *Annals of Surgery, 202(6),* 766–770.

Sitzmann, J.V. & Mueller, R. (1988). Enteral and parenteral feeding in the dysphagic patient. *Dysphagia, 3,* 38–45.

Smith, D., Hamlet, S., & Johns, L. (1990). Acoustic technique for determining timing of velopharyngeal closure in swallowing. *Dysphagia, 5(3),* 142–146.

Smith, G. K. & Farris, J. M. (1961). Re-evaluation of temporary gastrostomy as a substitute for nasogastric suction. *American Journal of Surgery, 102,* 168–175.

Smith O. (1934). Action potentials from single motor units in voluntary contractions. *American Journal of Physiology, 108,* 629–638.

Snyderman, C. H., & Johnson, J. T. (1988). Laryngotracheal separation for intractable aspiration. *Annals of Otology, Rhinology and Laryngology, 97,* 466–470.

Sonies, B. C., Baum, B. J., & Shawker, T. H. (1984). Tongue motion in elderly adults: Initial in situ observations. *Journal of Gerontology, 39* (3), 279–283.

Sonies B. C., Gottlieb E., Solomon B. I., Mathews K., & Huckabee M. L. (1996, October). *Simultaneous ultrasound and EMG study of swallowing,* Paper presented at the annual meeting of the Dysphagia Research Society, Aspen, CO.

Sonies, B., C. & Huckabee, M. L. (Eds.). (1995). From lab to clinic: Incorporating research into clinical practice. *American Speech-Language-Hearing Association Special Interest Division 13(Dysphagia), 4(3),* 2–16.

Sonies, B. C., Parent, L., Morrish, K., Baum, B. (1988). Durational aspects of the oral-pharyngeal phase of swallowing in normal adults. *Dysphagia, 3,* 1–10.

Spangler, P. F., Risley, T. R., & Bilyew, D. D. (1984). The management of dehydration and incontinence in nonambulatory geriatric patients. *Journal of Applied Behavioral Analysis, 17,* 397–401.

Splaingard, L. L., Hutchins, B., Sulton, L. D., & Chaundhuri, G. (1988). Aspiration in rehabilitation patients: Videofluoroscopy vs bedside clinical assessment. *Archives of Physical Medicine and Rehabilitation, 69,* 637–640.

Stanek, K., Hensley, C., & Van Riper, C. (1992). Factors affecting use of food and commercial agents to thicken liquids for individuals with swallowing disorders. *Journal of the American Dietetic Association, 92(4),* 488–490.

Stedman's medical dictionary (26th Ed.). (1995). Baltimore, MD: Williams & Wilkins.

Stellato, T. A., Danziger, L. H., Nearman, H. S., & Creger, R. J. (1984). Inadvertent intravenous administration of enteral diet. *Journal of Parenteral and Enteral Nutrition, 8*(4), 435–455.

Stern, J. S. (1986) Comparison of percutaneous endoscopic gastrostomy with surgical gastrostomy at a community hospital. *American Journal of Gastroenterology, 81*(12), 1171–1173. *92,* 488–490.

Stevens, K. M., & Newell, R. C. (1971). Cricopharyngeal myotomy in dysphagia. *Laryngoscope, 81,* 1616–1620.

Strand, E. A., Miller, R. M., Yorkston, K. M., & Hillel, A. D. (1996). Management of oral pharyngeal dysphagia symptoms in amyotrophic lateral sclerosis. *Dysphagia, 11*(2), 129–139.

Strodel, W. E., Lemmer, J. Exkhauser, F. Botham, M., & Dent, T. (1983). Early experience with endoscopic percutaneous gastrostomy. *Archives of Surgery, 118,* 449–453.

Strom, J. G., & Miller, J. W. (1990). Stability of drugs with enteral nutrient formulas. *Drug Intelligience and Clinical Pharmacy, 24,* 130–134.

Sukthankar, S. M., Reddy, N. P., Canilang, E. P., Stephenson, L., & Thomas, R. (1994) Design and development of portable biofeedback systems for use in oral dysphagia rehabilitation. *Medical Engineering and Physics, 16*(5), 430–5.

Sullivan, C. E. (1985). Obstructive sleep apnea. In M. H. Kryger (Ed.), *Clinics in chest medicine.* (pp. 633–650). Philadelphia: W. B. Saunders.

Sunderam, S. G., & Mankikar, G. D. (1983). Hyponatremia in the elderly. *Age and Ageing, 12,* 77–80.

Szczesniak, A. S. (1963). Classification of textural characteristics. *Journal of Food Science, 28,* 385–389.

Szczesniak, A. S. (1987). Correlating sensory with instrumental texture measurement—an overview of recent developments. *Journal of Texture Studies, 18,* 1–15.

Szczesniak, A. S. & Bourne, M. C. (1982). Unpublished data. In M. C. Bourne, *Food texture and viscosity: Concept and measurement* (p. 40). New York: Academic Press.

Takahashi, K., Groher, M. E., & Michi, K. (1994). Methodology for detecting swallowing sounds. *Dysphagia, 9,* 54–62.

Terry, P. B., & Fuller, S. D. (1989). Pulmonary consequences of aspiration. *Dysphagia, 3,* 179–183.

Thatcher, B. S., Ferguson, D. R., & Paradis, K. (1984). Percutaneous endoscopic gastrostomy: a preferred method of feeding tube gastrostomy. *American Journal of Gastroenterology, 79,* 748–750.

Torres, A., Serra-Battles, J., Ros, E., Piera, C., Puig de la Bellacasa, J., Cobos, A., Lomena, F., & Rodriguez-Roisin, R. (1992). Pulmonary aspiration of gastric contents in patients receiving mechanical ventilation: The effect of body position. *Annals of Internal Medicine,116*(7), 540–543.

Tremper, K. K., & Barker, S. J. (1989). Pulse oximetry. *Anesthesiology, 70,* 98–108.

Tuch B. E., Nielsen J. M. (1941) Apraxia of swallowing. *Bulletin of the Los Angeles Neurological Society. 6,* 52–53.

Tufts University. (1993). Does milk make mucus? *Diet & Nutrition Letter, 11*(8), 7.

U. S. Department of Health and Human Services. (1994, May 13). *Administration on Aging, Federal Register, 59(92)*. Washington, DC: Government Printing Office.

Varvares, M. A., Montgomery, W. W., & Hillman, R. E. (1995). Teflon granuloma of the larynx: Etiology, pathophysiology and management. *Annals of Otology, Rhinology and Laryngology, 104*, 511–515.

Veis, S., & Logemann, J. (1985). Swallowing disorders in persons with cerebrovascular accident. *Archives of Physical Medicine and Rehabilitation, 66*, 373–375.

Veldee, M. S., & Peth, L. D. (1992). Can protein-calorie malnutrition cause dysphagia? *Dysphagia, 7*, 86–101.

Warren, J. L., Bacon, E., Harris, T., McBean, A. M., Foley, D. J., & Phillips, C. (1994). The burden and outcomes associated with dehydration among US elderly. *American Journal of Public Health, 84*, 1265–1269.

Wasiljew, B.K., Ujiki, G. T., & Beal, J. M. (1982). Feeding gastrostomy: complications and mortality. *American Journal of Surgery, 143*, 194–195.

Watson, P. E., Watson, I. D., & Batt, R. D. (1980). Total body water volumes for adult males and females estimated from simple anthropometric measurements. *American Journal of Clinical Nutrition, 33(1)*, 27–39.

Waxman, M. J., Durfee, D., Moore, M., Morantz, R. A., & Koeller, W. V. (1990). Nutritional aspects and swallowing function of patients with Parkinson's disease. *Nutrition in Clinical Practice, 5*, 196–199.

Webster, M., Carey, L., & Ravitch, M. (1975). The permanent gastrostomy. *Archives of Surgery, 110*, 658–660.

Weisberger, E. C. (1991). Treatment of intractable aspiration using a laryngeal stent or obturator. *Annals of Otology, Rhinology and Laryngology, 100*, 101–107.

Welch, M.V., Logemann, J. A., Rademaker, A. W., & Kahrilas, P. J. (1993). Changes in pharyngeal dimensions effected by chin tuck. *Archives of Physical Medicine and Rehabilitation, 74(2)*, 178–181.

Whitney, E. N., & Cataldo, C. B. (1983). *Understanding normal and clinical nutrition.* New York, NY: West Publishing Company.

Wickline v. California, (1986). 192 Cal. App. 3d 1630, 239 Cal. Rptr. 810.

Wilke, W. L. (1993). *Consumer behavior* (3rd ed.). New York: John Wiley and Sons.

Wilkins, E. M. (1989). *Clinical practice of the dental hygienist* (6th ed.) Malvern, PA: Lea & Febiger.

Wilkins, S. A. (1964). Indications for section of the cricopharyngeus muscle. *American Journal of Surgery, 108*, 533–538.

Wilkinson, W., & Rickleman, J. (1982). Feeding gastrostomy. *American Journal of Surgery, 48*, 273–275.

Willig, T. N., Paulus, J., Laucau Saint Guily, J. Beon, C., & Navarro, J. (1994). Swallowing problems in neuromuscular disorders. *Archives of Physical Medicine and Rehabilitation, 75(11)*, 1175–1181.

Wilson, J. A., Pryde, A., White, A., Maher, L., Maran, A. G. D. (1995). Swallowing performance in patients with vocal fold motion impairment. *Dysphagia, 10*, 149–154.

Wolf, S. L. (1979). EMG biofeedback applications in rehabilitation. *Physiotherapy Canada, 31*, 65–72.

Wolf, S. L. (1994). Biofeedback. In J. A. Downey, S. J. Meyers, E. G.Gonzales, & J. S. Lieberman (Ed.)*The Physiological Basis of Rehabilitation Medicine, 2nd Ed.* (pp. 563–572). Stonneham, MA: Butterworth-Heinemann.

Woo, J. K., Van Hasselt, C. A., & Chan, H. S. (1992) Teflon injection for unilateral vocal cord paralysis and its effect on lung function. *Clinics in Otolaryngology, 17*(6), 497–500.

Ylvisaker, M. S., & Holland, A. L. (1985). Coaching, self-coaching and rehabilitation of head injury. In D. F. Johns (Ed.), *Clinical management of neurogenic communicative disorders* (2nd Ed., pp. 243–257). Boston: Little, Brown.

Ylvisaker, M., & Logemann, J. A. (1986). Therapy for feeding and swallowing following head injury. In M.Ylvisaker (Ed.), *Management of head injured patients.* San Diego, CA: Little, Brown.

Ylvisaker, M., & Weinstein, M. (1989). Recovery of oral feeding after pediatric injury. *Journal of Head Trauma Rehabilitation, 4,* 51–63.

Young, V. R. (1990). Amino acids and proteins in relation to the nutrition of elderly people. *Age and Ageing, 19*(4), S10–S24.

Young, V. R., Munro, H. N., & Fukagawa, N. (1989). Protein and functional consequences of deficiency. In A. Horowicz, D. M. Macfadyen, H. Munro, N. S. Scrimshaw, B. Steen, & T. F. Williams (Eds.), *Nutrition in the elderly* (pp. 65–84). Oxford: Oxford University Press.

Zaidi, N. H., Smith, H.A., King, S. C., Park, C., O'Neill, P. A., & Connolly, M. J. (1995). Oxygen desaturation on swallowing as a potential marker of aspiration in acute stroke. *Age and Ageing, 24,* 267–270.

Zenner, P. M., Losinski, D. S., & Mills, R. H. (1995). Using cervical auscultation in the clinical dysphagia examination in long-term care. *Dysphagia, 10,* 27–31.

Zimmer, J. G., Bentley, D. W., Valenti, W. M., & Watson, N. M. (1986). Systemic antibiotic use in nursing homes: A quality assessment. *Journal of the American Geriatrics Society, 34,* 703–710.

Index

t = table, *f* = figure

A

ADH secretion, increased in elderly, 162, 164–165
Aging, effect of on dehydration
  decreased ability to conserve free water and sodium, 165, 166*t*
  decreased perception of thirst in elderly, 165
  fluid loss in elderly, 164
  increased ADH secretion, 164–165
Airway protection and laryngeal valving, inadequate, 40–42
Alertness of patient, 222–223
American Dietetic Association (ADA), and National Dysphagia Diet Project, 209–210
American Hospital Association's Patient Bill of Rights, 252
American Speech-Language-Hearing Association
  Code of ethics of (*app*), 254
    preamble, 279–283
    principle of ethics I, 280–281
    principle of ethics II, 281
    principle of ethics III, 282
    principle of ethics IV, 282–283
  procedures and sanction of ethical violation, 253–254
  Statement of Practices and Procedures of the Board of Ethics (*app*), 285–291
Arytenoid adduction, 239
ASHA, *see* American Speech-Language-Hearing Association
Aspiration
  management of, 237–238
  as complication of enteral feeding, 181–184
    caused by body position, 183
    caused by tube position and reflux, 183
    effect of gastric emptying dysfunction caused by disease or injury, 183–184
    of oral secretions, 183
  risk of due to oropharyngeal dysphagia, 171–172
Aspiration pneumonia, risk of, 215–216
Assessment, skills for, 12*t*, 13–15
  information gathering, 13–15
  synthesizing information, 15
Auscultation, cervical, as biofeedback tool, 85–87

B

Backward chaining, 225–226
Bacteria flora, altered, risk of diarrhea from, 186
BE, *see* Board of Ethics of ASHA
Behavioral intervention approaches, 16
Bilateral submandibular gland excisions, 244
  duct relocation into tonsillar fossa, 244
Bilateral tympanic neurectomy, 244
Biochemical changes with aging, 156
Biofeedback modalities as treatment for dysphagia
  facilitating learning process, 54–56
  summary, 73–74
  surface electromyography (SEMG), 56–73

321